HORMONE CHEMISTRY

HORMONE CHEMISTRY

W. R. BUTT

Consultant Biochemist
Department of Clinical Endocrinology
United Birmingham Hospital

D. VAN NOSTRAND COMPANY LTD
LONDON

PRINCETON, NEW JERSEY   TORONTO

D. VAN NOSTRAND COMPANY LTD
Windsor House, 46 Victoria Street, London, SW1

D. VAN NOSTRAND COMPANY INC.
Princeton, New Jersey

VAN NOSTRAND REGIONAL OFFICES:
New York, Chicago, San Francisco

D. VAN NOSTRAND COMPANY (CANADA) LTD
Toronto

PRINTED IN GREAT BRITAIN BY BUTLER & TANNER LTD
FROME AND LONDON

PREFACE

The study of hormone chemistry may at first sight seem to be less spectacular than research in certain other scientific and medical fields. There have been several indications in the last fifty years or so, however, that the subject is of more than purely academic interest. Firstly there was the remarkable work of Banting and Best on the isolation of insulin and on its application to the treatment of diabetes. The characterization and recent synthesis of this hormone represent some of the most important advances in protein chemistry this century. Secondly the therapeutic usefulness of cortisone was first recognized some fifteen years ago. This stimulated a fascinating search for readily available raw material for the synthesis of this and related compounds. Thirdly we are now living in the midst of the 'population explosion'—in the eyes of some the most important social problem of the twentieth century. The subject of hormone chemistry can no longer be considered a backwater. Hormones are not only the necessities of patients attending an endocrine clinic: they are involved in the fundamental processes of life itself—the building of proteins, the control of fertility and in the nurture of the young. Here indeed is a fruitful field for chemical research.

Much of the early chemical work on hormones has now passed into history; it is so voluminous that only the merest outline can be sketched here. Recent work, which is the main concern of this book, is scattered in many publications both clinical and biological as well as chemical. As Thor Heyerdahl writes in *Aku Aku*: 'In order to penetrate ever further into their subjects, the host of specialists narrow their field and dig down deeper and deeper till they can't see each other from hole to hole. But the treasures their toil brings to light they place on the ground above.' It has been an important objective of this book to 'stay on top and piece all the different facts together' with adequate references for further reading.

In order to keep the book within reasonable size it has been possible to describe only the major mammalian hormones of the neurohypophysis, pituitary, adrenals, gonads, thyroid and pancreas. This means that mammalian hormones such as gastrin, and all the insect and plant hormones have had to be omitted. It so happens that the chemistry of some of these is particularly interesting and recent advances have been striking. Gastrin, which controls the secretion of acid in the stomach and the release of the digestive enzyme pepsin, has been recognized as a peptide containing 17 amino acids.[1] The last 4 acids in the sequence, Try-Met-Asp-Phe-NH$_2$, display the whole range of activity of the natural hormone, although the level of activity is less. Again, in the field of insect hormones some remarkable chemical findings have come to light. The sex-attractant of the silk worm, *Bombyx mori*, has been recognized as a 13-carbon fatty acid.[2] The remarkable fact about this substance is its biological sensitivity. A solution containing only 10^{-12} μg per ml will attract the male moth. It is calculated that probably only a molecule or two on the antennae are sufficient to excite the moth. It is thus probably the most active biological substance known.

These examples illustrate one of the main themes of this book, namely the relationship of structure to biological activity. The precise way by which hormones act is still largely hypothetical. The possibility that certain protein hormones may act by inducing enzymes in their target cells would explain their high biological activity.[3] The effect of certain reagents on biological activity, and the preparation of synthetic derivatives of simpler structure which show some or all of the biological activity help to define the active sites. Many examples are given of such approaches towards a better understanding of the mode of action and the relationship of chemical structure to activity.

Two general chapters are included in the text, one on protein and the other on steroid chemistry. These are designed to help the non-chemical reader to follow the subsequent chapters. There is a section on the statistics of biological assay since the use of accurate assays is essential in controlling any chemical work. Immunological assays are also described since they have become so important and are likely to become even more so in the future.

The clinical applications of hormone assay have only been referred to briefly. This is regretted but they could have been covered adequately only in a much larger book and it was considered that there are plenty of good clinical publications already available. Nevertheless it is hoped that the book will appeal to clinicians as well as to chemists and biochemists.

Progress in hormone research is so rapid that a book of this nature is never finished and only a cross-sectional view of the present state of our knowledge can be presented. The references are as up-to-date as possible and extend to about the middle of 1965.

My especial thanks go to Dr A. C. Crooke, the Director of the Department of Clinical Endocrinology. Without his guidance and encouragement over

[1] GREGORY, R. A., TRACY, H. J. and GROSSMAN, M. I. *Nature* **209**, 583 (1966); BENTLEY, P. H., KENNER, G. W. and SHEPPARD, R. C. *Nature* **209**, 583 (1966).
[2] BUTENANDT, A. *J. Endocrin.* **27**, ix (1963).
[3] BARKER, S. A. *Discovery* **26** (11), 30 (1965).

the last 15 years this book would never have been written. For much encouragement and constructive criticism I thank my colleague in the Department of Chemistry, University of Birmingham, Dr S. A. Barker. In the preparation of the text I have been particularly fortunate in having the co-operation of the Staff of the Endocrine Department. Many of the diagrams were drawn and the references checked by Miss Janet Stacey, while Dr Marion Bluck, Raymond Morris and Stuart Carrington have helped with the text and supplied much valuable information.

Finally I should like to thank my publishers, D. Van Nostrand Company, for their very helpful collaboration throughout.

WILFRID R. BUTT

January 1966

ACKNOWLEDGEMENTS

The author wishes to thank the editors of journals and the authors for permission to reproduce the following:

Journal of Chromatography, Table 1.3
Journal of Clinical Endocrinology, Fig. 11.14
Journal of Endocrinology, Table 5.1 and Fig. 5.1
Metabolism, Table 1.2.

CONTENTS

ABBREVIATIONS

The following abbreviations have been used without definition in the text:

ATP	Adenosine 5'-tri-phosphate	NAD(H$_2$)	Nicotinamide-adenine dinucleotide (reduced)
CM-cellulose	Carboxymethyl-cellulose	NADP(H$_2$)	Nicotinamide-adenine dinucleotide phosphate (reduced)
DEAE-cellulose	Diethylaminoethyl-cellulose		
DNA	Deoxyribonucleic acid	RNA	Ribonucleic acid
		Tris	2-Amino-2-hydroxy-methylpropane-1, 3-diol
DNP	2, 4-Dinitrophenyl		

Amino acids

Ala	Alanine	Lys	Lysine
Arg	Arginine	Met	Methionine
Asp(NH$_2$)	Asparagine	Orn	Ornithine
Asp	Aspartic acid	Phe	Phenylalanine
CyS	Cystine (half)	Pro	Proline
Glu	Glutamic acid	Ser	Serine
Glu(NH$_2$)	Glutamine	Thr	Threonine
Gly	Glycine	Try	Tryptophan
His	Histidine	Tyr	Tyrosine
Ile	Isoleucine	Val	Valine
Leu	Leucine		

1

THE PROTEIN HORMONES

Some of the most important hormones are proteins and this first chapter therefore will be concerned with certain general aspects of protein chemistry. Progress in the methods of isolation, identification and synthesis of these most complex of chemical compounds has been so rapid that it is clearly impossible to review the subject adequately here. Instead, some of the techniques which are of comparatively recent development or have been of particular usefulness in the study of hormones have been selected for special mention.

The isolation of a protein hormone is preceded by the identification of its physiological functions and classification of the hormones is based essentially on these properties. The biological properties of the hormones therefore will not be neglected in this book since without them much of the chemistry would be of merely academic, rather than of any practical value.

Origins

The glands which secrete protein or polypeptide hormones are listed in Table 1.1.

The *pituitary* gland contains an anterior and posterior lobe, the former producing a number of hormones which are proteins, glycoproteins or polypeptides and the latter secreting the peptides, oxytocin and vasopressin. An intermediate zone secretes a hormone originally termed intermedin, the melanophore-stimulating hormone. There has been a great deal of interest in recent years in a group of polypeptides which originate in the *hypothalamus* and control the release of certain of the pituitary hormones. There is much work still to be done on the identification of these compounds and on the discovery of new ones.

In the *pancreas* the structures known as the 'islets of Langerhans' produce insulin and glucagon, both polypeptides, which have been well characterized chemically.

TABLE 1.1

The protein hormones

Gland	Hormone	Type	Principal functions
Pituitary: anterior lobe	Corticotrophin	Polypeptide	Controls activity of adrenal cortex
	Gonadotrophins	Glycoprotein	Induce ovulation and spermatogenesis
	Thyrotrophin	Glycoprotein	Controls activity of thyroid gland
	Growth hormone	Protein	Controls growth of skeleton and tissue
	Prolactin	Protein	Influences growth of mammary glands, induces secretion of milk and maintains the mature corpus luteum
intermediate lobe	Melanophore stimulating hormone	Polypeptide	Disperses melanin granules in skin
posterior lobe	Vasopressin	Peptide	Acts as antidiuretic factor and vaso-constrictor with resulting pressor action
	Oxytocin	Peptide	Stimulates contractions of smooth muscle
Neurohypophysis	Various releasing factors	Probably peptides or polypeptides	Control release of various hormones from the anterior pituitary
Thyroid	Thyroglobulin	Protein	Stores thyroid hormones
	Calcitonin (probably)	Polypeptide	Regulates metabolism of calcium and phosphorus (antagonist to parathyroid hormone)
Parathyroid	Parathyroid hormone	Polypeptide	Regulates metabolism of calcium and phosphorus
Pancreas	Insulin	Polypeptide	Regulates metabolism of carbohydrate, fat and protein
	Glucagon	Polypeptide	Antagonist to insulin

The *thyroid* is one of the largest endocrine glands, and weighs approximately 20 g in adults. Although it does not secrete a protein hormone, it is mentioned now because the iodine-containing hormone, thyroxine, and related compounds are stored here in colloid on the protein, thyroglobulin. The small glands sometimes situated near the thyroid known as the *parathyroids* secrete a polypeptide, the parathyroid hormone, while another hormone, calcitonin, has been variously attributed to the parathyroid and thyroid glands.

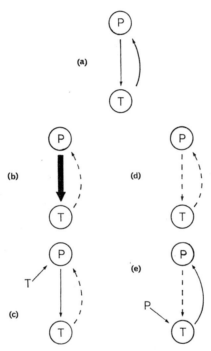

FIG. 1.1. 'Feed-back mechanisms
P = pituitary gland
T = target organ

(*a*) Normal function
(*b*) Failure of target organ to respond to trophic hormone leading to excess of the latter
(*c*) Condition (*b*) corrected by administration of target organ secretion
(*d*) Failure of pituitary leading to decreased secretion of target organ
(*e*) Condition (*d*) corrected by administration of pituitary hormone

'FEED-BACK' MECHANISMS   There is good evidence that besides being influenced by the central nervous system, the secretion of trophic hormones is affected by the secretions of the target glands. This has come to be called a 'feed-back' mechanism (Fig. 1.1). As the concentration of the hormones from the target gland rises in the blood, the secretion of the trophic hormone is inhibited, either by a mechanism involving the hypothalamus or by a direct action on the gland itself. Now the target gland secretion falls until at some critical level the release of the trophic hormone is permitted once more and the cycle recommences.

Composition of proteins

One of the greatest contributions to the study of the composition of proteins was the development of the ion-exchange column chromatographic method for the separation of amino acids from protein hydrolysates by Moore and Stein (71). The original method was very laborious, since it involved the collection of many fractions from the columns, followed by the analysis of each by the ninhydrin method, but nowadays this procedure is fully auto-mated. Details of the method and a discussion of its limitations may be found in textbooks on protein chemistry; the review of Tristram and Smith is worthy of study (106).

The amino acids, linked together by covalent peptide bonds into poly-peptide chains, make up the *primary structure* of the molecule. The *secondary structure* is concerned with the folding of the chains, e.g. into a helix. This is determined by such factors as hydrogen bonding, electrostatic forces or Van der Waals forces. Finally the helices may be linked together by other bonds, giving the protein its so-called *tertiary structure*.

The determination of the amino acid sequences therefore will reveal the primary structure of the molecule. The biological activity of the protein hormone often depends also on the secondary and tertiary structure and may well be destroyed by such changes as denaturation, the breaking of hydrogen bonding or the linkages involving groups in the side chains.

Structural analysis of proteins

END-GROUP ANALYSIS

(a) *Chemical methods*

N-TERMINUS   Great advances in our knowledge of the structure of protein and polypeptide hormones have stemmed from the introduction of the methods of end-group analysis of Sanger (92) and Edman (30, 73). The aim of these methods is to produce derivatives of the amino acid at the N-terminus which are stable during acid hydrolysis and are easily separated and identified.

In the former method the yellow dinitrophenyl (DNP) derivatives of α-amino acids are easily freed from the protein by acid hydrolysis, separated by extraction with ether and purified by chromatography. They can be quantitatively determined by spectrophotometry (38).

The general reaction of the N-terminal amino acid and the reagent, 1-fluoro-2,4-dinitrobenzene (FDNB), is shown in Fig. 1.2. Reaction occurs with other groups such as the phenolic group of tyrosine, the imidazole group of histidine and the ε-amino group of lysine; the —SH groups of cysteine tend to react as well. However, many of these derivatives are colourless, or are not extracted by ether and so do not interfere. Arginine is unusual in that its DNP-derivative is insoluble in ether.

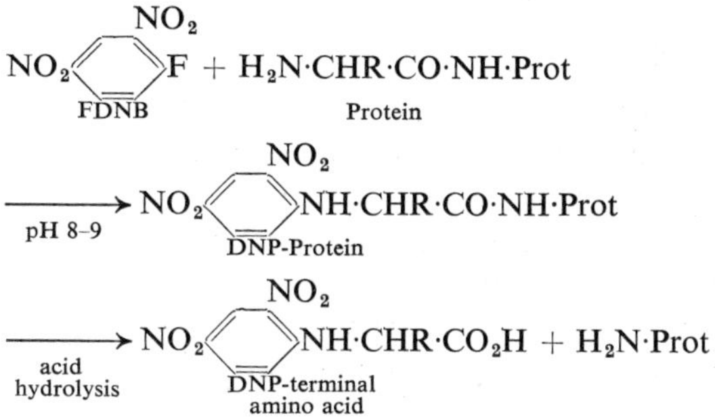

$$\text{NO}_2\text{—C}_6\text{H}_3(\text{NO}_2)\text{—F} + \text{H}_2\text{N·CHR·CO·NH·Prot}$$
FDNB   Protein

$$\xrightarrow[\text{pH 8–9}]{} \text{NO}_2\text{—C}_6\text{H}_3(\text{NO}_2)\text{—NH·CHR·CO·NH·Prot}$$
DNP-Protein

$$\xrightarrow[\substack{\text{acid}\\\text{hydrolysis}}]{} \text{NO}_2\text{—C}_6\text{H}_3(\text{NO}_2)\text{—NH·CHR·CO}_2\text{H} + \text{H}_2\text{N·Prot}$$
DNP-terminal amino acid

FIG. 1.2

In the second method amino groups react with phenyl isocyanate or phenyl isothiocyanate to give substituted urea or thiourea derivatives (Fig. 1.3). Catalytic reaction with acid leads to the release of the N-terminal residue as an ether-soluble hydantoin or thiohydantoin. It will be noted that the next amino acid in the polypeptide chain now appears as the new N-terminal residue; the reagent is particularly suitable therefore for the stepwise degradation of peptides.

$$\text{C}_6\text{H}_5\text{·NCS} + \text{H}_2\text{N·CHR'·CO·NH·CHR''·CO·NH·CHR'''·Prot}$$

$$\xrightarrow[\substack{\text{and}\\\text{acid hydrolysis}}]{\text{pH 9}} \text{H}_2\text{N·CHR''·CO·NH·CHR'''·Prot} +$$

$$\begin{array}{c}\text{CHR'}\\ \diagup\ \diagdown\\ \text{HN}\qquad\text{CO}\\ |\qquad\quad|\\ \text{S}=\text{C}\text{———}\text{N}\\ |\\ \text{C}_6\text{H}_5\end{array}$$
ether-soluble phenylthiohydantoin

FIG. 1.3

In a recent modification of the method, the reaction with phenylisothiocyanate is carried out in N-dimethyl-allylamine and trifluoroacetic acid buffer at pH 9·0 (74). Trifluoroacetic acid is used to split off the terminal amino acid and the final conversion to the thiohydantoin is effected with 30 per cent (v/v) ethanol in 0·1 N-HCl at pH 1·6–1·0. The derivatives are usually separated by the paper chromatographic systems of Sjöquist (103, 104). This method has been applied to the end-group analysis of thyroglobulin (27).

The glycoproteins form an important group of hormones and it must be remembered that steric effects of the carbohydrate moiety may influence reaction both with FDNB and phenyl isothiocyanate (74).

These two methods are complementary since in cases where one fails the other can usually be substituted. Thus serine gives an unstable thiohydantoin but the DNP derivative is easily separated and recognized. Conversely proline and glycine give labile DNP derivatives but stable thiohydantoins.

End-group analysis is not only the first stage in the structural analysis of a protein but gives information about the number of peptide chains and an indication of the purity of the protein. Frequently the N-terminal amino acid is essential for the biological activity of a protein hormone and knowledge of this is useful in the synthesis of active peptides.

C-TERMINUS   When a protein is heated in dry hydrazine at 100° for 6 hours the peptide bonds are disrupted and only the C-terminal residue yields a free amino acid (74). This method is not always applicable, cystine and tryptophan being almost completely destroyed.

(b) *Enzymic methods*

A number of enzymes are available which specifically attack proteins from the N- or C-terminus, splitting off the terminal residues one at a time. Carboxypeptidase A and aminopeptidase attack from the N-terminus, but some amino acids prove difficult, notably glycine, alanine, lysine and proline.

Carboxypeptidase B specifically cleaves basic amino acids from the C-terminus. Traces of contaminating enzymes such as trypsin and chymotrypsin can be inhibited by including di-isopropyl-phosphofluoridate in the incubation medium.

SPECIFIC SPLITTING OF PEPTIDE CHAINS

Stepwise degradation of a peptide chain by the phenylisothiocyanate method is satisfactory for a maximum of about eight residues, by which time the side reactions become troublesome. It is necessary therefore to split the protein into smaller peptide chains and determine the amino acid sequences of each.

The preliminary end-group analysis gives information about the number of peptide chains. Several may be held together only by secondary valencies; if so, they may be degraded by agents such as urea. In other cases two chains may be held together by the interchain disulphide bonds of cystine, as in insulin (p. 199), or a single chain protein may be crosslinked by intrachain disulphide bonds as in prolactin (p. 98).

A recent review of chemical methods for the selective cleavage of certain bonds in proteins contains information on such useful reagents as cyanogen bromide, which cleaves methionyl bonds in acid solution, and N-bromosuccinimide which attacks C-tryptophyl and C-tyrosyl bonds (113). Cleavage of the crosslinking disulphide bonds is often achieved by oxidation with performic acid (Fig. 1.4) but other residues such as tryptophan may be oxidized at the same time. Alternatively, reductive cleavage can be achieved by treatment with mercaptoethanol, thioglycollate or cysteine (37).

A number of enzymes are available for the non-random splitting of peptide chains. The most useful of these is trypsin which splits only the lysyl and

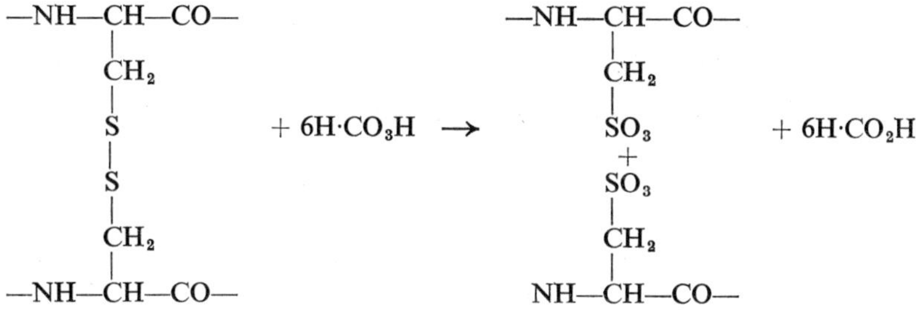

$$
\begin{array}{ccc}
\text{—NH—CH—CO—} & & \text{—NH—CH—CO—} \\
\quad | & & \quad | \\
\text{CH}_2 & & \text{CH}_2 \\
\quad | & & \quad | \\
\text{S} \quad + 6H\cdot CO_3H \rightarrow & & \text{SO}_3 \quad + 6H\cdot CO_2H \\
\quad | & & + \\
\text{S} & & \text{SO}_3 \\
\quad | & & \quad | \\
\text{CH}_2 & & \text{CH}_2 \\
\quad | & & \quad | \\
\text{—NH—CH—CO—} & & \text{NH—CH—CO—}
\end{array}
$$

FIG. 1.4

arginyl bonds. If the lysine residues are modified, e.g. by acetylation, they are no longer attacked by trypsin which then specifically cleaves the bonds next to arginyl residues. An example of the use of trypsin is given on p. 60 in the analysis of corticotrophin.

Other enzymes are less specific in their action but nevertheless have proved useful in certain respects. Pepsin is quite non-specific while α-chymotrypsin attacks tyrosyl, phenylalanyl and tryptophyl residues, i.e. those amino acids with aromatic side chains. It may hydrolyse others as well, including leucyl and methionyl bonds.

Synthesis of polypeptides

The history of the synthesis of peptides dates from around the turn of the century from the work of Curtius and Emil Fischer. Their methods were the only ones available for more than thirty years and they are still used today in conjunction with newer ones.

Recent advances in this field have been extremely rapid. Only a few years ago a peptide of ten or so amino acids would have been considered to be the largest molecule that could be synthesized. At the present time it seems possible theoretically to extend the peptide chain to any size required and already the corticotrophin molecule of 39 amino acids and the two chains of insulin with a total of 51 amino acids have been synthesized.

Several problems arise in the synthesis of peptides. Firstly, protective groups are required for masking the activity of the basic side chains of lysine and arginine. These protecting groups must be capable of being introduced by a simple reaction, and they must be easily removable again after the condensation procedure. Moreover they must show different reactivities towards various deblocking agents: there may be several protected functions in the synthesized intermediate, and selective unmasking of a particular group may be required for the elongation of the peptide chain.

Secondly the intermediates, containing the protecting groups, should be of the required solubility and preferably crystallizable. In this way they are easily separated from the reactants so that the final purity and the overall yield are satisfactory.

Finally there is the problem of racemization: if this occurs the product will most probably be inactive. The condensation processes available, with the exception of the azide method, are capable of causing some degree of racemization.

STEPS USED IN THE SYNTHESIS OF PEPTIDES

In the classical work of Curtius, peptide bonds were synthesized by the use of azides. N-benzoyl amino acids and peptide esters were converted to hydrazides which on exposure to nitrous acid gave the corresponding azides. These were coupled to amino acids or peptides to give the benzoyl peptides.

Fischer made use of amino acids protected by N-methoxy-carboxyl and N-ethoxy-carboxyl groups. Acid chlorides of these protected amino acids were prepared by the action of thionyl chloride, and they condensed readily with amino acid esters. The resulting peptide esters were saponified to the free N-alkoxy-carboxyl peptides but removal of the protecting groups was not possible. The difficulty was subsequently overcome by using the α-halogeno acyl group as the protecting agent. Again the protected amino acid was converted to the acid chloride, this time by the action of phosphorus pentachloride, and reaction with a second amino acid formed an N-α-halogeno-acyl-dipeptide ester (I). After removal of the ester group, exposure to ammonia gave the dipeptide (II). These steps are shown in the example in Fig. 1.5.

$$\text{ClCH}_2\text{·CO·Cl} + \text{H}_2\text{N·CH}_2\text{·CO}_2\text{C}_2\text{H}_5 \longrightarrow \text{ClCH}_2\text{·CO·NH·CH}_2\text{·CO}_2\text{C}_2\text{H}_5$$
amino acid ester

$$\xrightarrow[\substack{\text{saponified with}\\\text{NaOH}}]{} \text{ClCH}_2\text{·CO·NH·CH}_2\text{·CO}_2\text{H} \xrightarrow[\text{PCl}_5]{} \text{ClCH}_2\text{·CO·NH·CH}_2\text{·CO·Cl}$$

$$\xrightarrow[\text{H}_2\text{N·CH}_2\text{·CO}_2\text{C}_2\text{H}_5]{} \text{ClCH}_2\text{·CO·NH·CH}_2\text{·CO·NH·CH}_2\text{·CO}_2\text{C}_2\text{H}_5 \qquad \text{(I)}$$

$$\xrightarrow[\substack{\text{saponified with}\\\text{NaOH}}]{} \text{ClCH}_2\text{·CO·NH·CH}_2\text{·CO·NH·CH}_2\text{·CO}_2\text{H}$$

$$\xrightarrow[\text{NH}_3]{} \text{H}_2\text{N·CH}_2\text{·CO·NH·CH}_2\text{·CO·NH·CH}_2\text{·CO}_2\text{H} \qquad \text{(II)}$$

FIG. 1.5

The general method used for the synthesis of peptides may be summarized into four steps:

1. Preparation of a 'carboxyl component' by blocking the amino group of an amino acid or peptide with a group Y (III):

$$\text{H}_3\text{N}^+\text{·CHR'·CO}_2^- \longrightarrow \text{Y·HN·CHR'·CO}_2\text{H} \qquad \text{(III)}$$

2. Preparation of an 'amino component' by blocking the carboxyl group of another amino acid or peptide with a group Z (IV):

$$H_3N^+ \cdot CHR'' \cdot CO_2^- \rightarrow H_2N \cdot CHR'' \cdot CO_2Z \qquad \text{(IV)}$$

3. Activation of the first component with a group X and coupling with the second component to give a protected peptide (V):

$$\text{(III)} \rightarrow Y \cdot HN \cdot CHR' \cdot CO \cdot X$$

$$\xleftarrow{\text{(IV)}}$$

$$Y \cdot HN \cdot CHR' \cdot CO \cdot NH \cdot CHR'' \cdot CO_2Z + HX \qquad \text{(V)}$$

Less commonly the amino component is activated and coupled with the carboxyl component.

4. Removal of the blocking groups Y and Z from the intermediate to give a free peptide:

$$\text{(V)} \rightarrow H_3N^+ \cdot CHR' \cdot CO \cdot NH \cdot CHR'' \cdot CO_2^-$$

When the peptide chain is to be elongated only one of the blocking groups is removed and the resulting amino or carboxyl component is processed further.

Some of the protecting groups and coupling reactions used in the synthesis of polypeptide hormones will be described in the following two sections.

PROTECTING GROUPS

(a) *For amino groups*

Bergmann and Zervas in 1932 (9) described a procedure in which an amino group is protected by what they called a 'carbobenzoxy group'. This marked the beginning of modern peptide chemistry and none of the recent syntheses of peptide hormones have been accomplished without its use. The group is introduced under mild conditions without racemization or rupture of peptide bonds.

Derivatives of the general formula, $C_6H_5 \cdot CH_2 \cdot O \cdot CO \cdot NH \cdot CHR \cdot CO_2H$, are usually prepared by reaction of carbobenzoxy chloride with the corresponding amino acid in alkali. The group may be removed when required by catalytic reduction with hydrogen. There are many ways of carrying this out, a convenient and rapid method being by hydrogen bromide in acetic acid. In cases where catalytic reduction fails, sodium in liquid ammonia is often suitable. The great interest in the catalytic hydrogenation method is that the carbobenzoxy group can be removed selectively from peptides containing other protected groups such as N-t-butyloxycarbonyl, N-formyl, N-phthaloyl and N-tosyl. Sodium in liquid ammonia fails to differentiate the N-tosyl group however.

Modified carbobenzoxy groups have been widely studied. The p-nitrobenzyloxycarbonyl group is more rapidly removed by hydrogenolysis than the carbobenzoxy group and may be removed from peptides containing cysteine and is therefore sometimes particularly useful. However it is not easily removed by the hydrogen bromide method. It has been used for the synthesis of arginine vasopressin (47) and of a heptapeptide of insulin (101).

The p-phenylazocarbobenzoxy group is interesting in that it produces intensely yellow-coloured derivatives making separation easier (98). Moreover the derivatives are frequently easier to crystallize than other protected derivatives.

Limited use has been made of the phthaloyl group in the synthesis of peptide hormones. Excellent yields, with no racemization, have been claimed for the use of N-carboethoxy phthalimide (75) which gives phthaloyl amino acids in aqueous solution at room temperature. This protecting group may be removed by hydrazine: hydrazine acetate is used to remove the protecting group from the ε-amino group of lysine in the synthesis of α-melanophore-stimulating hormone (α-MSH, 94).

The group is particularly sensitive to alkali which opens the 5-membered ring to give phthalamic acid derivatives which are resistant to the action of hydrazine. However the group is resistant to catalytic hydrogenation which may sometimes be an advantage.

Derivatives of t-butanol have been introduced with great success for protecting amino groups and carboxylic acid groups as will be seen later. The t-butyloxycarbonyl (BOC) group (Fig. 1.6) is sometimes introduced by a rather complicated procedure but the effort is worthwhile since, when required, the group is removed quite easily by mild acid hydrolysis and the yields obtained are frequently better than those obtained by using other protective groups (4, 25, 69, 97).

$$(CH_3)_3 \cdot O \cdot CO \cdot NHR$$

Fig. 1.6 The t-butyloxycarbonyl group (BOC)

The synthesis of several BOC derivatives of amino acids is given by Riniker (88). Most derivatives are crystalline solids which dissolve readily in organic solvents.

The BOC group is removed smoothly by hydrolysis with anhydrous trifluoroacetic acid but catalytic hydrogenation and sodium in liquid ammonia have little effect.

This method is safe to use for peptides containing methionine, since the intermediate carbonium ion does not attack the S-atom, and also for those containing tryptophan (69). The chief disadvantage of the method is that BOC-chloride is difficult to prepare and store and therefore derivatives are often used (4, 69). Thus N-cyclopentyloxycarbonyl amino acids are relatively easily prepared from cyclopentylchloroformate and the amino acid dissolved in alkali.

The p-toluene sulphonyl (tosyl) group has been widely used, particularly by Li (87) and du Vigneaud (14, 62), and their associates. It is usually employed for blocking the ε-amino groups of lysine but it is also used for protecting the highly basic guanidino group of arginine (95). When introduced it is quite stable to acid or alkali at room temperature and to catalytic hydrogenolysis. Thus the selective removal of carbobenzoxy and other groups from amino functions elsewhere in the peptide is possible.

The method has been criticized because the removal of the tosyl group necessitates treatment with sodium in liquid ammonia. Low yields have been reported and there is the possibility of fragmentation of the peptide chain and cleavage of thioether linkages in methionine. However, Li's group report good recoveries (87) although yields tend to decrease as the number of protecting groups removed increases. An undue excess of sodium is evidently to be avoided in the reaction; it may be that some of the discrepancies in published yields result from differences in the experimental conditions used.

The use of the formyl group for protecting the ε-amino groups of lysine is another well-established method. In some cases the BOC and the tosyl group, which are both very bulky, may cause steric interference. The formyl group, although sometimes not as practical as the other groups, blocks the basic groups of lysine without any risk of this. It is introduced by treatment of the amino acid with formic acid in acetic anhydride at 5°–15° (100). The group is resistant to alkali but is readily removed by dilute acid. It is stable towards catalytic hydrogenation or to reduction by sodium in liquid ammonia. There are many examples of its use in the synthesis of polypeptide hormones, including that of α-MSH in which a derivative containing a formyl group protecting the lysine is as active as the natural hormone (55).

Some groups require special methods of protection, among which may be mentioned the guanidino group of arginine and the sulphydryl groups of cysteine.

As long ago as 1934, Bergmann et al. (10) protected the guanidino group by forming the nitro derivative:

$$\underset{\underset{NO_2}{\overset{|}{N}}\overset{|}{\underset{NH}{\overset{||}{C}}}}{\overset{H}{\overset{|}{}}}-\text{C}-\text{NH}-(\text{CH}_2)_3-\underset{\underset{CO_2^-}{|}}{\overset{\overset{NH_3^+}{|}}{\text{CH}}}$$

They showed that N^α-carbobenzoxy-N^w-nitroarginine gives unracemized arginine on catalytic hydrogenation. This method of protection has been used in the synthesis of several peptides related to corticotrophin.

Protection of the guanidino group may also be obtained because it is considerably more basic than the α-amino group and may be selectively protonated (46). The pK of the guanidino group is 12·5 while the α-amino group has a pK of 9 in amino acids and 8 or lower in peptides. There is no difficulty in removing the proton from the α-amino group while leaving the proton on the guanidino group, e.g. by the use of triethylamine. In this way no artifacts are formed as is often the case when other protecting groups have to be removed.

However some peptide salts containing arginine are very soluble and difficult to crystallize, so that their purification may be difficult. It is frequently advantageous to retain the arginine residues in some protected form throughout a synthesis and remove the blocking groups at the end.

An early method for the protection of the sulphydryl groups of cysteine was by the formation of the S-benzyl thioethers. Among the several methods available, S-benzylation occurs by reaction of cysteine with benzyl chloride in dilute ethanol containing sodium hydroxide (39). The protecting group is removed by sodium in liquid ammonia but it resists treatment with hydrogen bromide in acetic acid or catalytic hydrogenation. Examples of its use occur in syntheses of oxytocin and vasopressin.

Another method involves the protection of the sulphydryl with the triphenylmethyl (trityl) group. The reaction occurs smoothly at room temperature with trityl chloride in chloroform in the presence of triethylamine. The group is quickly removed under acidic conditions. The method has been applied to the synthesis of oxytocin (109) and of peptides related to corticotrophin (16).

(b) For carboxylic acid groups

Alkyl esters are often used for masking these groups but their use is limited as the alkaline conditions used for unmasking the carboxyl group involve the risk of racemization. Benzyl or p-nitrobenzyl or phenyl esters offer advantages over alkyl esters as they may be removed by reduction in sodium and liquid ammonia or by catalytic hydrogenation.

The p-nitrophenyl ester method was used successfully in the synthesis of oxytocin (13) and the 39-amino acid corticotrophin (96). To avoid possible racemization the amino acids are added to the amino end of the chain since the synthesis of p-nitrophenyl esters of acyl amino acids is relatively free from the possibility of racemization, but in the synthesis of a nitrophenyl ester of an acyl peptide racemization of the C-terminal amino acid is likely.

The esters are frequently prepared by the use of dicyclohexylcarbodiimide, a reagent that will be described later in connection with condensing agents (31, 89). The general reaction with p-nitrophenol and a protected amino acid is:

$$Z \cdot NH \cdot CHR \cdot CO_2H + HO \langle \rangle NO_2 + \langle \rangle N:C:N \langle \rangle$$

dicyclohexylcarbodiimide

$$\rightarrow Z \cdot NH \cdot CHR \cdot CO_2 \langle \rangle NO_2 + \langle \rangle NH \cdot CO \cdot NH \langle \rangle$$

There are some drawbacks to this most useful method. Structural changes may occur with some esters, particularly of arginine (15, 80), and slow racemization may occur if traces of alkali or tertiary amine are present (12, 49). Moreover the removal of the by-products of the reaction may be troublesome. A number of alternative reagents have been discussed by Anderson (5).

The t-butyl ester group (6, 107) has been used in several recent syntheses of polypeptide hormones (96). Acylamino acids or acylpeptides are treated with an excess of isobutylene in the presence of sulphuric acid or p-toluene sulphonic acid as catalyst. The product is isolated by treatment with aqueous alkali. Carbobenzoxy or other groups are used as amino-protecting groups. Thus in the preparation of t-butyl benzyloxycarbonyl-L-prolinate, benzyloxy-carbonyl-L-proline in methylene chloride and sulphuric acid is saturated with isobutylene. After 65 hours at room temperature sodium carbonate is added to neutralize the acids. The methylene chloride layer is separated, washed and concentrated and the desired product is crystallized.

Alternatively the t-butyl esters may be prepared from the silver salt of an N-acylamino acid by reaction with t-butyl iodide.

These esters are resistant to alkali, hydrazine and catalytic hydrogenation but they are readily cleaved by acid, e.g. trifluoroacetic acid.

COUPLING METHODS

The *azide* method of Curtius has already been mentioned and here it is only necessary to stress again its importance in modern syntheses: it is a method in which no racemization occurs. It is not suitable, however, for amino acids or peptides containing protecting groups which are sensitive to hydrazine.

In the *mixed anhydride* method acylamino acids or peptides react under anhydrous conditions with acid chlorides in the presence of a tertiary amine:

$$X \cdot NH \cdot CHR' \cdot CO_2H + R \cdot CO \cdot Cl \rightarrow X \cdot NH \cdot CHR' \cdot CO \cdot O \cdot CO \cdot R + HCl \quad (VI)$$

The mixed anhydride (VI) then reacts with the amino component:

$$(VI) + H_2N \cdot CHR'' \cdot CO_2Z \rightarrow X \cdot NH \cdot CHR' \cdot CO \cdot NH \cdot CHR'' \cdot CO_2Z$$
$$+ R \cdot CO_2H + CO_2$$

Unless the terminal amino acid is glycine there is an asymmetric carbon atom which is susceptible to racemization. The danger of racemization is reduced in non-polar solvents such as dimethyl formamide or tetrahydrofuran and in the absence of base (61, 107). In order to be soluble in non-aqueous media however the amino component cannot be a free amino acid or peptide but must be an ester.

Instead of using organic acids for the formation of mixed anhydrides, inorganic acids, particularly those based on phosphorus, have been widely studied. The important tetraethyl pyrophosphite method (6) has been applied to the syntheses of oxytocin and arginine vasopressin (28, 29). The reagent is added directly to the two fragments and the general reaction may be represented as:

$$X \cdot HN \cdot CHR' \cdot CO_2H + NH_2 \cdot CHR'' \cdot CO_2Y + (C_2H_5O)_2P \cdot O \cdot P(OC_2H_5)_2$$
$$\rightarrow X \cdot HN \cdot CHR' \cdot CONH \cdot CHR'' \cdot CO_2Y + 2(C_2H_5O)_2P \cdot OH$$

One of the most important condensing agents, *dicyclohexylcarbodiimide* (DCC), was described in the method of Sheehan and Hess (99). The two components couple directly and rapidly in high yield at room temperature in the presence of this reagent which takes up the elements of water to form diphenyl urea:

$$R' \cdot CO_2H + NH_2 \cdot R'' + C_6H_{11} \cdot N:C:N \cdot C_6H_{11}$$
$$\rightarrow R' \cdot CO \cdot NH \cdot R'' + C_6H_{11} \cdot NH \cdot CO \cdot NH \cdot C_6H_{11}$$

The reaction is not sensitive to moisture and may in fact be carried out in aqueous solution.

The only drawbacks to the method are firstly the tendency for some amino acids to form acyl urea derivatives and secondly racemization has been shown to occur occasionally. The former reaction occurs when the intermediate (VII)

$$R' \cdot CO_2H + C_6H_{11} \cdot N:C:N \cdot C_6H_{11} \rightarrow C_6H_{11} \cdot N:C \cdot NH \cdot C_6H_{11} \qquad \text{(VII)}$$
$$\overset{|}{CO_2R'}$$

undergoes an O→N shift to give:

$$C_6H_{11} \cdot N \cdot CO \cdot NH \cdot C_6H_{11}$$
$$\overset{|}{R' \cdot CO}$$

In cases where excessive acyl urea formation occurs the reagent 1,1'-carbonyl diimidazole (VIII) has proved useful. The reagent activates carboxyl groups and the products of the reaction are easily removed:

(VIII)

This reaction occurs at low temperature when the danger of racemization is negligible.

Racemization in the DCC procedure has been shown to occur in the synthesis of the pentapeptide His.Phe.Arg.Try.Gly. when the tripeptide His.Phe.Arg. is joined to Try.Gly. (56). This pentapeptide occupies positions 6–10 of the corticotrophin molecule.

Finally, carboxylic acid groups react rapidly with 3-unsubstituted isoxazolium salts (IX) under mild conditions to give enol esters (X).(114).

A particularly useful reagent is N-ethyl-5-phenyl-isoxazolium-3'-sulphonate (XI). A protected amino acid or peptide in acetonitrile or nitromethane containing triethylamine is added to a suspension of the reagent in the same solvent and stirred at 0° or room temperature until the reagent is dissolved. For the condensation the amino acid ester hydrochloride or peptide ester hydrochloride and triethylamine are added and stirred overnight at room temperature. The solvent is removed *in vacuo* and the secondary product (XII) is easily removed because of its solubility in water.

PURIFICATION OF INTERMEDIATES IN PROTEIN SYNTHESIS

In the early days of protein synthesis, the intermediates were nearly always purified by crystallization. Nowadays many other techniques are used including countercurrent distribution, zone electrophoresis, partition and ion-exchange chromatography and gel filtration.

Probably thin layer chromatography will be used much more in future since it is possible to employ systems in which lipophilic protecting groups are present whereas in many other systems they have to be split off before chromatography.

Racemization

This is still a problem in spite of the greatly improved methods available. It may be avoided by employing reactions involving *C*-terminal glycine which has no asymmetric centre.

The occurrence of racemization in a synthesis may be demonstrated by making use of the highly purified preparations of various enzymes that are available. Leucine amino peptidase is most widely used and complete digestion of the peptide into its constituent amino acids will only occur if L-amino acids are present. Configuration in acid hydrolysates can generally be determined by use of L-amino acid oxidase. Examples of these methods in connection with α-melanophore-stimulating hormone and corticotrophin are described by Schwyzer *et al.* (94).

SYNTHESIS OF POLYPEPTIDE HORMONES

An impressive number of polypeptide hormones has now been synthe-sized, examples of which will be found in the following chapters. In order to illustrate the use of the synthetic methods described in the preceding sections an actual example will now follow. This is the synthesis of the A chain of insulin reported by Katsoyannis (59).

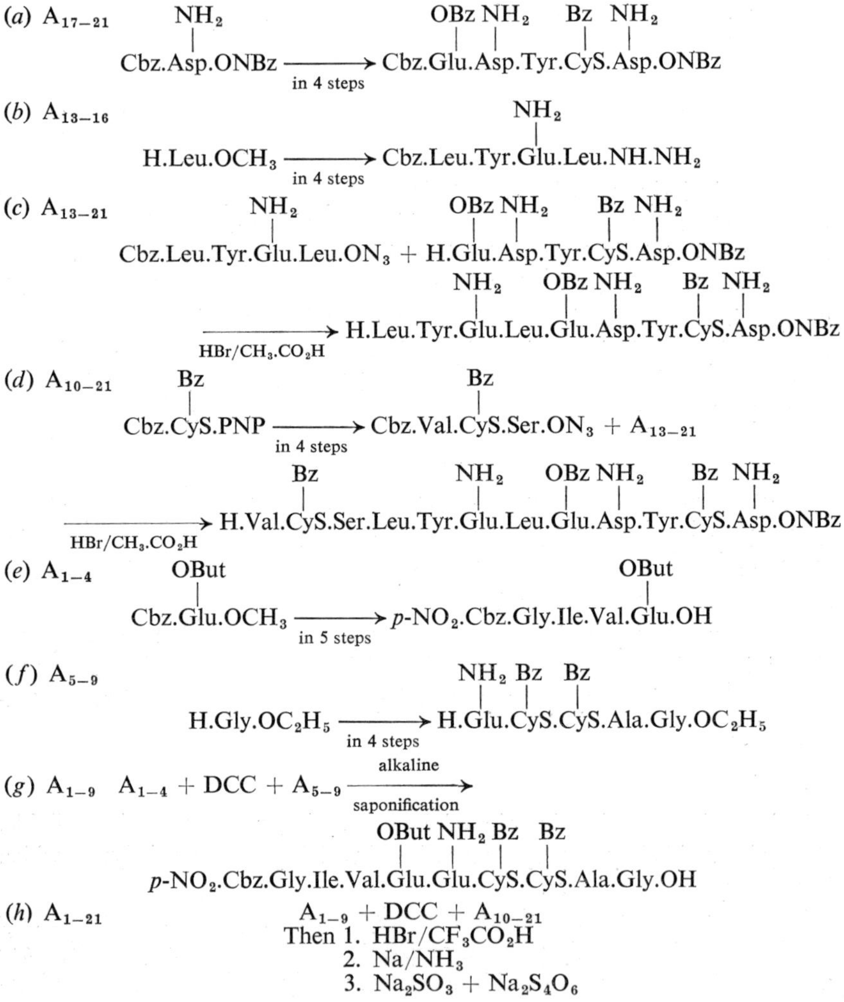

(a) A_{17-21}

$$\underset{\text{Cbz.Asp.ONBz}}{\overset{\displaystyle NH_2}{|}} \xrightarrow[\text{in 4 steps}]{} \text{Cbz.Glu.}\underset{|}{\overset{OBz}{}}\text{Asp.}\underset{|}{\overset{NH_2}{}}\text{Tyr.}\underset{|}{\overset{Bz}{}}\text{CyS.}\underset{|}{\overset{NH_2}{}}\text{Asp.ONBz}$$

(b) A_{13-16}

$$\underset{\text{H.Leu.OCH}_3}{} \xrightarrow[\text{in 4 steps}]{} \text{Cbz.Leu.Tyr.}\underset{|}{\overset{NH_2}{}}\text{Glu.Leu.NH.NH}_2$$

(c) A_{13-21}

$$\text{Cbz.Leu.Tyr.}\underset{|}{\overset{NH_2}{}}\text{Glu.Leu.ON}_3 + \text{H.}\underset{|}{\overset{OBz}{}}\text{Glu.}\underset{|}{\overset{NH_2}{}}\text{Asp.Tyr.}\underset{|}{\overset{Bz}{}}\text{CyS.}\underset{|}{\overset{NH_2}{}}\text{Asp.ONBz}$$

$$\xrightarrow[\text{HBr/CH}_3\text{.CO}_2\text{H}]{} \text{H.Leu.Tyr.}\underset{|}{\overset{NH_2}{}}\text{Glu.Leu.}\underset{|}{\overset{OBz}{}}\text{Glu.}\underset{|}{\overset{NH_2}{}}\text{Asp.Tyr.}\underset{|}{\overset{Bz}{}}\text{CyS.}\underset{|}{\overset{NH_2}{}}\text{Asp.ONBz}$$

(d) A_{10-21}

$$\text{Cbz.}\underset{|}{\overset{Bz}{}}\text{CyS.PNP} \xrightarrow[\text{in 4 steps}]{} \text{Cbz.Val.}\underset{|}{\overset{Bz}{}}\text{CyS.Ser.ON}_3 + A_{13-21}$$

$$\xrightarrow[\text{HBr/CH}_3\text{.CO}_2\text{H}]{} \text{H.Val.}\underset{|}{\overset{Bz}{}}\text{CyS.Ser.Leu.Tyr.}\underset{|}{\overset{NH_2}{}}\text{Glu.Leu.}\underset{|}{\overset{OBz}{}}\text{Glu.}\underset{|}{\overset{NH_2}{}}\text{Asp.Tyr.}\underset{|}{\overset{Bz}{}}\text{CyS.}\underset{|}{\overset{NH_2}{}}\text{Asp.ONBz}$$

(e) A_{1-4}

$$\text{Cbz.Glu.OCH}_3 \xrightarrow[\text{in 5 steps}]{} p\text{-NO}_2\text{.Cbz.Gly.Ile.Val.}\underset{|}{\overset{OBut}{}}\text{Glu.OH}$$

(f) A_{5-9}

$$\text{H.Gly.OC}_2\text{H}_5 \xrightarrow[\text{in 4 steps}]{} \text{H.}\underset{|}{\overset{NH_2}{}}\text{Glu.}\underset{|}{\overset{Bz}{}}\text{CyS.}\underset{|}{\overset{Bz}{}}\text{CyS.Ala.Gly.OC}_2\text{H}_5$$

(g) A_{1-9} $\quad A_{1-4} + \text{DCC} + A_{5-9} \xrightarrow[\text{saponification}]{\text{alkaline}}$

$$p\text{-NO}_2\text{.Cbz.Gly.Ile.Val.}\underset{|}{\overset{OBut}{}}\text{Glu.}\underset{|}{\overset{NH_2}{}}\text{Glu.}\underset{|}{\overset{Bz}{}}\text{CyS.}\underset{|}{\overset{Bz}{}}\text{CyS.Ala.Gly.OH}$$

(h) A_{1-21} $\qquad A_{1-9} + \text{DCC} + A_{10-21}$
Then 1. $\text{HBr/CF}_3\text{CO}_2\text{H}$
2. Na/NH_3
3. $\text{Na}_2\text{SO}_3 + \text{Na}_2\text{S}_4\text{O}_6$

FIG. 1.7

Abbreviations: Cbz　　carbobenzoxy
NBz　　p-nitrobenzyl
PNP　　p-nitrophenyl
But　　t-butyl ester
DCC　　dicyclohexylcarbodiimide

The chain consists of 21 amino acids (A_{1-21}) and the synthesis starts with the C-terminal pentapeptide (A_{17-21}). Asparagine is at the C-terminus and protection of its carboxyl group at first presented some difficulty. The problem was finally solved by using the p-nitrobenzyl (Nbz) group which is stable during treatment with hydrogen bromide and acetic acid, a deblocking process which it is necessary to use with peptides containing cysteine. The pentapeptide is gradually built up from Cbz-Asp(NH_2)–ONbz (Fig. 1.7a), the carbobenzoxy (Cbz) protecting group being removed at each step with hydrogen bromide and acetic acid before condensation with the next amino acid, always protected at the N-terminus by Cbz and at the C-terminus by the p-nitrobenzyl (or phenyl) group.

A similar procedure is adopted for the synthesis of the next tetrapeptide (A_{13-16}). Throughout, the C-terminal leucine is protected by a methyl group, which at the conclusion of the synthesis is converted to the hydrazide. The two peptides are then coupled to give the nonapeptide, A_{13-21}, the hydrazide of the tetrapeptide being first converted to the azide and the pentapeptide being decarbobenzoxylated by treatment with hydrogen bromide and acetic acid.

The Cbz protecting group is now removed from the nonapeptide which is

$$\overset{\displaystyle Bz}{\underset{\displaystyle |}{}}$$

then condensed with the protected tripeptide Cbz-Val-CyS-Ser-ON_3 giving the dodecapeptide, A_{10-21} (Fig. 1.7(d)).

Next the N-terminal peptides are prepared. The tetrapeptide, A_{1-4}, contains glutamic acid at its C-terminus. The γ-COOH group is protected by the t-butyl ester group which is stable during hydrogenolysis and during treatment with alkali. The synthesis therefore illustrates the useful selective deblocking achieved using this protecting group. The synthesis of the pentapeptide A_{5-9} is straightforward and the two fragments are condensed to give the nonapeptide A_{1-9} (Fig. 1.7(g)).

There now remains the final condensation of the N- and C-terminal peptides, achieved by using DCC as the condensing agent. Finally the protecting groups are removed by treatment with hydrogen bromide and trifluoroacetic acid for the t-butyl and p-nitrocarbobenzoxy groups and sodium in liquid ammonia for the S-benzyl and Nbz groups. The liberated sulphydryl groups are then converted to S-sulphonates by Na_2SO_3 and $Na_2S_4O_6$ and the product is purified by column chromatography.

BIOSYNTHESIS OF PROTEINS

All the recent work on the biosynthesis and structure of proteins shows that the sequence of amino acids is rigidly specified genetically. This was first suggested by Sanger from a consideration of the insulins (93). Protein hormones from various species may differ from one another by only a few amino acids, differences that are so slight that they may not be recognized by the ordinary methods of biological assay in mice or rats.

Vaughan and Steinberg (108) have reviewed the evidence for the specificity, and Fruton (40) the mechanisms, of the biosynthetic processes. The first step is considered to be the enzyme-catalysed reaction of free amino acids with ATP to form 5′-(aminoacylphosphoryl)-adenosine (Fig. 1.8) derivatives.

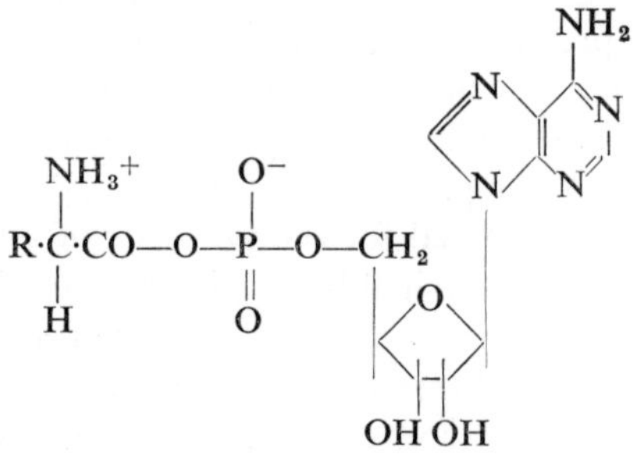

FIG. 1.8

These are subsequently linked to a specific low molecular weight RNA and are in turn transferred to a 'template' located on nucleoprotein particles (ribosomes) where the 'activated' amino acid units are joined together to form peptide chains.

Hormones with protein-anabolic action can influence the ability of ribosomes to assemble the activated amino acids and may also stimulate the synthesis of RNA, including messenger-RNA (63). These include such different hormones as growth hormone, insulin, oestrogens and testosterone and at first sight it may seem strange that they all affect the biosynthesis of protein. The probable explanation is that they exert their influence on RNA polymerase which may be of different structure in the cells of different tissues. Growth hormone, however, is able to influence the synthesis of protein in most tissues and must be assumed to have a more general action.

The genetic control of the biosynthesis of proteins is thought to be directed to the determination of the amino acid sequences of the peptide chains. It is on these sequences that the conformation of the chains depends and the functional integrity of the protein hormones in turn depends on at least some of the features of the secondary structure.

The complete characterization of a protein hormone must therefore include details of its amino acid sequence and the secondary and tertiary structure in addition to its biological properties. A battery of chemical, physical, biological and immunological tests is required. We have seen above how inadequate the ordinary methods of biological assay by themselves may be. Techniques such as the ultracentrifuge and moving boundary electrophoresis may give an indication of the purity of a protein hormone but not proof;

several hormones considered to be homogeneous by these techniques have been shown to be heterogeneous by other techniques such as starch gel electrophoresis (33). Some of the methods which are helpful in the characterization of protein hormones will now be considered in more detail.

Methods for the characterization of protein hormones

STARCH GEL ELECTROPHORESIS

The greatly improved resolution afforded by starch gel as a medium for electrophoresis was first demonstrated by Smithies (105). The technique has proved very useful for the investigation of protein hormones, particularly with discontinuous systems such as citric acid:tris-lithium hydroxide buffer at pH 8·1 in the gel and lithium hydroxide:boric acid at pH 8·5 in the electrode compartments (33).

Ferguson (32) has extended the scope of the technique beyond a test of homogeneity to include measurements of three parameters, the relation of *mobility to starch concentration,* the *retardation coefficient* and the *temperature coefficient.*

The gels examined varied in starch concentration from 10–22 per cent and by comparing the mobilities at the different concentrations an estimate of the mobility in free solution is obtained by extrapolation to zero concentration. The data obtained for various protein hormones compared with ovine prolactin as a standard are well fitted by the linear relation,

$$\log \frac{mx}{mp} = a' + b'S$$

where mx = mobility of the protein under investigation,
$\quad mp$ = mobility of the reference preparation,
$\quad S$ = concentration of the starch,
$\quad a'$ = a constant characteristic for each protein representing the logarithm of the ratio of its mobility to that of the reference preparation at zero starch concentration,
and b' = a constant characteristic for each protein representing the retardation of mobility resulting from the increasing starch concentration.

The value of b' largely reflects the molecular size, but molecular shape and the effects of adsorption may also be involved. Thus when b' is compared with the distribution coefficients obtained by gel filtration, i.e. with another measure of the molecular size of the protein, the correlation coefficient is not as highly significant as would be expected if only errors of measurement of both variables were present. No correlation is found between the relative mobility at zero concentration and the retardation coefficient (b') which suggests that the net charge does not substantially influence the value of b'.

Investigations of the temperature effects were made between 0° and 30°. The effects on mobility are in general less than those noted with changes in starch concentration and are presumably concerned with the effect on viscosity. Some values for the three parameters for several pituitary hormones are given in Table 1.2.

TABLE 1.2

Electrophoretic parameters for some of the pituitary hormones

Hormone	Species	Relative mobility (antilog $a + 0.174\,b$)	Relative retardation coefficient b	Temperature coefficient $b_t \times 10^3$	Molecular weight
β-MSH	Porcine	0·95	−0·70	0·31	2,177
Corticotrophin	Porcine	0·30	−0·52	−0·25	4,551
FSH	Human	1·63	0·84	−0·84	—
Prolactin	Bovine	1·19	0·49	−0·33	—
		1·12	0·02	0·14	26,000
		1·23	−0·02	−0·26	—
Prolactin	Ovine	1·36	0·51	−0·32	—
		1·00	0·00	0·00	23,300
		1·16	0·03	−0·28	—
Growth	Human	0·94	−0·01	−0·41	—
		0·99	−0·01	−0·18	27,100
		1·15	0·04	−0·21	—
Growth	Cetacean	0·24	1·04	7·92	39,900
Growth	Porcine	0·29	1·32	8·89	41,600

These parameters were calculated with reference to ovine prolactin. It should be noted that several hormones have more than one component and it is not certain that all these represent biologically active material, or that the molecular weights correspond to those of the active components.

The temperature coefficient, b_t, is calculated from the change in the logarithm of the relative mobility per degree C.

(From FERGUSON, K. A. *Metabolism* **13**, 985 (1964): reprinted by permission.)

The heterogeneity revealed by starch gel electrophoresis in protein hormones which appear homogeneous by other techniques is found to be due, not only to inactive contaminants but in many cases to different forms of the hormone. A good example is ovine prolactin where not only are some active forms of the hormone produced by modifications caused by the method of isolation but also different native forms of the hormone are demonstrated by examination of crude extracts. Smithies (105) was able to show that genetic polymorphism occurred with serum proteins but Ferguson and Wallace (33) in their extensive investigations of pituitary hormones were unable to conclusively demonstrate this to occur.

Gel filtration

The first separations of compounds by chromatographic systems dependent primarily on molecular size rather than on adsorption, partition or charge, made use of starch (64) or agar (84) columns. The most important advance in recent years however has been the introduction of artificially cross-linked dextrans as stationary phases (86). These compounds are marketed under the name of Sephadex (AB Pharmacia, Uppsala, Sweden), different grades of which are characterized by the degree of cross-linking. They swell in water or aqueous solutions and form gels that are able to discriminate against the entrance of molecules above a certain size. The degree of cross-linking is inversely related to the amount of water taken up—the water regain—and the grades at present available range from G-25 with a water regain (W_r) of between 1·9–2·5 g per g of dry gel to G-200 with a W_r of about 20 g per g. The former gel excludes molecules of molecular weight above 3,500–4,500 while the G-200 excludes those above 200,000.

The hydrophilic nature and the low adsorptive properties explain the marked success of these compounds in gel filtration (see 6a and 110a); they have been applied to the purification of each of the polypeptide and protein hormones, and numerous examples will be found in the succeeding chapters. Sanfelippo and Surak (91) have studied the behaviour of several pituitary hormones on Sephadex G-50 and have related their assumed molecular weights to their distribution coefficients, (K_d), between the solvent inside and outside the gel. Now in a column of Sephadex the volume of water outside the gel, the void volume V_0, can be determined by measuring the volume of liquid required to elute a substance that is completely excluded by the gel (e.g. haemoglobin). The volume inside the gel (V_i) can be calculated from the dry weight of the gel (a) and W_r since $V_i = aW_r$. The volume required to elute a given substance (V_e) depends on V_0, V_i and K_d:

$$V_e = V_0 + K_d V_i$$

i.e.
$$K_d = \frac{V_e - V_0}{V_i} \quad \text{or} \quad \frac{V_e - V_0}{aW_r}$$

As K_d approaches zero increasing exclusion of the solute from the internal solvent is indicated. Small molecules however will be retarded as they enter the gel and K_d increases to a maximum of 1. Values above 1 indicate that adsorption is also taking place.

The values of K_d obtained with the pituitary hormones in various solvents are given in Table 1.3. It is found that if K_d is plotted against the reciprocal of the logarithm of the molecular weight a linear relation exists:

$$K_d = \frac{k}{\log \text{M.W.}} - C$$

where C and k are constants. The values of k for the different solvents used were: (1) 7·25, (2) 4·24, (3) 14·48, (4) 11·90, (5) 2·23 and (6) 3·44. This formula can be used to predict the behaviour of a protein hormone of known molecular weight in these solvents.

TABLE 1.3*

Gel filtration of pituitary hormones (Ref. 91)

| Hormone | Species | K_d Solvent | | | | | | Molecular weight |
		1	2	3	4	5	6	
Corticotrophin	Porcine	0·95	1·0	—	0·87	—	0·30	3,500
TSH	Bovine	—	0·87	—	—	0·27	—	10,000
Luteotrophin	Equine	0·49	—	0·34	0·32	0·20	—	40,000
Growth	Bovine	—	—	0·25	—	—	0·07	45,000
FSH	Porcine	0·4	0·68	0·17	0·00	0·17	0·04	70,000

Solvents (1) 0·15 M-NaCl
      (2) 0·02 M-acetic acid
      (3) 0·1 M-HCl
      (4) 0·02 M-acetate in 0·1 M-$(NH_4)_2SO_4$, pH 4·0
      (5) 0·02 M-acetate, pH 5·5
      (6) 0·02 M-acetate in 0·3 M-KCl, pH 5·5

* Reprinted by permission from *J. Chromatog.* **13**, 148 (1964).

Porath (85) reports that glycoproteins containing sialic acid are poorly recovered from columns of Sephadex. A conformational change in structure, catalysed by the gel matrix, is suggested as the explanation rather than irreversible binding. However, it seems possible to use Sephadex columns satisfactorily for the recovery of several protein hormones which contain sialic acid, judging from the number of successful applications of the method that have been reported.

Sephadex is now available in a form suitable for thin layer chromatography which will extend its usefulness still further. Rapid and efficient separations of protein hormones labelled with fluorescein isothiocyanate from excess of the reagent and of antigen-antibody complexes from free antigen are possible (22).

Certain ionic groups have been introduced into Sephadex and the derivatives can be used as ion-exchange materials. They have a high capacity and a low degree of non-specific adsorption. At present the diethylaminoethylether derivative is available for anion exchange and a carboxymethylether and a sulphoether derivative for cation exchange experiments.

There is interest now in alternative materials for gel filtration, notably the polyacrylamide gels (72). A preparation, Biogel, is available commercially in several grades and preliminary work suggests that such material may be very useful in the purification of the glycoprotein, follicle stimulating hormone (3).

BIOLOGICAL ACTIVITY

There are some interesting differences in the biological activities of certain hormones of different species. The anterior pituitary secretes hormones in fish and in mammals that stimulate the thyroid gland and the gonads and that influence growth. It has been shown that the first of these, thyrotrophin, extracted from the pituitaries of fish stimulates the target organs in fish but does not have the same typical action in mammals (36). The corresponding mammalian hormones however are effective in fish. There are numerous other examples: here we may note that of the growth and gonadotrophic hormones; only the simian and human varieties are active in the human, but preparations from many species are active in rats or mice.

Fontaine (35), in attempting an explanation, suggests that the target organs become more and more specifically sensitive to the endogenous hormone in going from the lower to the higher orders. It is pointed out, however, that so little is known about the mechanism of action at the target organs that the most promising hypothesis for explaining the zoological specificity comes from a consideration of the structure of the hormones themselves. When thyrotrophin is extracted from various sources the most striking difference noted is between the amount of cystine in the fish and mammalian hormones, the fish containing the least. Now cystine is very important because of the fundamental part it plays in determining the tertiary structure of the molecule. It could be that during evolution the protein hormones tend to possess a more and more complicated and rigid tertiary structure. This may not change the type of biological activity but rather the capacity to act at the receptor site. In this respect it is interesting to note that there is apparently no zoological specificity with regard to corticotrophin, which has no disulphide bridges.

Another explanation of specificity may be that the protein contains an active centre, or core. The rest of the molecule which varies from species to species may mask the common active core and would have to be removed before the activity could be manifested. This may well be the case with regard to growth hormone which does not have a specific target organ.

Biological assay

A protein hormone is recognized essentially by its biological effects. The successful purification of a hormone therefore depends on the availability of reliable methods for detecting and quantifying these effects. Initially, detection may be all that is needed; many fractions obtained from chromatographic procedures, countercurrent distributions, etc., may have to be examined for biological activity and rapid, simple tests are required. Eventually, however, quantitative assays are necessary so that such factors as specific activity, yield and the level of the hormone in biological fluids may be assessed. An understanding of the basic principles of the design and analysis of biological assays, of their limitations and of the interpretation of the results is necessary for the chemist who is endeavouring to purify a protein hormone.

It is not possible to devote too much space here to a discussion of statistical methods: there are several textbooks on the subject (11, 34) and simplified methods have been published (17, 42). This is fortunate, because the more advanced treatises are difficult for the non-specialist, particularly as the nomenclature is not uniform. The methods described by Borth (17) are probably the most useful for the chemist since they include designs in which several unknown preparations, such as may be obtained during fractionations, are compared with a common standard.

GRADED RESPONSES AND 'ALL-OR-NONE' OR QUANTAL EFFECTS Biological assays are of two types, those in which an effect may be measured, e.g. the weight of an organ, the measurement of a chemical constituent, the number of a particular type of cell, etc., and those in which the end point depends on an all-or-none effect, e.g. the production of ova, an increase in weight above a certain threshold level counted as a positive response, survival or death etc.

In both types of assay the objective is to transform the results so that they vary in a linear fashion with increasing doses of the hormone. Then the dose-response lines of the unknown preparation and the standard preparation can be compared to give an estimate of relative potency.

The dosages are nearly always arranged on a logarithmic scale, successive doses increasing by two- to fivefold. Graded responses are used with no transformation except when the variation increases with the dose, as it often does, and then the responses are transformed to logarithms. The all-or-none effects are usually changed to percentage positive responses and then to probits which are obtained from published tables.

Before calculations are made it is often helpful to plot the mean responses against the log dosages. Then it is possible to see by eye whether any portion of the log dose-response curve obeys the equivalent of Beer's Law. If there is such a portion, the assay may then be likened to reading optical densities (the responses) several times (the number of animals at each dosage level) on a very bad spectrophotometer (the variation between responses within each dosage level). Calculation of the results therefore must take into account a number of factors which are not encountered in spectrophotometric methods.

TESTS OF VALIDITY Firstly there is the obvious test that the slope of the dose-response line (b) is significant. For a valid assay the index of significance of the combined slope of all the dose-response lines in the assay (g_c) must be less than 1 (for method of calculation see example, Appendix Table 1). If $g>1$ then b is not significantly different from zero and the fiducial limits are $\pm$ infinity.

When three or more doses are used of any one preparation, it is possible to test for *departure from linearity*. The method is shown in the example. Should the departure from linearity be significant, the offending portion of the line can usually be observed from the plotted results. Those responses outside the linear portion of the curve are then discarded before any further calculations are made.

The test for the *departure from parallelism* between the slopes of the dose-response lines of the various preparations being assayed is most important. Quantitative comparisons of potency are meaningless unless the lines are parallel. Departure from parallelism may be caused by the presence of toxic impurities or of impurities altering the rate of absorption of the hormone or because the substances being compared are different hormones. Therefore, this may be a very important test in the characterization of a hormone.

PRECISION   The error of the assay is conveniently expressed by the *index of precision* (λ), (42). In assays depending on graded effects, it is calculated by dividing the standard deviation of the responses (s) by the slope of the dose-response line (b): in quantal assays λ is the reciprocal of b. The precision of an assay is high when s is low and b is large. Thus it is clear that the lower the value of λ the more precise the assay. When λ is less than 0·2 the assay is suitable for all purposes but when it is above 0·4 the assay is hardly suitable for quantitative work.

INDEX OF DISCRIMINATION   Most protein hormones can be assayed by more than one method. The existence of qualitative differences between two preparations may be recognized by using a suitable pair of assays. Thus if one type of activity, X, is measured by the first assay and another activity, Y, by the second, the ratio of the potencies obtained by the two assays will be unity if the two preparations contain the same relative amounts of X and Y. The ratio will differ from unity when the relative amounts of X and Y differ in the two preparations. This ratio is termed the *index of discrimination* (43).

It must be noted that this index is calculated from two results, both subject to error. It is appropriate therefore to evaluate the statistical significance of the index from the data of the assays and a suitable method has been described (18).

COMPUTER PROGRAMMES FOR BIOLOGICAL ASSAYS   The importance of statistical methods in the design and analysis of biological assays is indicated by the fact that a special section of the Second International Congress of Endocrinology, London, 1964, was devoted to statistical methods. It was clear that the most notable advances have been in the preparation of computer programmes for biological assays. Particularly useful are programmes for covariant analysis. The precision of an assay is often improved considerably by taking into account a covariant factor, e.g. the ovarian weight in the assay for luteinizing hormone by the method depending on the depletion of ovarian ascorbic acid (see p. 105). The complete analysis of an experiment may take eight to ten hours of work for two persons, which is more time than is spent in performing the actual assay, but only two to three minutes of computer time (90).

There will undoubtedly be interesting new developments in this field within the next few years.

IMMUNOLOGICAL METHODS

Immunological methods are helpful in the study of several aspects of hormone chemistry. Besides providing one of the best tests for the purity of a protein, they may differentiate between hormones of various species which differ only slightly in structure, and they are extremely sensitive. It will also be seen later (pp. 34–36) how immunological techniques aid the cytologist and how they are used in the investigation of ultrastructure by means of the electron microscope (pp. 35–36).

THE PRODUCTION OF ANTIBODIES   To the ordinary reader, one of the confusing things about immunology is the variety of methods used for raising antibodies. The aim of all these methods is to produce the most potent antibody in the shortest possible time with the minimum amount of antigen— the purified antigen is nearly always in short supply.

The antigen is administered to the experimental animal, usually a rabbit, with a substance known as an adjuvant. This may be an antigen such as killed *tubercle bacilli*, or an inactive substance such as paraffin oil, lanolin, alum or bentonite. The best known are the adjuvants of Freund and Ramon (see 19) which have been employed for nearly all the investigations described in the succeeding chapters.

The courses and routes of administration vary between different laboratories almost as much as the adjuvants. Usually, however, subcutaneous or intraperitoneal routes are used initially and the titre of the antiserum is subsequently increased by 'booster' doses of antigen given intravenously. There is some evidence that the most sensitive route of administration is by intradermal injections in the footpads (52).

Protein hormones are not equally antigenic; the more foreign to the circulation of the experimental animal, the more antigenic the hormone will be. Thus protein hormones which do not vary much from species to species may be poor antigens. Then again, molecular size is important and some of the smaller polypeptides are not antigenic. However, as will be seen later, it may be possible to make even a steroid antigenic by attaching it as a hapten to a carrier protein (p. 252). The important point to note, however, is that a minor impurity in a protein hormone may be a much better antigen than the hormone itself, and so may give rise to the main antibody. There is usually less chance of this happening if the immunization is not prolonged for more than six to eight weeks and the experimental animal is not given too many courses of immunization. In the author's laboratory it has been found that with human chorionic gonadotrophin, three courses over a period of about a year are the most that can safely be carried out in each rabbit.

BIOLOGICAL INACTIVATION   At the very beginning of an immunological investigation it is important to know that the antibody is directed to the biologically active part of the hormone and not to some 'carrier protein' or inactive impurity. This information is obtained by investigating the capacity of the antiserum to neutralize the biological activity of the antigen. An effective dose of the hormone (antigen) is mixed with antiserum and the mixture is administered to the experimental animal. Alternatively, and this is probably a better method, the antigen and antibody are given at separate sites of injection, perhaps subcutaneously and intraperitoneally. Doses of 0·01 ml or less of the antiserum should effectively neutralize the activity contained in the minimum effective dose of antigen.

THE ANTIGEN-ANTIBODY REACTION   Full information on the chemistry of the antigen-antibody reaction and the methods of observing it will be found in textbooks on immunology (e.g. 19). Here we shall be concerned with certain techniques that have proved of value in relation to the protein hormones.

Gel diffusion and immunoelectrophoresis

There are several excellent reviews on these techniques (51, 78, 79). The double diffusion method in agar gel is particularly useful for observing reactions between antibodies and antigens from different species, the main types

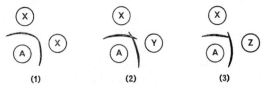

                              (1)   (2)   (3)

FIG. 1.9. Double diffusion in agar gel showing different types of precipitin pattern
A = antibody: X, Y and Z = antigens
(1) reaction of identity
(2) reaction of non-identity
(3) reaction of partial identity

of reaction being (1) of identity, (2) of non-identity and (3) of partial identity (see Fig. 1.9). Other types of reaction have been described subsequently by Ouchterlony (76, 77).

The combination of this technique with that of electrophoresis makes use of another distinctive property of the protein and has proved of immense value in following the purification of protein hormones.

Purified antigens can be measured quantitatively by the elegant method described by Gell (44) in which the patterns of precipitin lines given by dilutions of the unknown antigen are compared with those of the standard. When the antigen and antibody are not pure quantitative estimates may be obtained by an inhibition method (115). A purified preparation of the antigen is required as the standard, and a series of dilutions is set up against a similar series of dilutions of antibody, so that the minimum quantity of each which gives an observable precipitin line is found. Now when small quantities of antigen are mixed with the antiserum before the double diffusion, there will be insufficient antibody to react, i.e. the precipitin reaction is inhibited. By making suitable dilutions of the antigen being measured and comparing the degree of inhibition with that of known amounts of standard an estimate of potency is obtained. It will be noted that the end point depends only on the reaction between the purified antigen and excess antibody; any other immunological reaction between the preparation being assayed and the antiserum takes place independently and does not interfere with the end point.

Haemagglutination-inhibition reactions

Immunological reactions may be observed by attaching to the antigen a marker which may be a red cell or an inert particle such as latex, collodion or bentonite. In this way sensitivity is increased and it may be possible to observe reactions in systems in which soluble complexes form, which are not detectable by precipitation methods. The particles must of course be stable in saline or buffer and must not agglutinate spontaneously.

Red cells, usually from sheep, have been more widely used than any other particles and will be discussed first.

The first problem is concerned with the attachment of the antigen; a stable protein-cell linkage is required with a minimum of cross-linking of proteins or red cells. Several methods are available, the first—the tannic acid method—being the most widely used.

(a) TANNIC ACID METHOD   In this method, originally described by Boyden (20), washed sheep cells are exposed to a dilute solution of tannic acid. Some of the phenolic groups of the acid become attached to the amino groups on the surface of the red cells while others remain free. The antigen is now added and when incubated at 37° it becomes attached through the tannic acid to the cell surface. Probably steric factors prevent cell-cell linkages which would cause spontaneous agglutination.

Tanned cells, sensitized with antigen in this way, are not stable for very long and the antigen slowly leaches off the cell. The stability is improved by treating the cells with formalin before tannic acid (111); they may then be kept in suspensions for long periods or freeze-dried without losing reactivity.

(b) BIS-DIAZOTIZED BENZIDINE METHOD (50)   In this method the diazotization is carried out in an ice-bath, the diazo solution being added to a mixture of the antigen and the red-cell suspension. Benzidine is usually used in the diazotization reaction but *o*-dianisidine is also satisfactory. The method has been applied to insulin (7) and corticotrophin (68).

(c) 1,3-DIFLUORO-4,6-DINITROBENZENE METHOD (66)   This reagent gives the best results when used with cells that have been treated with formalin. It is dissolved in dioxan and added to the cells in buffer at pH 8.4 when reaction proceeds at 37° for thirty minutes. The cells are then incubated with the antigen for ninety minutes at 37°.

The method has been applied to human chorionic gonadotrophin (41).

(d) PYRUVIC ALDEHYDE METHOD (65)   This reagent has proved most satisfactory for stabilizing red cells. Since amino and other groups on the cell surfaces are conjugated, the cell becomes somewhat more lipophilic and inactive towards coupling agents which depend on a free amino group (e.g. method (c)). Coupling agents which react primarily with peptide bonds, such as tannic acid however may still be used. Some protein hormones may be attached directly to the cells which have been treated with pyruvic aldehyde and this method has proved most satisfactory for human chorionic gonadotrophin (23). The cells are incubated with the antigen at low ionic strength, at a pH sufficiently low to produce enough cationic amino groups to form an ionic link with the carboxyl groups of the cell surface but not enough to form cell-protein-cell linkages. The initial cell-protein interaction is ionic, but secondary forces seem to be involved causing the protein to be firmly held by the cell.

Provided a preservative is added, such cells remain stable in suspension at 4° for several weeks.

TITRATION OF ANTISERUM   After the cells have been sensitized they are washed several times with normal rabbit serum in saline or buffer and are stored as an approximately 2 per cent suspension with sodium azide or merthiolate as preservative. All available binding sites on the cell surface should by now be occupied and when added to antiserum reaction should only occur between antibody in the serum and antigen on the cells which causes agglutination (Fig. 1.10). Non-specific agglutinins and complement are removed from the antiserum before carrying out the titration by absorption with washed red cells and treatment at 56° for thirty minutes respectively. Then suitable dilutions are set up as shown and the final concentration of antiserum which causes agglutination is termed the titre.

INHIBITION REACTION   In this stage of the method the antiserum is used at a concentration slightly greater than the titre. The addition of quite small amounts of antigen will reduce the concentration of antibody to less than the titre so that when the sensitized cells are added no agglutination will occur. By using a series of dilutions of antigens, both of standards and unknowns,

Titration of antiserum

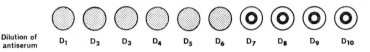

Dilution of
antiserum D_1 D_2 D_3 D_4 D_5 D_6 D_7 D_8 D_9 D_{10}

Inhibition reaction

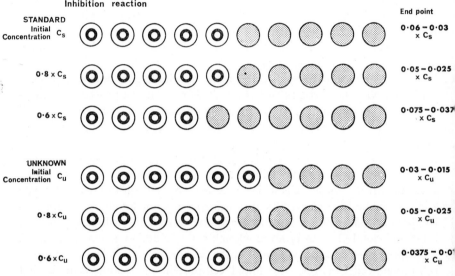

FIG. 1.10. D_1, D_2, etc, are doubling dilutions of antiserum. The lowest concentration causing agglutination is D_6 and is termed the 'titre'. D_5 would be suitable for the inhibition experiments.

C_s and C_u are the initial concentrations of standard and unknown antigens respectively used in the inhibition experiments. Doubling dilutions of C_s and C_u are used in each row. The end point of the standard, i.e. the minimum concentration inhibiting agglutination, is between 0.05 and $0.0375 \times C_s$: the end point of the unknown is between 0.03 and $0.025 \times C_u$.

The potency of the unknown compared with the standard is:

$$\frac{(0.05 \times 0.0375)^{\frac{1}{2}}}{(0.03 \times 0.025)^{\frac{1}{2}}} \times 100 \times \frac{C_s}{C_u}, \text{ i.e. } 158 \times \frac{C_s}{C_u} \%.$$

The lower limit is:

$$\frac{0.0375}{0.03} \times 100 \times \frac{C_s}{C_u} = 125 \times \frac{C_s}{C_u} \%.$$

The upper limit is:

$$\frac{0.05}{0.025} \times 100 \times \frac{C_s}{C_u} = 200 \times \frac{C_s}{C_u} \%.$$

the minimum amounts causing inhibition of the agglutination can be estimated and hence the relative potencies. A simple method of performing this is shown in Figure 1.10.

OTHER PARTICLES   Latex particles of uniform size are available and may be sensitized by mixing with protein antigen. Although they tend to agglutinate

spontaneously they have been used successfully for human chorionic gonadotrophin (p. 132) and growth hormone (60). Bentonite (2), bismuth tannate (83)
and barium sulphate (45) have also been suggested but they do not appear to
have been widely used.

Although these particles can be obtained in a more uniform state than red
cells, they appear to be even less stable in the presence of extracts of biological
fluids. Undoubtedly some purely chemical system would be desirable but at
the moment a completely satisfactory one has not been described.

Complement fixation

Some protein hormones can be estimated by the well-established method of
complement fixation. A fairly simple micro-method has been described for
human chorionic gonadotrophin (21) and another for growth hormone (60).
In some other systems anti-complementary factors present in serum or
tissue may prove troublesome.

Radioimmunoassay

The course of an immunological reaction can conveniently be observed if a
radioactive tracer is attached to the antigen. Radioactive iodine, ^{131}I, is often
used for proteins containing tyrosine. It can be introduced by an iodine

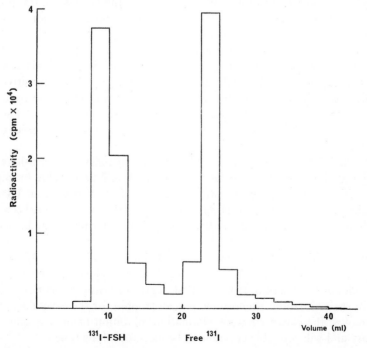

FIG. 1.11. Separation of ^{131}I-labelled FSH from free ^{131}I on column of Sephadex G-25

monochloride method (116) or by the method of Hunter and Greenwood (see p. 86). Here the hormone is exposed to radiation and oxidizing agent for a very short period and non-specific protein such as albumin is added to reduce radiation damage further. The excess ^{131}I is easily removed by gel filtration through Sephadex G-25 or G-50. A typical separation of labelled follicle stimulating hormone from free iodine is shown in Figure 1.11.

The titration of antiserum and the displacement of labelled antigen bound to antibody by the addition of unlabelled antigen form the basis of the quantitative immunoassay (see Fig. 1.12). There are several ways of separating the ^{131}I-labelled antigen that is bound to antibody from that which is displaced. Electrophoresis has been used for insulin (116) and growth hormone (58), while precipitation of the antigen–antibody complex by the addition of an anti γ-globulin serum has been described for growth hormone (53) and human chorionic gonadotrophin (112). The amount of labelled hormone displaced from the complex is related to the concentration of unlabelled antigen present in the system (Fig. 1.12).

Comparison of these methods

The sensitivities of the methods differ considerably, the radioimmunoassay being by far the most sensitive and the agar gel methods the least. It is possible to make a direct comparison of the methods since human chorionic gonadotrophin has been estimated by each.

Approximately 10 i.u. per ml is detected by the agar gel double diffusion method (24) while the sensitivity of haemagglutination methods has been variously reported, but is usually about 0·5–1·0 i.u. per ml. The sensitivity can be increased by decreasing the concentration of antiserum, or by adding slightly more sensitized cells, but the end points become less clear. The latex agglutination and complement fixation methods are of the same order of sensitivity.

The radioimmunoassay however is at least ten times more sensitive: certainly 0·06 i.u. per ml can be detected and it should be possible to improve upon this. In the best preparations this would represent about 0·004 μg protein per ml; the analogous method for growth hormone has been more highly developed and as little as 0·00007 μg of this hormone may be detected (58).

When sensitivity is the main factor the method of choice is clearly the radioimmunoassay. It is probably the only method which gives reliable results for determinations in serum. If the highest degree of sensitivity is not required, e.g. in the estimation of chorionic gonadotrophin for the early diagnosis of pregnancy, the cheaper haemagglutination-inhibition method is quite satisfactory and will probably continue to be used for a long time.

(1) Titration of antiserum:

$$AS + AGI^* \longrightarrow \boxed{AS - AGI^*}$$

(labelled antigen bound to antibody)

(2) Displacement of labelled antigen by unlabelled antigen:

$$AG + AS + AGI^* \longrightarrow \boxed{AS - (AG + \{1 - p\}AGI^*)} + p.AGI^*$$

(antigen-antibody complex) (labelled antigen displaced)

The unlabelled antigen displaces a proportion (p) of the labelled antigen from the antigen-antibody complex. The proportion, p, is related to the amount of unlabelled antigen and the measurement of p forms the basis of the quantitative immunoassay.

(3) Separation of free and bound labelled antigen, e.g. by:

(a) electrophoresis

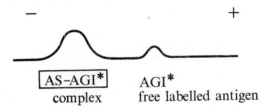

or (b) precipitation of antibody complex by an anti γ-globulin.

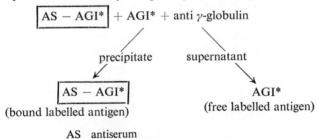

AS   antiserum
AG   unlabelled antigen
AGI*   antigen labelled with ^{131}I

FIG. 1.12. The radioimmunoassay of hormones

Cellular origin of the protein hormones

Methods for the investigation of the cellular origin of the protein hormones include histochemical techniques and electron microscopy. Here we shall be concerned with a summary of some of the histochemical techniques—mainly

D

because the nomenclature of the cell types is confusing and so many systems exist—and with immunological methods applied to electron microscopy.

HISTOCHEMICAL TECHNIQUES

Three principal cell-types are recognized in the anterior pituitary:

Acidophils   which contain cytoplasmic granules and stain with acidic dyes.
Basophils   which contain cytoplasmic granules and stain with basic dyes.
Chromophobes which contain no specific granules and do not stain. The
                hormones are secreted by the acidophils and basophils only.

A most important advance to pituitary cytology was the introduction of the periodic acid-Schiff (PAS) reaction (70). By use of this reagent it is possible to investigate those proteins containing carbohydrate and to show that they, follicle stimulating, luteinizing and thyroid stimulating hormones, are products of the basophils (81). These cells have been called *mucoid* cells and they are subdivided by many different systems of nomenclature. In some species, but not the human, no fewer than five different cell types (α, β, γ, δ, ε) may be recognized (54).

Then again by use of performic acid and alcian blue (1) in conjunction with PAS the mucoid cells have been divided into two distinct types, a red R cell in which the PAS-positive granule is not extracted by performic acid, and a blue S cell whose granule contains a high percentage of cystine. The S cells contain two types of cell, S^1 and S^2; the S^1 type stains a pure phthalocyanine blue and the S^2, the larger cell, a deep purplish blue.

The acidophils consist of a single cell type (α) which is rich in tyrosine. It is the source of growth hormone and prolactin, two hormones relatively rich in tyrosine. These cells are conveniently recognized by a diazotization-coupling method for tyrosine (48). However, studies on the pituitary of the mouse by the electron microscope indicate that even the α cells may be subdivided into those secreting growth hormone and those secreting prolactin (8).

FLUORESCENT-ANTIBODY TECHNIQUES

In 1950 Coons and Kaplan (26) described a technique whereby the cellular origin of a protein hormone (the antigen) could be located by staining with an antibody to this hormone which had been labelled with a fluorescent indicator.

The early methods of labelling were rather laborious and time-consuming and included extensive dialysis and absorption with tissue proteins. These techniques have been greatly improved: usually the γ-globulin fraction of the antiserum is treated with fluorescein isothiocyanate in alkaline solution and then the excess reagent is removed by filtration through Sephadex gels. The gel filtration saves much time that was previously taken up by dialysis; it may still be advisable to treat the labelled antiserum with non-specific tissue proteins, such as powdered liver, before use however (57).

A double-layer technique is sometimes employed whereby an antiserum to the hormone antibody is labelled with fluorescein instead. If the hormone antibody is raised in a rabbit an antiserum to rabbit γ-globulin is required, which is often raised in a goat or horse. The section is first treated with the antibody to the hormone and secondly with the labelled anti γ-globulin in order to locate the first antibody and therefore the antigen.

Other fluorescent indicators have been used, notably rhodamine. An interesting use of both indicators has been reported (67). Antibody to thyrotrophin was labelled with rhodamine and antibody to corticotrophin with fluorescein. Since rhodamine gives a pinkish, orange fluorescence and fluorescein is green, the stained sites can be differentiated. Should both labels appear at the same sites, as in this instance, further differentiation is possible by first blocking the sites of origin of one hormone by treatment with unlabelled antibody. Subsequent treatment with the labelled antibody should give no staining, but treatment with labelled antiserum to the second hormone will give positive staining if the sites of origin are really different.

ELECTRON MICROSCOPY

In order to extend the labelled-antibody method to the sub-cellular level sufficient electron-density must be conferred on the antibody molecule, without inactivating it, to render it visible in the electron microscope.

One of the most promising methods is by use of ferritin, a crystalline protein of molecular weight 460,000 containing 23 per cent ferric hydroxide-phosphate micelles. Under the electron microscope the crystals exhibit a characteristic micellar arrangement on the corners of a roughly square lattice.

There are several reagents available for coupling ferritin to antibody: these include m-xylylene diisocyanate, toluene 2,4-diisocyanate and p,p'-difluoro-m,m'-dinitrodiphenyl sulphone (110).

The method of Singer and Schick (102) has proved satisfactory in the author's laboratory. Ferritin in phosphate buffer at pH 7·5 is cooled in ice and then added to the reagent, toluene 2,4-diisocyanate. The mixture is stirred in ice for 25 minutes and any sediment is removed by centrifugation. After a further hour in ice the γ-globulin antibody is added in borate buffer at pH 9·5 and the mixture is brought to 37°. After one hour at 37° it is dialysed against 0·1 M-ammonium carbonate and finally phosphate buffer at pH 7·5.

The two functional —NCO groups of the reagent are of different reactivity. The group in the *ortho* position is sterically hindered and less reactive than that in the *para* position. In the first stage of the reaction the *para* group preferentially combines with the ferritin while the *ortho* group remains substantially unreacted. The second stage of the procedure is carried out under different conditions when the γ-globulin reacts with this latter group. A disadvantage of the xylylene diisocyanate reagent is that the two functional groups are equally reactive.

This is potentially a very powerful method but relatively little work has been reported using hormones. Ferritin is an excellent marker for electron microscopy but because of its size it may alter the immunological activity and there may be steric hindrance. It would be worth while investigating alternative labels for the antibody; mercury might prove very suitable (82).

REFERENCES

1 ADAMS, C. W. M. and SWETTENHAM, K. V. *J. Path. Bact.* **75,** 95 (1958).
2 AGAR, J. A. M., HUTT, M. S. R. and SMITH, G. *Nature, Lond.* **184,** 478 (1959).
3 AMIR, S. M., BARKER, S. A., BUTT, W. R. and CROOKE, A. C. *Nature, Lond.* **209,** 1092 (1966).
4 ANDERSON, G. W. *Metabolism* **13,** 1026 (1964).
5 ANDERSON, G. W., BLODINGER, J. and WELCHER, A. B. *J. Amer. chem. Soc.* **74,** 5309 (1952).
6 ANDERSON, G. W. and MCGREGOR, A. C. *J. Amer. chem. Soc.* **79,** 6180 (1957).
6a ANDREWS, P. *Biochem. J.* **91,** 222 (1964); **96,** 595 (1965).
7 ARQUILLA, E. R. *Ciba Fdn Colloq. Endocr.* **14,** 146 (1962).
8 BARNES, B. G. *Endocrinology* **71,** 618 (1962).
9 BERGMANN, M. and ZERVAS, L. *Ber. dt. chem. Ges.* **65,** 1192 (1932).
10 BERGMANN, M., ZERVAS, L. and RINKE, H. *Hoppe-Seyler's Z. physiol. Chem.* **224,** 40 (1934).
11 BLISS, C. I. In *The Statistics of Bioassay.* Academic Press, New York (1952).
12 BODANSKY, M. *Ann. N. Y. Acad. Sci.* **88,** 655 (1960).
13 BODANSKY, M. and DU VIGNEAUD, V. *J. Amer. chem. Soc.* **81,** 5688 (1959).
14 BODANSKY, M., MEIENHOFER, J. and DU VIGNEAUD, V. *J. Amer. chem. Soc.* **82,** 3195 (1960).
15 BODANSKY, M. and SHEEHAN, J. C. *Chemy Ind.* 1268 (1960).
16 BOISSONNAS, R. A., GUTTMANN, ST., JAQUENOUD, P.-A., SANDRIN, ED. and WALLER, J.-P. *Helv. chim. Acta* **44,** 123 (1961).
17 BORTH, R. *Acta endocr. Copenh.* **35,** 454 (1960).
18 BORTH, R., LINDER, A. and LUNENFELD, B. *Acta endocr. Copenh.* **31,** 192 (1959).
19 BOYD, W. C. In *Fundamentals of Immunology*, 3rd edn., Wiley-Interscience, London (1956).
20 BOYDEN, S. V. *J. exp. Med.* **93,** 107 (1951).
21 BRODY, S. and CARLSTROM, G. *Lancet* ii, 99 (1960).

22 BUTT, W. R. Unpublished observations.
23 BUTT, W. R., CROOKE, A. C. and CUNNINGHAM, F. J. *Biochem. J.* **81,** 596 (1961).
24 BUTT, W. R., CROOKE, A. C. and CUNNINGHAM, F. J. *Ciba Fdn Colloq. Endocr.* **14,** 310 (1962).
25 CARPINO, L. A. *J. Amer. chem. Soc.* **79,** 4427 (1957).
26 COONS, A. H. and KAPLAN, M. H. *J. exp. Med.* **91,** 1 (1950).
27 DOPHEIDE, T. A. A. and TRIKOJUS, V. M. *Nature, Lond.* **201,** 1128 (1964).
28 DU VIGNEAUD, V., GISH, D. T. and KATSOYANNIS, P. G. *J. Amer. chem. Soc.* **76,** 4751 (1954).
29 DU VIGNEAUD, V., RESSLER, C., SWAN, J. M., ROBERTS, C. W. and KATSOYANNIS, P. G. *J. Amer. chem. Soc.* **76,** 3115 (1954).
30 EDMAN, P. *Acta chem. scand.* **4,** 283 (1950).
31 ELLIOTT, D. F. and RUSSELL, D. W. *Biochem. J.* **66,** 49P (1957).
32 FERGUSON, K. *Metabolism* **13,** 985 (1964).
33 FERGUSON, K. and WALLACE, A. L. C. *Recent Prog.Horm. Res.* **19,** 1 (1963).
34 FINNEY, D. J. In *Statistical Method in Biological Assay*, Griffin, London (1952).
35 FONTAINE, Y. A. *Nature, Lond.* **202,** 1296 (1964).
36 FONTAINE, M. and FONTAINE, Y. A. *Gen. comp. Endocr.* Suppl. 1, 63 (1962).
37 FRAENKEL-CONRAT, H. In *Comprehensive Biochemistry* (edited by M. Florkin and E. H. Stotz) Vol. 7, Part 1, p. 56, Elsevier, Amsterdam (1963).
38 FRAENKEL-CONRAT, H., HARRIS, J. I. and LEVY, A. L. In *Methods of Biochemical Analysis* (edited by D. Glick) Vol. II, p. 359, Wiley-Interscience, New York (1955).
39 FRANKEL, M., GERTNER, D., JACOBSON, H. and ZILKHA, H. *J. chem. Soc.* 1390 (1960).
40 FRUTON, J. S. In *The Proteins* (edited by H. van Neurath) Vol. I, 2nd edn., p. 189, Elsevier, Amsterdam (1963).
41 FULTHORPE, A. J., PARKE, J. A. C., TOVEY, J. E. and MONCKTON, J. C. *Br. med. J.* i, 1049 (1963).
42 GADDUM, J. H. *J. Pharm. Pharmacol.* **6,** 345 (1953).
43 GADDUM, J. H. In *Polypeptides which Stimulate Plain Muscle*, p. 133, Livingstone, Edinburgh (1955).
44 GELL, P. G. H. *J. clin. Path.* **10,** 67 (1957).
45 GILBOA-GARBER, N. and NELKEN, D. *Nature, Lond.* **197,** 158 (1963).
46 GISH, D. T. *Metabolism* **13,** 1075 (1964).
47 GISH, D. T. and DU VIGNEAUD, V. *J. Amer. chem. Soc.* **79,** 3579 (1957).
48 GLENNER, G. C. and LILLIE, R. D. *J. Histochem. Cytochem.* **7,** 416 (1959).
49 GOODMAN, M. and STUEBEN, K. C. *J. org. Chem.* **26,** 3347 (1961).
50 GORDON, J., ROSE, B. and SEHON, A. H. *J. exp. Med.* **108,** 37 (1958).

51 GRABAR, P. In *Immunological Methods* (edited by J. F. Ackroyd), p. 79, Blackwell, Oxford, (1964).

52 GRUMBACH, M. M. and KAPLAN, S. L. *Ciba Fdn Colloq. Endocr.* **14**, 63 (1962).

53 HARTOG, M., GRAAFAR, M. A. and FRASER, R. *Lancet* ii, 376 (1964).

54 HERLANT, M. *C. R. Acad. Sci. Paris* **248**, 1033 (1959).

55 HOFMANN, K. *Metabolism* **13**, 1079 (1964).

56 HOFMANN, K., WOOLNER, M. E., SPUHLER, G. and SCHWARTZ, E. T. *J. Amer. chem. Soc.* **80**, 1486 (1953).

57 HOLBOROW, E. J. In *Immunological Methods* (edited by J. F. Ackroyd), p. 155, Blackwell, Oxford (1964).

58 HUNTER, W. M. and GREENWOOD, F. C. *Biochem. J.* **91**, 43 (1964).

59 KATSOYANNIS, P. G. *Metabolism* **13**, 1057 (1964).

60 KEELE, D. K. and WEBSTER, J. *Proc. Soc. exp. Biol. Med.* **106**, 168 (1961).

61 KENNER, G. W. *Symposium on Peptide Chemistry* p. 103. The Chemical Society, London (1955).

62 KIMBROUGH, R. D. and DU VIGNEAUD, V. *J. biol. Chem.* **236**, 778 (1961).

63 KORNER, A. *Biochem. J.* **92**, 449 (1964).

64 LATHE, G. H. and RUTHUEN, C. R. J. *Biochem. J.* **62**, 665 (1956).

65 LING, N. R. *Biochem. J.* **77**, 12P (1960).

66 LING, N. R. *Immunology* **4**, 49 (1961).

67 MCGARRY, E. E., AMBE, L., NAYAK, R., BIRCH, E. and BECK, J. C. *Metabolism* **13**, 1154 (1964).

68 MCGARRY, E. E., BALLANTYNE, A. and BECK, J. C. *Ciba Fdn Colloq. Endocr.* **14**, 273 (1962).

69 MCKAY, F. C. and ALBERTSON, N. F. *J. Amer. chem. Soc.* **79**, 4686 (1957).

70 MCMANUS, J. F. A. *Nature, Lond.* **158**, 202 (1946).

71 MOORE, S. and STEIN, W. H. *J. biol. Chem.* **192**, 663 (1951).

72 MORRIS, C. J. O. R. and MORRIS, P. In *Separation methods in Biochemistry* p. 393, Pitman, London (1964).

73 NEFKENS, G. H. L. *Nature, Lond.* **185**, 309 (1960).

74 NIALL, H. and EDMAN, P. *J. gen. Physiol.* **45**, Suppl. 185 (1962).

75 NIV, C.-I. and FRAENKEL-CONRAT, H. *J. Amer. chem. Soc.* **77**, 5882 (1955).

76 OUCHTERLONY, O. *Lancet* i, 346 (1949).

77 OUCHTERLONY, O. *Acta path. microbiol. scand.* **32**, 231 (1953).

78 OUCHTERLONY, O. *Prog. Allergy* **5**, 1 (1958).

79 OUDIN, J. In *Methods in Medical Research* Vol. 5, p. 335, Year Book Publishers, Chicago (1952).

80 PAUL, R., ANDERSON, G. W. and CALLAHAN, F. M. *J. org. Chem.* **26**, 3347 (1961).

81 PEARSE, A. G. E. and VAN NOORDEN, S. *Can. med. Ass. J.* **88**, 462 (1963).

82 PEPE, F. A. *J. biophys. biochem. Cytol.* **11**, 515 (1961).

83 PICK, E. and NELKEN, D. *Nature, Lond.* **197**, 157 (1963).
84 POLSON, A. *Biochim. biophys. Acta* **50**, 565 (1961).
85 PORATH, J. *Metabolism* **13**, 1004 (1964).
86 PORATH, J. and FLODIN, P. *Nature, Lond.* **183**, 1657 (1959).
87 RAMACHANDRAN, J., CHUNG, D. and LI, C. H. *Metabolism* **13**, 1043 (1964).
88 RINIKER, B. *Metabolism* **13**, 1032 (1964).
89 ROTHE, M. and KUNITZ, F.-W. *Justus Liebigs Annln Chem.* **609**, 88 (1957).
90 SAKIZ, E. and GUILLEMIN, R. *Endocrinology*, **72**, 804 (1963).
91 SANFELIPPO, P. M. and SURAK, J. G. *J. Chromatog.* **13**, 148 (1964).
92 SANGER, F. *Biochem. J.* **39**, 507 (1945).
93 SANGER, F. *Adv. Protein Chem.* **7**, 1 (1952).
94 SCHWYZER, R., COSTOPANAGIOTIS, A. and SIEBER, P. *Helv. chim. Acta* **46**, 870 (1963).
95 SCHWYZER, R. and LI, C. H. *Nature, Lond.* **182**, 1669 (1958).
96 SCHWYZER, R. and SIEBER, P. *Nature, Lond.* **199**, 172 (1963).
97 SCHWYZER, R., SIEBER, P. and KAPPELER, H. *Helv. chim. Acta* **42**, 2622 (1959).
98 SCHWYZER, R., SIEBER, P. and ZATSKO, K. *Helv. chim. Acta* **41**, 491 (1958).
99 SHEEHAN, J. C. and HESS, G. P. *J. Amer. chem. Soc.* **77**, 1067 (1955).
100 SHEEHAN, J. C. and YANG, D.-D. H. *J. Amer. chem. Soc.* **80**, 1154 (1958).
101 SHIELDS, J. E. and CARPENTER, F. H. *J. Amer. chem. Soc.* **83**, 3066 (1961).
102 SINGER, S. J. and SCHICK, A. F. *J. biophys. biochem. Cytol.* **9**, 519 (1961).
103 SJÖQUIST, J. *Acta chem. scand.* **7**, 448 (1953).
104 SJÖQUIST, J. *Biochim. biophys. Acta* **41**, 20, 1960.
105 SMITHIES, O. *Biochem. J.* **61**, 629 (1955).
106 TRISTRAM, G. R. and SMITH, R. H. *Adv. Protein Chem.* **18**, 227 (1963).
107 VAUGHAN, J. R. *J. Amer. chem. Soc.* **74**, 6137 (1952).
108 VAUGHAN, J. R. and STEINBERG, D. *Adv. Protein Chem.* **14**, 115 (1959).
109 VELLUZ, L., AMIARD, G., BARTOZ, J., GOFFINET, B. and HEYNES, R. *Bull. Soc. chim. Fr.* 1464 (1956).
110 VOGT, A. and KOPP, R. *Nature, Lond.* **202**, 1350 (1964).
110a WHITAKER, J. R. *Analyt. Chem.* **35**, 1950 (1963).
111 WIDE, L. and GEMZELL, C. A. *Ciba Fdn Colloq. Endocr.* **14**, 296 (1962).
112 WILDE, C. E., ORR, H. A. and BAGSHAWE, K. D. *Nature, Lond.* **205**, 191 (1965).
113 WITKOP, B. and RAMACHANDRAN, L. K. *Metabolism* **13**, 1016 (1964).
114 WOODWARD, R. B., OLOFSON, R. A. and MAYER, H. *J. Amer. chem. Soc.* **83**, 1010 (1961).
115 WRIGHT, S. T. C. *Nature, Lond.* **183**, 1282 (1959).
116 YALOW, R. I. and BERSON, S. A. *J. clin. Invest.* **39**, 1157 (1960).

2

NEUROHYPOPHYSIAL HORMONES

The supposition that the hypothalamus exerts a controlling influence over the secretions of the pituitary gland was strongly suggested by the work of Marshall some thirty years ago (for review see 61). The pituitary stalk connecting the median eminence of the tuber cinereum with the anterior pituitary gland contains a minute portal system of blood vessels (Fig. 2.1). Various nerve tracts in the hypothalamus probably release humoral substances into these portal vessels by which they are carried down into the anterior pituitary to regulate the secretion of hormones.

The evidence for this comes from extensive work on sectioning of the pituitary stalk and from transplantation of the pituitary (3, 42, 43). It is also believed that the hormones of the posterior pituitary gland are not formed in the gland but in the hypothalamus and are liberated from the nerve endings directly into the blood vessels of the posterior lobe (81).

The substances responsible have come to be known as 'releasing factors' (RF) and they appear to be peptides or polypeptides. Techniques for the study of such compounds have advanced rapidly in the last few years and already there is good evidence for the existence of releasing factors for corticotrophin (CRF), luteinizing hormone (LRF) and thyrotrophin (TRF) in addition to the octapeptides, oxytocin and vasopressin which have been isolated from the posterior pituitary.

Corticotrophin releasing factor

The existence of CRF activity has been demonstrated by both *in vitro* and *in vivo* methods (37, 38). Thus when extracts containing CRF are incubated with pituitary tissue corticotrophin is released and may be recognized by standard methods of assay. CRF may be assayed *in vivo* by the measurement of corticosteroids in the plasma of rats whose endogenous CRF has been blocked pharmacologically.

There are major differences of opinion, however, regarding the region of the hypothalamus from which the CRF is released. The anatomical sites of hypothalamic lesions which have been reported to block the discharge of corticotrophin following stress extend from the posterior hypothalamus (mammillary body region) to the anterior hypothalamus (medium eminence) (Fig. 2.1). Brodish (13) studied the effect of various lesions of the hypothalamus in rats and concluded that the entire region of the ventral hypothalamus, extending from the optic chiasm to the mammillary bodies was involved.

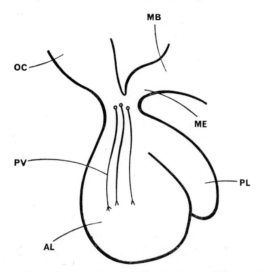

Fig. 2.1. Diagram illustrating section through pituitary and base of hypothalamus

OC	optic chiasma	AL	anterior lobe
PV	portal vessels	PL	posterior lobe
ME	median eminence	MB	mammillary body

It has been established that vasopressin possesses CRF activity although it is not considered to be the natural neurohormone (78, 89). Thus it has a corticotrophin-like effect in dogs but no CRF activity at similar dosage levels (2).

Two distinct peptides, or families of peptides, possess CRF activity. One is related structurally to lysine vasopressin and contains cysteine and no methionine: this is termed β-CRF. The other (α-CRF) is related to α-melanophore-stimulating hormone (α-MSH) and contains methionine (34, 36, 39, 79, 80). In addition to all the amino acids in α-MSH it also contains threonine, alanine and leucine (64, 80). Schally et al. (80) further subdivide α-CRF into α_1, the form extracted from porcine posterior pituitary lobes to distinguish it from α_2, the form extracted from whole pituitary glands.

EXTRACTION

The peptides are extracted by acid-acetone at pH 1·5 and the corticotrophin and MSH are largely removed by adsorption on oxycellulose (80). Protein is removed by precipitation with trichloroacetic acid and the active material is precipitated by ammonium sulphate.

The CRF can be separated from other peptides by chromatography on carboxymethyl cellulose at pH 4·6 with a gradient to pH 7·0. The α and β forms are then separated by countercurrent distribution in the system n-butanol–0·03 M-p-toluene sulphonic acid (77, 79). The α-CRF is then largely separated from the α-MSH which it still contains by further chromatography on carboxymethyl cellulose, while the β-CRF is separated in a similar fashion from the vasopressin.

STRUCTURE

There is a possibility that the α_2-CRF isolated from whole pituitary glands (80) is an artifact produced from α-MSH. The amino acid sequences appear to be similar: there is probably a change of structure at the N-terminus which is responsible for the appearance of CRF activity.

A provisional partial amino acid sequence for β-CRF is:

$$\text{(Acetyl)Ser-Tyr-C}\overset{\lceil}{\text{y}}\text{S-Phe-His-(Asp,Glu)-C}\overset{\rceil}{\text{y}}\text{S-(Pro,Val)-Lys-Gly(NH}_2\text{)}$$
$$\underset{\text{NH}_2}{\mid}\ \underset{\text{NH}_2}{\mid}$$

A number of synthetic peptides related to vasopressin and oxytocin exhibit CRF activity. Two of these which show enhanced CRF activity and decreased pressor activity are: (23)

$$\text{His-Ser-C}\overset{\lceil}{\text{y}}\text{S-Tyr-Ile-Glu(NH}_2\text{)-Asp(NH}_2\text{)-C}\overset{\rceil}{\text{y}}\text{S-Pro-Leu-Gly(NH}_2\text{)}$$

$$\text{His-Ser-C}\overset{\lceil}{\text{y}}\text{S-Tyr-Phe-Glu(NH}_2\text{)-Asp(NH}_2\text{)-C}\overset{\rceil}{\text{y}}\text{S-Pro-Lys-Gly(NH}_2\text{)}$$

Luteinizing hormone releasing factor

The introduction of the sensitive ovarian ascorbic acid depletion assay for luteinizing hormone (see page 105) has facilitated research into the purification of LRF.

Substances with LRF activity have been isolated from extracts of ovine, bovine and rat hypothalamus (35, 63, 65, 76). These extracts made in acetic acid are purified by gel filtration on Sephadex G-25 and by chromatography on carboxymethyl cellulose. In this way a polypeptide has been separated that is distinct from vasopressin, MSH and CRF. It appears to have a molecular weight of between 1,200 and 1,600 as judged by its behaviour on Sephadex and it contains aspartic acid, glutamic acid, glycine, alanine, lysine, histidine, arginine, threonine, proline, leucine and serine with traces of tyrosine and phenylalanine (76).

Follicle stimulating hormone releasing factor

The evidence for the existence of a *follicle stimulating releasing factor*, FSH-RF, is less well established and certainly there is no information as to its chemical nature. Relatively crude extracts of rat or bovine stalk-median eminence were first used to demonstrate this type of activity (53, 54, 63). When the extracts are purified by gel filtration through Sephadex G-25, the LRF and the FSH-RF are eluted together near vasopressin. Neither vasopressin itself however, nor oxytocin, are active enough to account for the FSH-releasing activity. More careful fractionations of acetic acid extracts of sheep median eminence on long columns of Sephadex G-25 suggest that LRF and FSH-RF are separable, the latter being eluted ahead of the LRF (22).

Thyrotrophin releasing factor

Relatively small lesions in the anterior hypothalamus or suprachiasmatic region are claimed to block the release of thyrotrophin although the importance of this area as a site for the production of TRF has been questioned (6). There is more general agreement that more posterior lesions of the median eminence block the release of thyrotrophin under all conditions.

Early claims to have isolated a canine hypothalamic TRF (83) were not confirmed by later work (66). However there is now evidence by *in vivo* (88) and by *in vitro* (40) experiments for the existence of such a factor in hypothalamic extracts from sheep.

The factor has been purified by gel filtration and by chromatography on carboxymethyl cellulose although the latter method does not always give consistent results (35, 55). An active peptide has been isolated after gel filtration and high-voltage electrophoresis. It contains asparagine, glutamic acid, glycine, isoleucine, leucine, serine, threonine and valine (82), and its retention volume on gel filtration is similar to that of CRF and α-MSH.

The effect of TRF appears to be specific and is not given by LRF or CRF. Preincubation of pituitary tissue with small doses of thyroxine inhibits the subsequent *in vitro* effect of TRF (40). This parallels what is considered to be the *in vivo* mechanism whereby thyroxine inhibits the secretion of thyrotrophin by a feedback mechanism acting, at least partly, on the pituitary.

The mode of action of TRF is unknown. Whether it releases pre-formed thyrotrophin or whether it participates in the processes of biosynthesis and release is not clear.

Oxytocin and vasopressin

These hormones occur in the hypothalamus bound specifically to the carrier protein, neurophysin, of molecular weight 25,000–30,000 (17, 86). The fine structure of the gland has been studied by means of the electron microscope and although single molecules of neurophysin would be too small to be visible, aggregates of a few molecules may be observed. At high magnification ($\times$ 100,000 or more) microvesicles with diameter 50–100Å are visible and these may represent aggregates of the neurophysin complex (59). The mode of binding is thought to be an anionic association between the cationic free terminal amino groups of the cystine residues of the peptides and the free carboxyl groups in the protein (33).

The active peptides are dissociated from the neurophysin by a variety of methods including acid hydrolysis, electrodialysis and precipitation and they may be recombined *in vitro*. They are not separated from the carrier protein by simple dialysis against water, ultracentrifugation or by salting-out procedures.

A very mild method of hydrolysis is by use of dilute formic acid at room temperature (52). Complete dissociation occurs on Sephadex G-25 in 0·05 N-formic acid. The protein itself, isolated by this means, contains five bands when submitted to electrophoresis in starch gel.

In another method vasopressin is separated from neurophysin by use of DEAE-cellulose. Vasopressin passes through the column in 0·02 M-ammonium acetate at pH 5·5 while neurophysin is retained; it is then eluted in 0·2 M-ammonium acetate pH 5·5 (84).

BIOSYNTHESIS

After the infusion of ^{35}S-labelled cysteine to dogs, relatively pure labelled vasopressin has been isolated from the hypothalamus and the neurohypophysis (71) which suggests that the peptide is synthesized there. Evidence is also available for its synthesis *in vitro*. For this purpose the intact hypothalamus and neurohypophysis were removed from guinea pigs, and when incubated under appropriate conditions in the presence of [^{35}S]cysteine or [^{3}H]tyrosine labelled vasopressin was formed (84). The synthesis also occurred with slices of the median eminence but not with the infundibular stem or process.

STRUCTURE

The isolation of oxytocin and vasopressin as pure hormones was achieved by du Vigneaud and his co-workers (60, 85).

The amino acid sequence of oxytocin was established as:

$$\overline{\text{CyS}}\text{-Tyr-\textbf{Ile}-Glu(NH}_2\text{)-Asp(NH}_2\text{)-}\overline{\text{CyS}}\text{-Pro-\textbf{Leu}-Gly(NH}_2\text{)}$$

CyS-Tyr-**Ile**-Glu(NH$_2$)-Asp(NH$_2$)-CyS-Pro-**Leu**-Gly(NH$_2$)
 1   2   3   4   5   6 7 8   9

and its formula was confirmed by synthesis (12, 24). The hormone is an octapeptide with a 20-membered cyclic disulphide ring which is branched by a tripeptide side chain. The synthetic compound has the same biological activity as the natural in both experimental animals and in the human. Its isoelectric point is at pH 7·7 and the pK of the phenolic group is 10·2.

There are two forms of vasopressin which differ only in one amino acid at position 8 which may be arginine or lysine:

$$\overline{\text{CyS}}\text{-Tyr-}\textbf{Phe}\text{-Glu(NH}_2)\text{-Asp(NH}_2)\text{-}\overline{\text{CyS}}\text{-Pro-}\textbf{Arg}\text{-Gly(NH}_2)$$
$$123456789$$

Arginine vasopressin

$$\overline{\text{CyS}}\text{-Tyr-}\textbf{Phe}\text{-Glu(NH}_2)\text{-Asp(NH}_2)\text{-CyS-Pro-}\textbf{Lys}\text{-Gly(NH}_2)$$
$$123456789$$

Lysine vasopressin

Phenylalanine has replaced the isoleucine of oxytocin at position 3 but the essential difference between these vasopressins and oxytocin lies in the amino acid at position 8 where the non-polar leucine of oxytocin is replaced by the strongly charged arginine or lysine.

The iso-electric point of arginine vasopressin is at pH 10·9 and the pK of the phenolic group is 9·75.

Arginine vasopressin is found in many species including man, while the lysine form occurs in the pig (47) and the hippopotamus (49). The peccary, however, which is believed to be more closely related to pigs than is the hippopotamus, prefers arginine vasopressin (74, 75) and sometimes has both arginine and lysine forms (28). Domestic pigs show comparable antidiuretic responses to either vasopressin so preference for lysine is puzzling.

The neurohypophysis of the chicken contains oxytocin but the vasopressor antidiuretic principle differs from the mammalian, being arginine vasotocin:

$$\overline{\text{CyS}}\text{-Tyr-}\textbf{Ile}\text{-Glu(NH}_2)\text{-Asp(NH}_2)\text{-CyS-Pro-}\textbf{Arg}\text{-Gly(NH}_2)$$
$$123456789$$

This peptide contains the ring of oxytocin but the side chain of arginine vasopressin. It occurs also in other birds, in reptiles and in amphibia. It has been synthesized by Katsoyannis and du Vigneaud (56).

BIOLOGICAL ACTIVITY

Oxytocin stimulates contraction of the smooth muscles, particularly of the uterus, both *in vivo* and *in vitro*.

Vasopressin causes constriction of arterioles and capillaries with a resultant pressor action; it acts as an antidiuretic factor probably by increasing the re-absorption of water by the renal tubules.

There is a certain amount of overlapping of these actions, which is not really surprising in view of their close structural similarity. They also play a role in a variety of functions such as parturition, milk-ejection and the transport of sperm (14, 45, 47).

Vasotocin possesses a remarkable ability to promote water permeability of the isolated toad bladder and to increase the transport of sodium through frog skin *in vitro* (4, 73). It is far more effective in this respect than either oxytocin or vasopressin.

Sawyer (75) has traced the interesting history of the possible evolution of these neurohypophysial hormones through fish, amphibia, birds and mammals.

It appears that arginine vasotocin is the most primitive hormone, persisting in all vertebrates except the elasmobranchs and the mammals. Its function in fish is not clear, but in amphibia and birds it is an antidiuretic hormone. Any change in the molecule markedly reduces its antidiuretic activity in amphibia so that any mutation would be deleterious.

Now in birds and reptiles, arginine vasopressin is also an effective antidiuretic agent and therefore in the reptilian ancestors of the mammals the survival of a mutation resulting in the appearance of arginine vasopressin would not be deleterious; the substitution of phenylalanine for isoleucine at position 3 would not destroy the antidiuretic efficiency.

It will be remembered that arginine vasotocin contains the ring structure of oxytocin. In birds it acts to stimulate contraction of the oviduct and ovipositor which is essentially an oxytocic effect. In mammals also it has a potent oxytocic and milk-ejecting action. Arginine vasopressin however has not. Oxytocin itself is present in birds and in the course of evolution assumed a similar function in mammals when it acquired a new activity, that of milk ejection. Thus the control of water excretion and stimulation of the uterus and mammary gland are functions of two distinct neurohypophysical principles in mammals. The separation of these functions would have been difficult if arginine vasotocin were present in mammals since it has effects which are similar to both principles.

BIOASSAY

An international standard (the 3rd) is available for oxytocic, vasopressor and antidiuretic substances. The unit is defined as the activity of 0·5 mg of the standard.

There are numerous methods of assay. A commonly used method for oxytocin employs the isolated uterus of the rat or guinea-pig (9, 31, 32, 50); another depends on the lowering of the blood pressure in the chicken (18), and a third on the ability of oxytocin to bring about the ejection of milk from the primed mammary gland of a rabbit (20). Pure oxytocin possesses about 500 i.u per mg by each of these methods of assay.

Vasopressin may be assayed by its pressor or antidiuretic actions in anaesthetized rats (21). A very sensitive method, particularly for vasotocin, depends on the transport of water or sodium across isolated frog bladders (4).

The potency of arginine vasopressin by these procedures is about 400 i.u. per mg while lysine vasopressin is less active at 250 i.u./mg.

EXTRACTION

The hormones may be extracted from posterior pituitary powders by acetic acid (70) or by percolation through Celite by means of 70 per cent ethanol and gradually-increasing concentrations of water and acetic acid (70, 72).

A method which has been applied to the extraction of oxytocin and vasopressin from many species is based on the concentration of the neurophysin-peptide complex (1). This is extracted in acetic acid and the protein is precipitated with sodium chloride. Dissociation of the complex is then effected by treatment with trichloroacetic acid which precipitates the protein.

Crude extracts from the hypothalamus contain not only oxytocin and vasopressin but at least three other substances, 5-hydroxytryptamine, noradrenaline and substance P described by Eliasson et al. (26), which interfere with estimations made by the normal methods. Lederis (58) has described methods of removing these substances by paper chromatography in n-butanol–acetic acid–water (5:1:4 by volume). Other methods include chromatography on carboxymethyl cellulose (87) or Dowex 50 X2 resin in ammonium formate (70), countercurrent distribution in s-butanol–0·05 per cent acetic acid (87) and electrophoresis in 0·5 M-acetic acid at 1,000–1,500 volts. Rapid separations are possible by thin layer chromatography on cellulose in the system n-butanol–acetic acid–water (6:2:2 by vol). The respective R_F values of lysine and arginine vasopressins and of oxytocin are 0·1–0·2, 0·25–0·40 and 0·6–0·8 (27).

Methods for the extraction and determination of these peptides in blood have been described (29, 44, 46). Proteins are precipitated from heparinized plasma by adding ten volumes of acetone. The supernatant is distilled under vacuum until all the solvent is removed and the residue is washed with ether. Standard methods of assay may then be used.

STRUCTURE AND BIOLOGICAL ACTIVITY

Many synthetic analogues have been prepared and tested for biological activity, and certain tentative conclusions can be drawn regarding the relationships of structure to biological activity (48).

The ring of five amino acids closed by the S—S linkage appears to be essential for biological activity since reduction of the bond abolishes activity (30).

It may be that the S—S bonds are important in the binding of the hormones to sulphydryl groups of a protein in the kidney and that this binding is reversed when the bond is reduced (65a, 82a). *In vitro* experiments with reagents such as *N*-ethyl maleimide and oxidized and reduced glutathione which block sulphydryl groups support the concept (5).

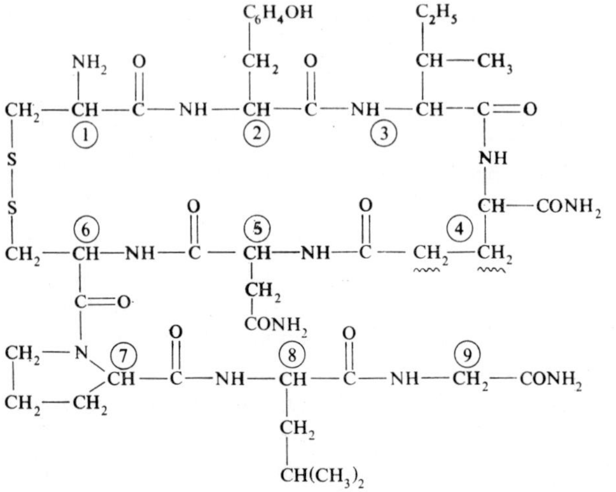

Isoglutamic acid isomer of oxytocin

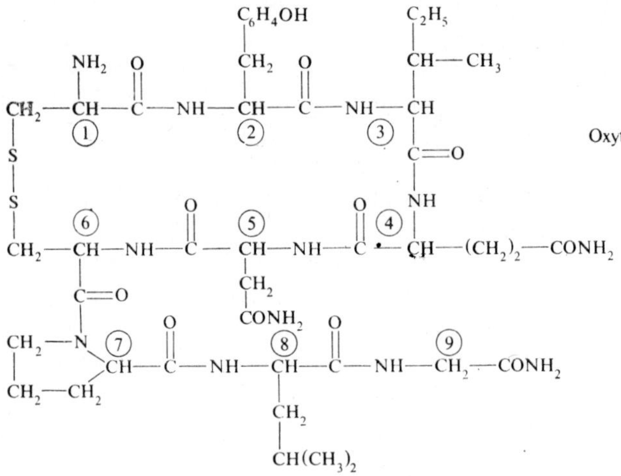

Oxytocin

FIG. 2.2

The size of the ring is of great importance and the activities disappear if the size is reduced or enlarged. An example is the isomer of oxytocin containing isoglutamic instead of glutamic acid where the ring is enlarged from 20 to 22 members (Fig. 2.2) (68). When an extra amino acid is introduced into the ring between positions 2 and 3, inactive or even inhibitory compounds result (7, 8, 11, 41) (Table 2.1). On the other hand if the three amino acids in the side chain of oxytocin are removed, the ring structure itself is only a fraction as active as the whole (67).

TABLE 2.1

The activity of peptides related to oxytocin with an extra amino acid between positions 2 and 3

Inhibitory	CyS-Tyr-**Tyr-Ile**-Glu(NH$_2$)-Asp(NH$_2$)-CyS-Pro-**Lys**-Gly(NH$_2$)
Low activity	CyS-Tyr-**Tyr-Phe**-Glu(NH$_2$)-Asp(NH$_2$)-CyS-Pro-**Lys**-Gly(NH$_2$)
Inactive	CyS-Tyr-**Tyr-Phe**-Glu(NH$_2$)-Asp(NH$_2$)-CyS-Pro-**Leu**-Gly(NH$_2$)
Inhibitory	CyS-Tyr-**Tyr-Ile**-Glu(NH$_2$)-Asp(NH$_2$)-CyS-Pro-**Leu**-Gly(NH$_2$)
Low activity	CyS-Tyr-**Ile-Ile**-Glu(NH$_2$)-Asp(NH$_2$)-CyS-Pro-**Leu**-Gly(NH$_2$)

There has been a great deal of work published on the effect of substituting individual amino acids for others at different positions in the peptides.

Replacement of tyrosine at position 2 by phenylalanine causes loss of all types of oxytocic activity but the product is by no means completely inert. Thus although the phenolic group of tyrosine contributes to the activity it is not essential (10). As may be expected from an inspection of the structural formulae, isoleucine at position 3 favours oxytocic activity, while phenylalanine favours vasopressor activity and markedly reduces oxytocic. Substitution of 3-isoleucine for 3-valine or 3-leucine reduces the activity of oxytocin but peptides with other substituents such as tyrosine or tryptophane in this position have little or no activity (25). It is interesting that the 3-valine oxytocin, although only about one sixth as active as the natural hormone, contains relatively less pressor-antidiuretic activity and is in a sense therefore a purer oxytocin. The 3-leucine derivative however has relatively more vasopressor and less oxytocic activity.

The glutamic and aspartic acids at positions 4 and 5 seem to be important since substitution by isoglutamic acid or by asparagine gives inert peptides.

The substituent at position 8 has a marked effect on activity. Substitution of isoleucine or valine for the leucine of oxytocin does not appreciably decrease oxytocic activity but, as may be expected from the structure of the natural hormone, an 8-arginine or 8-lysine (giving the vasotocins) reduces oxytocic activity considerably whilst it enhances the vasopressor activity (11). The basicity of the amino acid in this position appears to be important. Arginine gives the most active vasopressin; lysine is somewhat less basic and the derivative is less active. Histidine is much less basic and leucine is neutral and they give correspondingly less active derivatives.

The replacement of glycinamide at position 9 by sarcosinamide reduces oxytocic activity considerably, although this varies somewhat in different

E

tests (15). The free amino group at the other end of the molecule however does not appear to be required for most of the biological activities. Desamino-oxytocin (1β-mercaptopropionic acid oxytocin, Fig. 2.3) in which the free amino group of the half-cystine residue at position one is replaced by hydrogen has been synthesized (51). It has considerably higher uterine-contracting, antidiuretic and avian depressor activity than oxytocin itself, but the rat pressor activity is lower (16). Similar changes in activity occur in 8-lysine vasopressin by the substitution of the free amino group by hydrogen (16, 57).

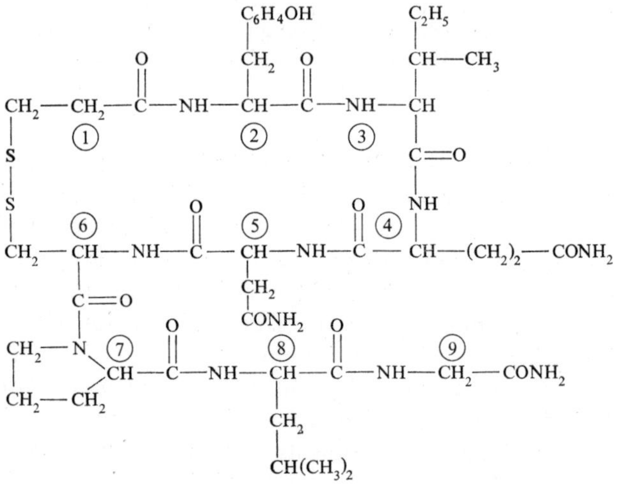

FIG. 2.3

Certain derivatives may act as inhibitors. Thus 2-*O*-methyl tyrosine oxytocin inhibits the uterine stimulating effect of oxytocin *in vitro* (69). There are also examples of analogues with extended peptide chains which act as inhibitors (see Table 2.1).

The effect of structure on other functions, including CRF activity, has been studied. Although the peptide 1-(histidine-serine-cystine)-8-lysine vasopressin has weak vasopressor activity its relative CRF activity is greater (23, 62). This indicates that CRF and vasopressor activities are not linked together and that the CRF activity is not dependent on its vasopressor activity.

Craig *et al.* (19) have suggested that overall conformation plays an important part in relation to the specific activity of these peptides. They have demonstrated by dialysis experiments that the peptide tail in oxytocin is folded more closely to the body than in vasopressin where the repulsion of the two positive groups would be expected to hold the tail in extended form.

References

1 ACHER, R., LIGHT, A. and DU VIGNEAUD, V. *J. biol. Chem.* **233,** 116 (1958).
2 ANDERSEN, R. N. and EGDAHL, R. H. *Endocrinology* **74,** 538 (1964).
3 BENOIT, J. and ARSENMACHER, I. *Archs. Anat. microsc. Morph. exp.* **42,** 334 (1953).
4 BENTLEY, P. J. *J. Endocr.* **26,** 295 (1963).
5 BENTLEY, P. J. *J. Endocr.* **30,** 103 (1964).
6 BEUGEN, L. VAN and VAN DER WERFF TEN BOSCH, J. J. *Abstr. 1st. Int. Congr. Endocr.,* Copenhagen, p. 95 (1960).
7 BEYERMAN, H. C. and BONTEKOE, J. S. *Recl Trav. chim. Pays-Bas Belg.* **79,** 1044 (1960).
8 BEYERMAN, H. C., BONTEKOE, J. S. and KOCH, A. C. *Rec. Trav. chim.* **79,** 1034 and 1039 (1960).
9 BISSET, G. W. and WALKER, J. M. *J. Physiol., Lond.* **126,** 588 (1954).
10 BODANSKY, M. and DU VIGNEAUD, V. *J. Amer. chem. Soc.* **81,** 6072 (1959).
11 BOISSONNAS, R. A., GUTTMANN, ST., BERDE, B. and KONGETT, H. *Experientia* **17,** 1 and 377 (1961).
12 BOISSONNAS, R. A., GUTTMANN, ST., JAQUENOUD, P.-A. and WALLER, J.-P. *Helv. chim. Acta* **38,** 1491 (1955).
13 BRODISH, A. *Endocrinology* **73,** 727 (1963).
14 CALDEYRO-BARCIA, R. *Acta endocr., Copenh.* Suppl. 34, 41 (1960).
15 CASH, W. D., MAHAFFEY, L. M., BUCK, A. S., NETTLETON, D., ROMAS, C. and DU VIGNEAUD, V. *J. mednl pharm. Chem.* **5,** 413 (1962).
16 CHAN, W. Y. and DU VIGNEAUD, V. *Endocrinology* **71,** 977 (1962).
17 CHAUVET, J., LENCI, M.-T. and ACHER, R. *Biochim. biophys. Acta* **38,** 266 (1960).
18 COON, J. M. *Arch. int. Pharmacodyn. Thér.* **62,** 79, 1939.
19 CRAIG, L. C., HARFENIST, E. J. and PALADINI, A. C. *Biochemistry* **3,** 764 (1964).
20 CROSS, B. A. and VAN DYKE, H. B. *J. Endocr.* **9,** 232 (1953).
21 DEKANSKI, J. *Br. J. Pharmac. Chemother.* **7,** 567 (1952).
22 DHARIWAL, A. P. S., NALLAR, R., BATT, M and McCANN S. M. *Endocrinology* **76,** 290 (1965).
23 DOEFFNER, W., STURMER, E. and BERDE, B. *Endocrinology* **72,** 897 (1963).
24 DU VIGNEAUD, V., RESSLER, C., SWAN, J. M., ROBERTS, C. W. and KATSOYANNIS, P. G. *J. Amer. chem. Soc.* **76,** 3115 (1954).
25 DU VIGNEAUD, V., WINESTOCK, G., MURTI, V. S., HOPE, D. B. and KIMBROUGH, R. D. *J. biol. Chem.* **235,** PC64 (1960).
26 ELIASSON, R., LIE, L. and PERNOW, B. *Br. J. Pharmac. Chemother.* **11,** 137 (1956).
27 FERGUSON, D. R. *J. Endocr.* **39,** 119 (1965).

28 FERGUSON, D. R., HELLER, H., LEDERIS, K. and PICKFORD, M. *Gen. comp. Endocr.* **2,** 605 (1962).

29 FITZPATRICK, R. J. In *Oxytocin* (edited by R. Caldeyro-Barcia and H. Heller), Pergamon Press, London (1960).

30 FONG, C. T. O., SILVER, L., CHRISTMAN, D. R. and SCHWARTZ, I. L. *Proc. natn Acad. Sci. U.S.A.* **46,** 1273 (1960).

31 GADDUM, J. H. *Br. J. Pharmac. Chemother.* **8,** 321 (1953).

32 GADDUM, J. H., PEART, W. S. and VOGT, M. *J. Physiol., Lond.* **108,** 467 (1949).

33 GINSBERG, M. and IRELAND, M. *J. Endocr.* **30,** 131 (1964).

34 GUILLEMIN, R. *J. Physiol. Paris* **55,** 7 (1963).

35 GUILLEMIN, R. *Metabolism* **13,** 1206 (1964).

36 GUILLEMIN, R. *Recent Prog. Horm. Res.* **20,** 89 (1964).

37 GUILLEMIN, R., HEARN, W. R., CHEEK, R. and HOUSHOLDER, D. E. *Endocrinology* **60,** 488 (1957).

38 GUILLEMIN, R. and SCHALLY, A. V. *Endocrinology* **65,** 555 (1959).

39 GUILLEMIN, R., SCHALLY, A. V., LIPSCOMBE, H. S., ANDERSEN, R. N. and LONG, J. M. *Endocrinology,* **70,** 471 (1962).

40 GUILLEMIN, R., YAMAZAKI, E., GARD, D. A., JUTISZ, M. and SAKIS, E. *Endocrinology* **73,** 564 (1963).

41 GUTTMAN, ST., JAQUENOUD, P. A., BOISSONNAS, R. A., KONZETT, H. H. and BERDE, B. *Naturwissenschaften* **44,** 632 (1957).

42 HARRIS, G. W., *Br. med. Bull.* **6,** 345 (1950).

43 HARRIS, G. W. and JACOBSOHN, D. *Proc. R. Soc. B.* **139,** 263 (1952).

44 HAWKER, R. W. *J. clin. Endocr.* **18,** 54 (1958).

45 HAWKER, R. W. In *Modern Trends in Human Reproductive Physiology* Vol. 1 (edited by H. M. Carey), p. 1, Butterworths, London (1963).

46 HAWKER, R. W. and ROBERTS, V. S. *Br. vet. J.* **113,** 459 (1957).

47 HELLER, H. *Acta endocr., Copenh.* Suppl. 34, 51 (1960).

48 HELLER, H. In *Comparative Endocrinology* Vol. 1 (edited by U. S. von Euler and H. Heller), p. 25, Academic Press, New York (1963).

49 HELLER, H. and LEDERIS, K. *J. Physiol. Lond.* **151,** 47P (1960).

50 HOLTON, P. *Br. J. Pharmac. Chemother.* **3,** 328 (1948).

51 HOPE, D. B., MURTI, V. V. S. and DU VIGNEAUD, V. *J. biol. Chem.* **237,** 1563 (1962).

52 HOPE, D. B., SCHACTER, B. A. and FRANKLAND, B. T. B. *Biochem. J.* **93,** 7P (1964).

53 IGARASHI, M. and MCCANN, S. M. *Endocrinology* **74,** 446 (1964).

54 IGARASHI, M., NALLAR, R. and MCCANN, S. M. *Endocrinology* **75,** 901 (1964).

55 JUTISZ, M. *C.R. Acad. Sci. (Paris)* **256,** 2925 (1963).

56 KATSOYANNIS, P. G. and DU VIGNEAUD, V. *J. biol. Chem.* **233,** 1353 (1958).

57 KIMBOROUGH, R. D., CASH, W. D., BRADA, L. A., CHAN, W. Y. and DU
    VIGNEAUD, V. *J. biol. Chem.* **238**, 1411 (1963).
58 LEDERIS, K. *Gen. Comp. Endocr.* **1**, 80 (1961).
59 LEDERIS, K. *Z. Zellforsch. mikrosk. Anat.* **65**, 847 (1965).
60 LIVERMORE, A. H. and DU VIGNEAUD, V. *J. biol. Chem.* **180**, 365 (1949).
61 MARSHALL, F. H. A. *Biol. Rev.* **17**, 68 (1942).
62 MARTINI, L. *Metabolism* **13**, 1211 (1964).
63 MCCANN, S. M., RAMIREZ, V. D. and IGARISHI, M. *Metabolism* **13**, 1177
    (1964).
64 PRIVAT DE GARILHE, M., GROS, C., PORATH, J., LINDNER, E. B. *Experientia*
    16, 414 (1960).
65 RAMIREZ, V. D., NALLAR, R. and MCCANN, S. M. *Proc. Soc. exp. Biol.
    Med.* **115**, 1072, 1964.
65a RASMUSSEN, H. S., SCHWARTZ, I. L., SCHOESSLER, M. A. and HOCHSTER,
    G. *Proc. natn. Acad. Sci. U.S.A.* **46**, 1278 (1960).
66 REICHLIN, S., BOSHANS, R. L. and BROWN, J. G. *Endocrinology* **72**, 334,
    1963.
67 RESSLER, C. *Proc. Soc. exp. Biol. Med.* **92**, 725 (1956).
68 RESSLER, C. and du VIGNEAUD, V. *J. Amer. chem. Soc.* **79**, 4511 (1957).
69 RUDINGER, J. and KREJČI, I. *Experientia* **18**, 595 (1962).
70 RUMSFELD, H. W. and PORTER, J. I. *Endocrniology* **70**, 62 (1962).
71 SACHS, H. *J. Neurochem.* **5**, 296 (1960).
72 SAFFRAN, M., CAPLAN, B. U., MISHKIN, S. and MUHLSTOCK, B. *Endo-
    crinology* **70**, 43 (1962).
73 SAWYER, W. H. *Endocrinology* **66**, 112 (1960).
74 SAWYER, W. H. *Recent Prog. Horm. Res.* **17**, 437 (1961).
75 SAWYER, W. H. *Endocrinology* **75**, 981 (1964).
76 SCHALLY, A. V. and BOWERS, C. Y. *Endocrinology* **75**, 608 (1964).
77 SCHALLY, A. V. and BOWERS, C. Y. *Metabolism* **13**, 1190 (1964).
78 SCHALLY, A. V., BOWERS, C. Y. and LOCKE, W. *Amer. J. med. Sci.* **248**,
    79 (1964).
79 SCHALLY, A. V. and GUILLEMIN, R. *Proc. Soc. exp. Biol. Med.* **112**, 1014
    (1963).
80 SCHALLY, A. V., LIPSCOMBE, H. and GUILLEMIN, R. *Endocrinology* **71**,
    164 (1962).
81 SCHARRER, E. and SCHARRER, B. *Recent Prog. Horm. Res.* **10**, 183 (1954).
82 SCHREIBER, V., RYBÁK, M., ECKERTOVÁ, A., JIRGL, V., KOČÍ, J., FRANC,
    Z. and KMENTOVÁ, V. *Experientia* **18**, 338 (1962).
82a SCHWARTZ, I. L., RASMUSSEN, H. S., SCHOESSLER, M. A., SILVER, L.
    and FONG, C. T. O. *Proc. natn. Acad. Sci. U.S.A.* **46**, 1288 (1960).
83 SHIBUSAWA, K., SAITO, S., NISHI, K., YAMAMOTO, T., TOMIZAWA, K.
    and ABE, C. *Endocr. jap.* **3**, 116 (1956).
84 TAKABATAKE, Y. and SACHS, H. *Endocrinology* **75**, 934 (1964).

85 TURNER, R. A., PIERCE, J. G. and DU VIGNEAUD, V. *J. biol. Chem.* **191,** 21 (1951).

86 VAN DYKE, H. B., CHOW, B. F., GREEP, R. O. and ROTHEN, R. *J. Pharmac. exp. Ther.* **74,** 190, 1947.

87 WARD, D. N., WALBORG, E. E., LIPSCOMBE, H. S. and GUILLEMIN, R. *Acta endocr., Copenh.* **40,** 283 (1962).

88 YAMAZAKI, E., SAKIZ, E. and GUILLEMIN, R. *Experientia* **19,** 480 (1963).

89 YATES, F. E. and URQUHART, J. *Physiol. Rev.* **42,** 359 (1962).

3

CORTICOTROPHIN

Corticotrophin (adrenocorticotrophin, ACTH) is the hormone which controls the growth and function of the adrenal cortex. It also possesses a number of extra-adrenal effects which include fat-mobilizing (adipo-kinetic) and melanophore-stimulating activities (24).

Source

Corticotrophin is believed to be produced and stored in the basophilic cells of the anterior pituitary. Evidence obtained by the use of the fluorescent antibody technique supports this concept. Cruickshank and Currie (12) thus demonstrated that staining occurred in some granules of the basophils. However they showed that their antisera were non-specific since preliminary treatment of the sections with unlabelled antibody did not block the subsequent staining with labelled antibody. Moreover pre-absorption of the antiserum with antigen did not abolish the staining capacity. Nevertheless, similar work was reported in the carefully controlled studies by Leznoff et al. (64) which supported their general conclusions. Antiserum was raised to both bovine and human corticotrophin which reacted specifically to corticotrophin and melanophore-stimulating hormone (MSH) which, as will be seen later, forms a portion of the corticotrophin molecule. Fluorescent staining was located in some of the basophils, not only in the anterior, but also in the posterior lobes. The latter staining was considered unlikely to be due to MSH since the cross-reaction with MSH would be too weak to account for the degree of staining.

Similar work by Pearse and van Noorden (76) confirmed that the fluorescent staining was confined to the mucoid cells of the R type (see page 34). In most glands some of the R cells in the posterior lobe were stained, but usually these were less than half the number present. No fluorescein-labelled antibody was attached to the S_1 or S_2 cells.

55

Although the granules of the *R* cells stain with periodic acid-Schiff's reagent the degree of staining does not correlate well with the fluorescent staining. This is not surprising since corticotrophin is not a glycoprotein. Thus Currie and Davies (13) showed no direct correlation between the changes in PAS staining after extraction with trichloroacetic acid and the amount of corticotrophin extracted.

As a result of their investigations with the trichloroacetic acid method, these workers suggested that corticotrophin is stored in two chemical forms, the first being of low molecular weight, dialysable, extractable by trichloroacetic acid and accounting for about 30 per cent of the total activity, and the second being a protein or bound to protein.

Stability

The loss of corticotrophic activity in intact glands is not rapid, but if they are to be stored before extraction, freezing and drying from the frozen state is necessary. Good results have been obtained by drying with acetone but Dixon and Stacke-Dunne (21) have shown that a change in chemical structure occurs during this procedure and this should be borne in mind when structural work is required.

EXTRACTION OF CORTICOTROPHIN

Progress was made in the 1940s towards the isolation, from ovine and bovine pituitaries, of corticotrophin preparations which were apparently pure proteins of molecular weight about 20,000. Subsequently it was shown that these preparations could be digested with pepsin without loss of activity; Cortis-Jones *et al.* (10) showed that the active principle could be ultrafiltered without hydrolysis, and that its molecular weight was certainly less than 20,000 and probably nearer to 12,000.

A major advance came when it was shown that the active principle could be adsorbed on to oxycellulose (2) from weakly-acid solution and eluted by stronger acid. The preparation of pure polypeptides with high corticotrophic activity soon followed.

In order to distinguish preparations obtained without hydrolysis from those obtained following enzymic hydrolysis, the former have been termed 'corticotrophin A' and the latter, 'corticotrophin B'. Subsequently it has been necessary to subdivide corticotrophin A into A_1, A_2, α_1 etc., since several different chemical forms of the hormone have been obtained.

Biological properties

The direct effect of corticotrophin on the adrenal gland is to increase its weight or to maintain its weight in hypophysectomized animals and to promote the production of corticosteroids. The latter effect can be observed *in vitro* and is the basis of a method of assay described by Saffran and Schally (80). A commonly-used *in vivo* method of assay originally described by Sayers *et al.* (81) is based on the depletion of ascorbic acid in the adrenals of hypophysectomized rats.

In addition there are numerous extra-adrenal effects that were originally considered to be due to impurities but that are now established as intrinsic properties of the hormone. These have been discussed in an authoritative review by Engel (24).

Some of these extra-adrenal effects of corticotrophin are:

(a) *adipo-kinetic*: it stimulates the mobilization of free fatty acids. In addition it stimulates the release of free fatty acids from adipose tissue.
(b) *carbohydrate metabolism:* it has a hypoglycaemic action and improves the tolerance of the rat for intravenous glucose.
(c) *protein metabolism:* it reduces the rate of formation of urea from amino acids infused intravenously.
It also has melanophore-stimulating activity and this will be described at greater length later in this chapter.

The mode of action of corticotrophin has been studied extensively. The increased production of steroid hormones from the adrenal cortex stimulated by corticotrophin is believed to result from increased supplies of $NADPH_2$. An attractive theory has been proposed (41a) which ascribes the initiation of the process to the production from ATP of adenosine-3',5'-monophosphate which activates phosphorylase. There is a good deal of experimental evidence to support this theory. Glycogen is then converted to glucose-1-phosphate at an increased rate and this in turn to glucose-6-phosphate which is metabolized by dehydrogenation. Consequently increased amounts of $NADPH_2$ are formed and serve as a source of energy for a number of steps in steroidogenesis.

Standard preparation

The third international standard preparation is now available (4). It was prepared from porcine pituitaries by extraction in acetic acid, precipitation by ethyl ether, adsorption and elution from oxycellulose and freeze-drying.

Its potency varies according to the route of administration. Collaborative assays were therefore by both subcutaneous and intravenous routes. In the adrenal ascorbic acid depletion method the respective potencies were 99·9 i.u./mg and 32–35 i.u./mg. It has also been standardized by the assay depending on thymus involution and by the *in vitro* method (80).

The potency of the pure corticotrophins is between 80 and 150 i.u. per mg assayed by the ascorbic acid depletion method. The human hormone was originally believed to be less active than the bovine, ovine or porcine polypeptides, but more recent observations suggest that this is not so (Table 3.1).

TABLE 3.1

The biological activities of corticotrophin and MSH of various species. The results are collected from figures quoted in References 49, 74 and 86 in addition to.
LI, C. H. *Recent Prog. Horm. Res.* **18**, 1 (1962) and NEY, R. L., OGATA, E., SHIMIZU, N., NICHOLSON, W. E. and LIDDLE, G. W. *Proc. Second Int. Congr. Endocr.* 1184 (1964)

	Corticotrophin			MSH		
Type	Cortico-trophin i.u./mg	MSH U/g in vitro	Cortico-trophin i.u./mg	MSH U/g in vitro	Type
Porcine	85	1.3×10^8		$0.4-1.0 \times 10^{10}$	Porcine (β)
Ovine	106	1.0×10^8	0.02	3.8×10^9	Ovine (β)
Bovine	140	0.5×10^8	0.02	9.7×10^9	Bovine (β)
Human	133	1.2×10^8		3.3×10^9	Human (β)
Synthetic (1–39)	90	1.0×10^8	0.03	8.3×10^9	Synthetic (β)
				1.2×10^9	Equine (β)
			0.04	1.2×10^{10}	All species (α)
			0.17	1.46×10^{10}	Synthetic (α)

METHODS OF PREPARATION

(a) OVINE GLANDS   The preparation of a pure polypeptide hormone from ovine glands was reported in 1954 (72). The glands were extracted in an acetone-acid mixture and, in a later modification (71), adsorbed and eluted from oxycellulose. Further purification was by salt fractionation, electrophoresis on starch at pH 11·1 and chromatography on the carboxylic acid ion-exchange resin Amberlite IRC-50 (XE-97) equilibrated with 0·05 M-NaHCO$_3$. Active material was eluted by a salt gradient to 0·15 M-NaHCO$_3$. Finally the polypeptide was purified by countercurrent distribution using 500 transfers in s-butanol–0·2 per cent trichloroacetic acid (K for α-corticotrophin = 0·719). The product, α-corticotrophin triacetate, possessed 150 units per mg and 12 mg were obtained from one kilogramme of whole pituitaries.

Careful studies were reported to demonstrate the purity of the product. It was homogeneous as judged by countercurrent distribution in s-butanol–0·1 per cent trichloroacetic acid, by partition chromatography in phosphate–cellosolve mixtures, by zone electrophoresis at several pHs and by end group analysis. In addition biological assays showed no other biological contaminants.

The preparation was called α-*corticotrophin* to distinguish it from corticotrophin A obtained from porcine glands which differed slightly in composition.

A relatively simple method giving a product of reasonably high potency employed 0·1 N-HCl for extraction (79). After adjustment of the pH to 5·6 the extract was heated at 85° to coagulate most of the proteins. Treatment with oxycellulose was followed by chromatography on IRC-50 and the product contained about 100 units/mg and the yield was 50 mg per kilogramme of wet glands.

Li's group (7) have described a more efficient method than their earlier one using chromatography on carboxymethyl cellulose and gel filtration on Sephadex G-50. It is interesting that the distribution in s-butanol–0·1 per cent trichloroacetic acid differed from the previously described behaviour ($K = 0.29$ compared with 0·41). The reason for this is not clear but is probably related to the use of oxycellulose in the earlier method.

A method similar to that employed by Li *et al.* (72) for ovine glands has been used for the preparation of *bovine* corticotrophin (68).

(b) PORCINE GLANDS A highly purified preparation, called *corticotrophin A*, was obtained by White (91). Further investigations of the method revealed several forms of corticotrophin A (21). Crude extracts were adsorbed and eluted from oxycellulose and then fractionated on the resin IRC-50 (XE-64) in phosphate buffer at pH 6·7. Several peaks were revealed by the ninhydrin reaction and these were labelled A_1, A_2, etc., A_1 having the largest retention volume. Corticotrophin A_1 was completely converted to A_2 after standing at pH 11·3 overnight. When fresh-frozen glands were used instead of acetone-dried glands the proportion of A_2 to A_1 decreased. The potency of A_1 was between 30 and 40 i.u./mg.

Bell *et al.* (5) succeeded in separating porcine corticotrophin into several components (labelled α_1, α_2, β, γ etc.) by countercurrent distributions. After 200 transfers in 6 per cent acetic acid containing 3·5 per cent NaCl–n-butanol the β fraction ($K = 0.95$) which accounted for 33 per cent of the total activity was removed and re-cycled for 720 transfers. At this stage it was judged to be pure by the shape of the distribution curve. The α and γ fractions were also redistributed and after 400–500 transfers fractions $\alpha_1(K = 12\text{–}14)$, $\alpha_2(K = 4.5)$, $\alpha_3(K = 1.5\text{–}2.0)$, $\gamma_1(K = 0.35)$, $\gamma_2(K = 0.16)$ and $\gamma_3(K = 0.27)$ were isolated. From ultracentrifugal data the molecular weight was judged to be 4,500.

(c) HUMAN GLANDS Lee (62) used an acetic acid extract from acetone dried glands which was subsequently purified by the oxycellulose method. It was then fractionated on DEAE-cellulose at 5° using gradient elution to 0·2 M-ammonium acetate (pH 5·5) through a mixing flask containing 0·005 M-ammonium acetate at pH 7·0. The major fraction was next purified on carboxymethyl-cellulose with stepwise elution from 0·05 M-(pH 5·9) to 0·25 M-(pH 6·9) ammonium acetate. The fraction containing corticotrophin was judged to be homogeneous but the active material was found to be unstable. When prepared it contained 26 i.u./mg.

Currie and Davies (13) extracted the hormone in 2·5 per cent trichloroacetic acid or water acidified to pH 5·4 and thereby obtained a low molecular weight corticotrophin. The extract was ultrafiltered and then purified by gel filtration on Sephadex G-25 followed by Sephadex G-50. The final product

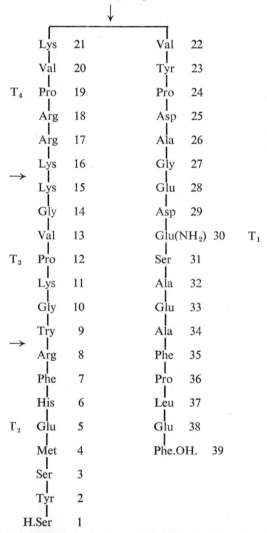

Fig. 3.1. Amino acid sequence of human corticotrophin. The peptides T_1, T_2, T_3 and T_4 are obtained by hydrolysis with trypsin: three minor fragments are obtained from T_4.

behaved as a single component in the ultracentrifuge and the calculated molecular weight was 3,200. About 6·8 per cent of the original activity in the trichloroacetic acid extract was recovered, but the specific activity was low (it contained about 10 i.u./mg.).

STRUCTURE

The methods that have been used for establishing the structure of the purified corticotrophins are similar to those developed by Sanger for insulin. After selective hydrolysis with proteolytic enzymes—usually trypsin, chymotrypsin and pepsin—the peptide fragments are isolated, being separated by paper chromatography or electrophoresis. The amino acid composition and the N- and C-terminal amino acids are then determined, from which the complete structure can be gradually assembled.

Tryptic digestion of human corticotrophin splits the hormone into four major and three minor fragments, Fig. 3.1 (62). These are separated by electrophoresis in pyridine-acetate buffer at pH 6·5 followed by paper chromatography. The final sequences of the constituent amino acids are shown in the figure.

Similar methods have been used to determine the amino acid sequences of ovine (70), bovine (69) and porcine (5,53) corticotrophins.

These hormones are all straight-chain polypeptides containing 39 amino acids and calculated to have molecular weights of about 4,500. Proline residues occur at the 12th, 19th and 24th positions, and so limit the opportunity for helix formation in this region.

The structures of ovine, bovine and porcine corticotrophins differ only in the amino acids in positions 25–33 (Fig. 3.2). The ovine and bovine have an identical composition but the arrangement of amino acids is different. The porcine hormone differs not only in arrangement but in containing leucine instead of serine at position 31. The positions of the amino acids in this part of the molecule are difficult to determine and in fact at the time of writing there is still some doubt about the sequence in human corticotrophin.

Porcine	Asp-Gly-Ala-Glu-Asp-Glu(NH$_2$)-Leu-Ala-Glu
Ovine	Ala -Gly-Glu-Asp-Asp-Glu -Ala -Ser -Glu(NH$_2$)
Bovine	Asp-Gly-Glu-Ala -Glu-Asp -Ser -Ala-Glu(NH$_2$)
Human	Asp-Ala-Gly-Glu-Asp-Glu(NH$_2$)-Ser -Ala-Glu
	25 26 27 28 29 30 31 32 33

FIG. 3.2. Amino acids 25–33 in various corticotrophins.

Melanophore stimulating hormone (MSH)

BIOLOGICAL ACTIVITY

Although MSH has been recognized for over forty years, its function in mammals is obscure. It is believed to be formed in the intermediate lobe of the pituitary and is detectable in blood and urine.

In some pathological conditions, notably in cases of adrenocortical insufficiency, marked darkening of the skin occurs presumably due to the excessive secretion of MSH. In hypopituitarism on the other hand, lack of the hormone leads to lightening of the skin, which burns easily on exposure to sunlight. The function of the hormone may therefore be to maintain the melanophores in a somewhat darkened state to provide protection from sunlight. There is no evidence however that the dark and white skinned races secrete different quantities of MSH and the difference in colour depends on other, probably, genetic factors.

Biological assay

MSH brings about darkening of the skin of frogs or tadpoles both *in vivo* and *in vitro* within about 60 minutes. The change in colour can be measured quantitatively and developed as an assay for MSH (87).

The biological activities of MSH from various species are given in Table 3.1, p. 58.

METHODS OF EXTRACTION

The preparation of a homogeneous peptide from *porcine* posterior pituitary powder was described by Lee and Lerner (61). The original powder possessed 3×10^7 units of MSH activity per g. It was extracted in a mixture of acetone and acetic acid at 50° and after precipitation from salt it was adsorbed on oxycellulose. After elution and countercurrent distribution (s-butanol–0·5 per cent w/v trichloroacetic acid) it was fractionated by electrophoresis on paper in pyridine-acetate buffer at pH 4·5. The product possessed $1–2 \times 10^{10}$ U per g and the recovery was between 10 and 40 per cent.

The product was homogeneous as judged by electrophoresis at pH values between 1·4 and 12·2 and its isoelectric point was 10·5–11·0. Countercurrent distribution in s-butanol–0·5 per cent w/v trichloroacetic acid showed that 95 per cent of the preparation moved as one component with $K = 2·1$ but there was some loss of activity during this distribution. The preparation was called α-MSH and is distinguished from the β-MSH from which it may be separated by countercurrent distribution in the same solvents. The partition coefficient (K) for β-MSH is 0·6.

Porcine β-MSH has also been purified after adsorption on oxycellulose by chromatography on the ion-exchange resin Zeo-Karb 225 in 0·2 M-ethylenediamine–0·1 M-acetic acid (19), or by zone electrophoresis on starch at pH 4·9 followed by countercurrent distribution (32, 33).

β-MSH from *bovine* glands is prepared by similar methods. In zone electrophoresis on starch it has a slightly greater cathodic mobility than the porcine hormone and its partition coefficient in s-butanol–0·5 per cent w/v trichloroacetic acid is 0·52 compared with 0·6 for porcine β-MSH (34).

The separation of *equine* α- and β-MSH is possible by countercurrent distribution in the system 0·1 per cent acetic acid–n-butanol–pyridine (11 : 5 : 3 by vol.), the partition coefficient for α being 1·5 and for β being 0·09 (23). The behaviour of equine and bovine β-MSH is similar in this solvent system, in s-butanol–0·5 per cent w/v trichloroacetic acid and in starch zone electrophoresis.

Dixon (19) has described a method suitable for the preparation of MSH from human glands. After initial extraction in KCl at pH 5·5 and salt precipitation the active fraction was adsorbed on to oxycellulose. Most of the active material was next passed unretarded through a carboxylic acid resin and was further purified by distribution in the system 1·2 M-urea–0·2 M-ethylenediamine–0·1 N-acetic acid. The product was homogeneous in high voltage electrophoresis between pH 3·5 and 6·4. It was slightly more basic than porcine β-MSH.

STRUCTURE

The amino acid sequences of the various preparations of MSH and, for comparison, of corticotrophin are shown in Figure 3.3 (21, 38, 39, 40, 41, 61).

It will be observed that α-MSH has thirteen amino acids and has the same structure regardless of source. These thirteen amino acids are identical to those in corticotrophin, except that the *N*-terminal serine has an acetyl group and the *C*-terminal valine is an amide. The structure of β-MSH varies from species to species and contains eighteen amino acids except in the human when it contains twenty-two.

The effect of chemical reagents on biological activity of corticotrophin and MSH

OXIDATION-REDUCTION   Treatment of corticotrophin with hydrogen peroxide gives a biologically inactive product which can be distinguished chromatographically from untreated corticotrophin (21, 27). Reduction of the oxidized product with thiol compounds completely restores the biological activity and the product is chromatographically identical to the original (17). The oxidation-reduction centre is the thio-ether grouping of methionine (16, 49).

This interesting property of reversible inactivation has been shown for α-MSH (49) and also for parathyroid hormone (78).

OXIDATION WITH PERIODATE   Periodate reacts with the *N*-terminal serine and destroys corticotrophic activity irreversibly (18, 30), but the MSH activity and other extra-adrenal activities such as the fat-mobilizing and ketogenic remain (25). This suggests that the *N*-terminal serine is important with regard to corticotrophic activity; further evidence for this has been obtained by modifying the terminal serine. Oxidation with periodate followed by reduction with borohydride gives a glycolloyl residue ($HO.CH_2.OH$) in place of serine

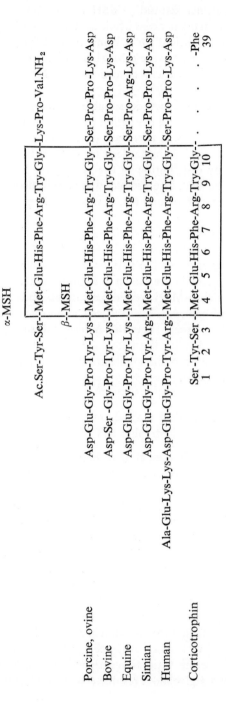

Fig. 3.3. Amino acid sequences in α- and β-MSH illustrating the common heptapeptide which occupies positions 4–10 of corticotrophin.

(8, 20). This results in a marked loss of adrenal-stimulating activity but some extra-adrenal activities remain. Conversion of serine to glycine however gives a peptide which is as active as the natural hormone in adrenal-stimulating activity and is somewhat more active in its hypoglycaemic effect (22, 60).

GUANIDINATION   Geschwind and Li (31) used O-methyl isourea to convert free amino groups to guanidine groups. Probably three of the four lysine residues were affected and corticotrophic activity was retained.

ACETYLATION   The acetylation of the N-terminal serine of corticotrophin has been studied extensively (31, 89). Waller and Dixon (89) were careful to ensure the specificity of their reaction since the usual methods of acetylation would affect the ε-amino groups of the four lysine residues as well. The method was based on earlier work (35) in which the protected pentapeptide t-butyloxy carboxyl-Ser-Tyr-Ser-Met-α-methyl-γ-benzyl-Glu was treated with hydrogen bromide in acetic acid. This removed the butyloxy carboxyl group and on adjusting the pH to above 7·0 N-acetyl-Ser-Tyr-O-acetyl-Ser-Met-α-methyl-γ-benzyl-Glu was obtained as a result of an O → N acyl shift.

When N-acetyl corticotrophin was prepared, it contained less than 10 per cent of the activity of untreated corticotrophin. This supports the work quoted above showing that the free amino group is essential for corticotrophic activity. The MSH activity was increased five to ten times however by this N-terminal acetylation when assayed on isolated frog skin.

SUCCINYLATION   In this procedure corticotrophin was treated with succinyl anhydride at pH 9·0 and the excess was removed by dialysis (66). The product migrated during electrophoresis as an anion, although the untreated hormone migrated as a cation. Reaction occurred at the N-terminus and at the ε-amino group of lysine and it is therefore not surprising that the potency dropped considerably. However the MSH activity dropped also, although the hepta-peptide sequence from positions 4 to 10 in the molecule—a sequence which is common to corticotrophin and MSH—is not disturbed in this reaction. This implies that the lysine next to the C-terminal glycine or the N-terminal serine may influence the MSH activity.

ALKALI   MSH shows interesting behaviour in that it may be boiled for ten minutes in 0·1 N-sodium hydroxide with retention of activity. When given to frogs *in vivo* the treated hormone produces both a *potentiation* and a *prolongation* of skin-darkening compared with the original hormone (57). The prolongation effect is seen also *in vitro* It has been shown (63) that race-mization of the arginine and phenylalaline residues occurs during this reaction.

ENZYMIC HYDROLYSIS   Reference has been made to the common sequence of amino acids between positions 1 and 24 in the corticotrophins of different species. Small differences in the arrangements and the constituent amino acids occur between positions 25 and 33, and it may be inferred therefore that these amino acids are not essential for biological activity. That this is so has been shown by subjecting corticotrophin to hydrolysis with pepsin (6, 11).

F

The C-terminal peptide of 11 amino acids was released from porcine or ovine corticotrophin and the N-terminal portion (positions 1–28) retained all the corticotrophic activity. Subsequent studies involving partial hydrolysis with dilute acid showed that the first 24 amino acids also retained activity.

In contrast, aminopeptidase which attacks the N-terminal serine and the next amino acid, tyrosine, destroys most of the biological activity (92). This is consistent with the results of chemical attack at the N-terminus.

Structure and activity of corticotrophin and MSH

The most striking similarity in structure between all preparations of corticotrophin and MSH is in the heptapeptide Met-Glu-His-Phe-Arg-Try-Gly which occupies positions 4–10 of the molecule.

This provides an explanation for the intrinsic MSH activity of corticotrophin. However, corticotrophin possesses only about 1 per cent of the activity of α-MSH (see Table 3.1) and it has been suggested that the free N-terminal serine of corticotrophin, which is essential for its corticotrophic activity, may also be one of the factors which inhibits the potential MSH activity of the corticotrophin molecule.

More information regarding the relationship of structure and activity arises from an investigation of related synthetic peptides. This is contained in the next section.

SYNTHETIC PEPTIDES

The smallest peptide related to corticotrophin with biological activity is the tetrapeptide, His-Phe-Arg-Try (75). This sequence of amino acids occurs in positions 6–9 in the molecules of both corticotrophin and MSH. The potency is only one millionth of that of authentic MSH and no other types of activity are reported (Fig. 3.4).

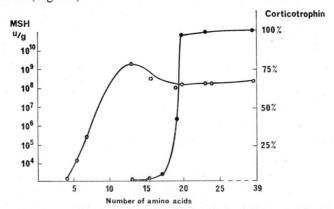

FIG. 3.4. The biological activities of peptides of different chain lengths: MSH activity o—o as u./g, corticotrophic activity •—• as percentage of natural hormone

The pentapeptide, His-Phe-Arg-Try-Gly was synthesized by the carbo-benzoxy-DCC procedure (45) and is weakly active in assays for MSH ($1 \cdot 5$–$3 \cdot 0 \times 10^4$ U per g) and it stimulates lipolysis in rabbits *in vitro* (88). When glutamic acid is attached to the N-terminus, the lipolytic activity is ten times greater, and a further tenfold increase in activity is obtained by the addition of methionine to give a heptapeptide. This heptapeptide occupies positions 4–10 in the corticotrophin molecule and also occurs in all types of MSH. The MSH activity is appreciable and has been estimated to be between $2 \cdot 8 \times 10^5$ and $1 \cdot 4 \times 10^6$ U per g (see Fig. 3.4).

The next peptide obtained by adding serine at the N-terminus is also active in assays for MSH (43). Addition of the next two amino acids gives a decapep-tide which serves as a key compound in the synthesis of larger peptides in the methods used by Li's group. This peptide has been synthesized from the partially protected hexapeptide Glu-His-Phe-Arg-Try-Gly and the carbo-benzoxy-protected tetrapeptide Z-Ser-Tyr-Ser-Met-NH.NH_2 by the azide procedure. The resulting derivative was crystallized and de-blocked by sodium in liquid ammonia (77).

The first indication of corticotrophic activity occurs in the peptide amide containing the first thirteen amino acids of corticotrophin (29, 48). The activity is less than $0 \cdot 1$ i.u. per mg by the *in vivo* adrenal ascorbic acid depletion test and by the steroidogenic activity in rats, but nevertheless is significant. The MSH potency now approaches that of natural α-MSH and it may be noted that the chemical structure is identical except for the lack of the acetyl group on the N-terminal serine.

Similar low corticotrophic activity is found in the hexadecapeptide con-taining amino acids 1–16 of corticotrophin (84), but a sharp rise to 6 i.u. per mg by the *in vitro* steroidogenic method occurs with the next peptide (amino acids 1–17) (67). This compound has also been shown to be active in man. It has high MSH activity both *in vivo* and *in vitro* and is as active as corticotrophin itself in the perirenal adipose tissue assay in rabbits (77).

The nonadecapeptide (amino acids 1–19) was synthesized by Li's group (73) and contained 40 i.u. by the *in vitro* assay for corticotrophin and was also highly active *in vivo*; the next peptide (amino acids 1–20) is the first to contain the full corticotrophic activity of the natural hormone (51). When this peptide is protected (as the triacetate decahydrate) it is inert in assays for cortico-trophin but contains $4 \cdot 2 \times 10^8$ U MSH per g. When hydrolysed in $0 \cdot 5$ N-HCl the corticotrophic activity is 111 i.u. per mg but the MSH activity falls slightly to $1 \cdot 1 \times 10^8$ per g.

Full corticotrophic activity is also reported for the peptide with the first 23 amino acids of corticotrophin (50). When protected with N^ε-formyl lysine, N-acetyl and amide groups there is only slight activity, but again, marked MSH activity *in vivo* and *in vitro* (2×10^8 u. per g). On hydrolysis in $0 \cdot 5$ N-HCl to the free peptide full corticotrophic activity is obtained (103–116 i.u. per mg). It is active *in vivo* in animals and in man (9, 14).

The tetracosapeptide (amino acids 1–24) has also been synthesized (56), and its effects in man are comparable to those of natural corticotrophin (55, 58, 90).

The first total synthesis of a complete corticotrophin with the amino acid sequence of porcine β-corticotrophin was reported by Schwyzer and Sieber (85). They formed peptide bonds mainly by means of active esters (e.g. *p*-nitrophenyl esters) while amino and carboxyl functions were protected by blocking groups derived from t-butanol which can be removed in the last stages of synthesis without destruction of sensitive peptides. This is essential since corticotrophin is sensitive to attack by the reactions needed to remove some of the other common protecting groups. The synthesis started from position 39 with L-phenylalanine t-butyl ester and proceeded stepwise by the addition of one appropriately substituted amino acid *p*-nitrophenyl ester after another until the protected pentadecapeptide occupying positions 25–39 of the corticotrophin molecule was obtained.

The octapeptide (amino acids 17–24) was added by the method of mixed anhydrides and the product was hydrogenated and condensed with the azide of the protected hexapeptide (11–16). After purification and further hydrogenation, condensation with the decapeptide (amino acids 1–10) followed by the DCC method.

The purification of all intermediates and the final product was by the method of countercurrent distribution and sometimes by thin layer chromatography on silica gel. The final biological activity was 110 i.u. per mg and the polypeptide was effective in man (4a).

Several syntheses of α-MSH have been reported (36, 47, 52, 82). The earlier ones depended on the use of the classical protecting groups such as carbobenzoxy, but the yields were small. In a later synthesis (82) t-butanol derivatives were used as protecting groups which are easily removed at the end and high yields resulted.

A similar general method has been used in a recent synthesis of β-MSH (83). Five peptides were used here, the first containing the three *N*-terminal amino acids, protected as shown:

$$
\begin{array}{c}
\text{OBut*} \\
|\\
\text{BOC*—Asp—Ser—Gly—ONBz*}\\
\phantom{\text{BOC*—}}1\phantom{\text{sp—}}2\phantom{\text{er—}}3
\end{array}
$$

---

* Abbreviations: BOC = t-butoxy-carbonyl
But = t-butyl
NBz = *p*-nitrobenzyl
Z = carbobenzoxy

The second, a tetrapeptide, contained a trityl (CPh$_3$—) group at the N-terminus:

$$\overset{\overset{\displaystyle BOC}{\displaystyle |}}{\underset{\underset{\displaystyle 4 \quad\; 5 \quad\; 6 \quad\; 7}{}}{CPh_3\text{—}Pro\text{—}Tyr\text{—}Lys\text{—}Met\text{—}OMe}}$$

Condensation of these peptides with the removal of the trityl group in 75 per cent acetic acid gave the crystalline heptapeptide methyl ester (amino acids 1–7).

Next the dipeptide:

$$\overset{\overset{\displaystyle OBut}{\displaystyle |}}{\underset{\underset{\displaystyle 8 \quad\; 9}{}}{Z^*\text{—}Glu\text{—}His\text{—}NH.NH_2}}$$

was condensed with the tetrapeptide:

$$\overset{\overset{\displaystyle NO_2}{\displaystyle |}}{\underset{\underset{\displaystyle 10 \quad\;\; 11 \quad\;\; 12 \quad\;\; 13}{}}{Z\text{—}Phe\text{—}Arg\text{—}Try\text{—}Gly\text{—}OMe}}$$

to yield the hexapeptide (amino acids 8–13). This was condensed with the pentapeptide:

$$\overset{\overset{\displaystyle BOC \quad\;\; OBut}{\displaystyle |\qquad\;\; |}}{\underset{\underset{\displaystyle 14 \quad\;\; 15 \quad\;\; 16 \quad\;\; 17 \quad\;\; 18}{}}{Z\text{—}Ser\text{—}Pro\text{—}Pro\text{—}Lys\text{—}Asp\text{—}OBut}}$$

giving the undecapeptide (amino acids 8–18). Finally this was condensed with the hydrazide of the heptapeptide (amino acids 1–7), the release of the β-MSH from the protected octadecapeptide being accomplished by reaction with trifluoroacetic acid for one hour at room temperature. It was identical in biological activity to naturally occurring β-MSH (0·1 of synthetic α-MSH).

PEPTIDE STRUCTURE AND BIOLOGICAL ACTIVITY

It seems that the amino acids which are essential for corticotrophic activity must be present in the first 13 amino acids of the peptide chain since this peptide is the first to show some activity. Hofmann considers that the rise in activity which occurs as the chain is lengthened is due to increased binding to the receptors (42). The arginyl-arginine moiety which is located in positions 17 and 18 is probably of major importance in this respect, as is valine in position 20, in view of the significant increase in activity which occurs on lengthening the chain from 19 to 20 amino acids.

The MSH activity increases from the very low activity of the tetrapeptide to the full activity of the natural hormone when the chain includes 13 amino acids. It is then found that various chemical changes may occur without loss of activity. Thus the glutamyl residue may be changed to glutaminyl and the lysine to ε-formyl lysine.

The *N*-acetylation of the terminal serine in MSH is, however, important. Thus α-MSH without the *N*-acetyl group has only 7 per cent of the full activity (42). It will be remembered that corticotrophin which has a free *N*-terminal serine has only low MSH activity but this is increased considerably by *N*-acetylation.

The replacement of methionine by α-amino butyric acid decreases the activity of synthetic α-MSH considerably (46). However, since the activity is not completely destroyed, this indicates that methionine is not absolutely essential for biological activity as was thought at one time.

Another very interesting observation concerns the replacement of L-isomers by D-isomers. Although the pentapeptide His-Phe-Arg-Try-Gly has only a fraction of the activity of natural MSH, this activity remains when the L-arginine is replaced by D-arginine (42) or the L-phenylalanine is replaced by D-phenylalanine. Furthermore if all the L-amino acids are replaced by D-amino acids, the resulting peptide has no darkening property itself but lightens skin that has previously been darkened by the L-peptide (37). The D-peptide has no influence on the darkening effect by other agents such as caffeine, however; this suggests that their mode of action on the melanophores is different, and that the D-peptide behaves like a competitive inhibitor specifically to peptides which involve the active sequence in their molecule.

Corticotrophin and MSH in biological fluids

Corticotrophin and MSH can be extracted and concentrated from urine and blood by the use of acid-acetone, by adsorption on benzoic acid (54), on the carboxylic acid ion-exchange resin IRC-50 (93) or on oxycellulose (15). The latter method is reported to give almost 95 per cent recovery from blood.

The concentration of corticotrophin in normal blood is less than 1 m.u. per 100 ml, so that very sensitive methods of assay are required. Espiner *et al.* (26) have reported that the transplanted gland of a sheep may be used to measure amounts between 0·005 and 0·05 m.u., but this technique is obviously not generally available (26). Probably the method of choice is that of Lipscombe and Nelson (74) in which the increased secretion rate of corticosterone in the adrenal vein of hypophysectomized rats is measured 5 minutes after the injection of the test material into the jugular vein.

IMMUNOLOGICAL METHODS

Preparations of corticotrophin from several species are antigenic. None of the antisera produced so far contain precipitins however, but haemagglutination and ^{131}I methods may be used to study cross-reactions and for quantitative measurements.

Human, bovine and porcine corticotrophins are immunologically identical (59). Cross-reactions also occur between the different forms of corticotrophin that have been isolated, i.e. α_1, α_2, β, γ_1, γ_2 and δ_1 (3) but not between the synthetic preparations containing less than 24 amino acids. Both natural and synthetic α-MSH show some cross reaction but the β form does not.

Methods of immunoassay are now being developed. The ^{131}I method will probably be the method of choice because of its high sensitivity.

A number of synthetic peptides have been investigated for antigenicity (3). These are all related to the N-terminus and contain 13, 16, 20 or 23 amino acids. In each, the glutamic acid is replaced by glutamine, the ε-amino groups of lysine are protected by formyl groups, the N-terminus by an acetyl group and the C-terminal carboxyl is aminated. These peptides are active in tests for MSH but are devoid of corticotrophic activity. They are each antigenic as judged by skin hypersensitivity and by anaphylactic sensitivity, however, and the larger peptides also show haemagglutinating properties. It is interesting to note that if the protecting groups are removed from the 23-amino acid peptide it becomes fully active as corticotrophin but becomes non-antigenic. This may be because it becomes bound to its receptor molecules and thus fails to reach the sites of antibody production (44).

PEPTIDES WHICH AFFECT FAT METABOLISM

Certain peptides which affect lipids have been known to exist for some time, e.g. 'Astwood's peptides I and II' (1, 28 and see 79a and 79b). Recently Li (65) has noted that during the fractionation of corticotrophin from ovine glands a polypeptide more acidic than corticotrophin is separated and affects fat metabolism. It contains 59 amino acids and has a molecular weight of 6,900 with glutamic acid rather than serine at the N-terminus and lysine instead of phenylalanine at the C-terminus. Its purity has been established by column chromatography, gel filtration, zone and disc electrophoresis, countercurrent distribution and sedimentation studies.

It has very low corticotrophic activity and this is not potentiated by boiling with sodium hydroxide as is corticotrophin. It affects the mobilization of fat *in vivo* and the liberation of free non-esterified fatty acids *in vitro* (foot-pad technique). The term 'lipotrophin' has been proposed for this peptide.

Another form of ovine lipotrophin, called β-lipotrophin, has now been isolated (65a). The final step in the purification of this compound was chromatography on the ion-exchange resin IRC-50 equilibrated with 0·01 M-ammonium acetate at pH 4·6. The complete amino acid sequence of the 90 residues has been worked out and it is of interest that the residues in positions 47–53 are Met-Glu-His-Phe-Arg-Try-Gly, present in this sequence also in corticotrophin and MSH of various species. Furthermore, the sequence in positions 37–58 is identical to that of human β-MSH except that amino acid residues in positions 42 and 46 are serine and lysine instead of glutamic acid and arginine.

REFERENCES

1 ASTWOOD, E. B., BARRETT, R. J. and FRIESEN, H. *Proc. natn. Acad. Sci. U.S.A.* **47,** 1525 (1961).

2 ASTWOOD, E. B., RABEN, M. S., PAYNE, R. W. and GRADY, A. B. *J. Amer. chem. Soc.* **73,** 2969 (1951).

3 AXELROD, A. E., TRAKETELLIS, A. C. and HOFMANN, K. *Nature, Lond.* **197,** 146 (1963).

4 BANGHAM, D. R., MUSSETT, M. V. and STACKE-DUNNE, M. P. *Bull. Wld Hlth Organ.* **27,** 395 (1962).

4a BARTHE, P., DESAULLES, P. A., SCHÄR, B. and STÄHELIN, M. *Nature, Lond.* **202,** 908 (1964).

5 BELL, P. H. *J. Amer. chem. Soc.* **76,** 5565 (1954).

6 BELL, P. H., HOWARD, K. S., SHEPHERD, R. G., FINN, B. M. and MEISEN-HELDER, J. H. *J. Amer. chem. Soc.* **78,** 5059 (1956).

7 BIRK, Y. and LI, C. H. *Biochim. biophys. Acta* **82,** 430 (1964).

8 BORIGHT, H., ENGEL, F. L., LEBOVITZ, H. F., KOSTYO, J. L. and WHITE, J. E. *Biochem. J.* **83,** 15 (1962).

9 BRADLOW, H. L., FUKUSHIMA, D. K., GALLAGHER, T. F., HELLMAN, L., HOFMANN, K., LI, C. H., ROSENFELD, R. S., SPENCER, H. and ZUMOFF, B. *J. clin. Endocr.* **23,** 792 (1963).

10 CORTIS-JONES, B., CROOKE, A. C., HENLEY, A. A., MORRIS, C. J. O. R. and MORRIS, P. *Biochem. J.* **46,** 173 (1950).

11 COLE, R. D., LI, C. H., HARRIS, J. I. and PON, N. G. *J. biol. Chem.* **219,** 903 (1956).

12 CRUIKSHANK, B., and CURRIE, A. R. *Immunology* **1,** 13 (1958).

13 CURRIE, A. R. and DAVIES, B. M. A. *Acta endocr. Copenh.* **42,** 69 (1963).

14 DANOWSKI, T. S., HOFMANN, K., YAJIMA, H. and MOSES, C. *Metabolism* **10,** 835 (1961).

15 DAVIES, B. M. A. *Acta endocr. Copenh.* **45,** 55 (1964).

16 DEDMAN, M. L., FARMER, T. H. and MORRIS, C. J. O. R. *Biochem. J.* **78,** 348 (1961).

17 DIXON, H. B. F. *Biochim. biophys. Acta* **18,** 599 (1955).

18 DIXON, H. B. F. *Biochem. J.* **62,** 25P (1956).

19 DIXON, H. B. F. *Biochim. biophys. Acta* **37,** 38 (1960).

20 DIXON, H. B. F. *Biochem. J.* **83,** 91 (1962).

21 DIXON, H. B. F. and STACKE-DUNNE, M. P. *Biochem. J.* **61,** 483 (1955).

22 DIXON, H. B. F. and WEITKAMP, L. R. *Biochem. J.* **84,** 462 (1962).

23 DIXON, J. S. and LI, C. H. *Gen. comp. Endocr.* **1,** 161 (1961).

24 ENGEL, F. L. *Vitams Horm.* **19,** 189 (1961).

25 ENGEL, F. L. and ENGEL, M. G. *Endocrinology* **62,** 150 (1958).

26 ESPINER, E. A., BEAVEN, D. W. and HART, D. S. *J. Endocr.* **27,** 267 (1963).

27 FARMER, T. H. and MORRIS, C. J. O. R. *Nature, Lond.* **178,** 1465 (1956).

28 FELTS, P. W. and MORGAN, H. E. *Endocrinology* **74,** 504 (1964).

29 FLÜCKIGER, E. W. *Acta endocr. Copenh.* Suppl. 51, 333 (1960).

30 GESCHWIND, I. I. *Endocrinology* **63,** 449 (1958).

31 GESCHWIND, I. I. and LI, C. H. *Biochim. biophys. Acta* **25,** 171 (1957).

32 GESCHWIND, I. I., LI, C. H. and BARNAFI, L. *J. Amer. chem. Soc.* **78,** 4494 (1956).

33 GESCHWIND, I. I., LI, C. H. and BARNAFI, L. *J. Amer. chem. Soc.* **79,** 620 (1957).

34 GESCHWIND, I. I., LI, C. H. and BARNAFI, L. *J. Amer. chem. Soc.* **79,** 1003 (1957).

35 GUTTMANN, ST. and BOISSONNAS, R. A. *Helv. chim. Acta* **41,** 1852 (1958).

36 GUTTMANN, ST. and BOISSONNAS, R. A. *Helv. chim. Acta* **42,** 1257 (1959).

37 HANO, K., KOIDA, M., KUBO, K. and YAJIMA, H. *Biochim. biophys. Acta.* **90,** 201 (1964).

38 HARRIS, J. I. *Biochem. J.* **71,** 451 (1959).

39 HARRIS, J. I. *Nature, Lond.* **184,** 167 (1959).

40 HARRIS, J. I. and LERNER, A. B. *Nature, Lond.* **179,** 1346 (1957).

41 HARRIS, J. I. and ROOS, P. *Biochem. J.* **71,** 434 (1959).

41a HAYNES, R. C., SUTHERLAND, E. W. and RALL, T. W. *Recent Prog. Horm. Res.* **16,** 121 (1960).

42 HOFMANN, K. *Brookhaven Symposium in Biology* **13,** 184 (1960).

43 HOFMANN, K. *VIth Int. Cong. Biochem.* Abst. 2, 101 (1964).

44 HOFMANN, K. *Metabolism* **13,** 1275 (1964).

45 HOFMANN, K., THOMPSON, T. A., WOOLNER, M. E., SPÜHLER, G., YAJIMA, H., CIPERA, J. D. and SCHWARTZ, E. T. *J. Amer. chem. Soc.* **82,** 3721 (1960).

46 HOFMANN, K., WELLS, R. D., YAJIMA, H. and ROSENTHALER, J. *J. Amer. chem. Soc.* **85,** 1546 (1963).

47 HOFMANN, K., WOOLNER, M. E., SPÜHLER, G., THOMPSON, J. A. and SCHWARTZ, E. T. *J. Amer. chem. Soc.* **80,** 6458 (1958).

48 HOFMANN, K. and YAJIMA, H. *J. Amer. chem. Soc.* **83,** 2289 (1961).

49 HOFMANN, K. and YAJIMA, H. *Recent Prog. Horm. Res.* **18,** 41 (1962).

50 HOFMANN, K., YAJIMA, H., LIU, T.-Y. and YANAIHARA, N. *J. Amer. chem. Soc.* **84,** 4475 (1962).

51 HOFMANN, K., YAJIMA, H., LIU, T.-Y., YANAIHARA, N., YANAIHARA, C. and HUMAS, J. L. *J. Amer. chem. Soc.* **84,** 4481 (1962).

52 HOFMANN, K., YAJIMA, H. and SCHWARTZ, E. T. *J. Amer. chem. Soc.* **82,** 3732 (1960).

53 HOWARD, K. S., SHEPHERD, R. G., EIGNER, E. A., DAVIES, D. S. and BELL, P. H. *J. Amer. chem. Soc.* **77,** 3419 (1955).

54 IBAYASHI, H., FUJITA, T., MOTOHASHI, K., YOSHIDA, S., OHSAWA, N., MURAKAWA, S., YOKATA, T. and OKINAKA, S. *J. clin. Endocr.* **21,** 140 (1961).

55 JENNY, P. M. A., MÜLLER, A. F. and MACH, R. S. *Schweiz. med. Wschr.* **93**, 766 (1963).

56 KAPPELER, H. and SCHWYZER, R. *Helv. chim. Acta* **44**, 1136 (1961).

57 LANGREBE, F. W. and MITCHELL, G. M. *Q. Jl. exp. Physiol.* **39**, 11 (1964).

58 LANDON, J., JAMES, V. H. T. and STAMP, T. C. B. *Biochem. J.* **90**, 20P, 1964.

59 LARON, Z., ARIE, B. Z. and ASSA, A. *Acta endocr. Copenh.* Suppl. 89, 4 (1964).

60 LEBOVITZ, H. E. and ENGEL, F. L. *Endocrinology* **73**, 573 (1963).

61 LEE, T. H. and LERNER, A. B. *J. biol. Chem.* **221**, 943 (1956).

62 LEE, T. H., LERNER, A. B. and BUETTNER-JANUSCH, V. *J. Amer. chem. Soc.* **81**, 6084 (1959).

63 LERNER, A. B. and LEE, T. H. *Vitams. Horm.* **20**, 337 (1962).

64 LEZNOFF, A., FISHMAN, J., TALBOT, M. McGARRY, E. E., BECK, J. C. and ROSE, B. *J. clin. Invest.* **49**, 1930 (1962).

65 LI, C. H. *Nature, Lond.* **201**, 924 (1964).

65a LI, C. H., BARNAFI, L., CHRÉTIEN, M. and CHUNG, D. *Nature, Lond.* **208**, 1093 (1965).

66 LI, C. H. and BERTSCH, L. *J. biol. Chem.* **235**, 2638 (1960).

67 LI, C. H., CHUNG, D., RAMACHANDRAN, J. and GORUP, B. *J. Amer. chem. Soc.* **84**, 2460 (1962).

68 LI, C. H. and DIXON, J. S. *Science* **124**, 934 (1956).

69 LI, C. H., DIXON, J. S. and CHUNG, D. *J. Amer. chem. Soc.* **80**, 2587 (1958).

70 LI, C. H., GESCHWIND, I. I., COLE, R. D., RAACKE, L. D., HARRIS, J. I. and DIXON, J. S., *Nature, Lond.* **176**, 687 (1955).

71 LI, C. H., GESCHWIND, I. I., DIXON, J. S., LEVY, A. L. and HARRIS, J. I. *J. biol. Chem.* **213**, 171 (1955).

72 LI, C. H., GESCHWIND, I. I., LEVY, A. L., HARRIS, J. I., DIXON, J. S., Pon, N. G. and PORATH, J. O. *Nature, Lond.* **173**, 251 (1954).

73 LI, C. H., MEIENHOFER, J., SCHNABEL, E., CHUNG, D., LO, T.-B. and RAMACHANDRAN, J. *J. Amer. chem. Soc.* **83**, 4449 (1961).

74 LIPSCOMBE, H. S. and NELSON, D. H. *Endocrinology* **71**, 13 (1962).

75 OTSUKA, H. and INOVE, K. *Bull. chem. Soc. Japan* **37**, 289 (1964).

76 PEARSE, A. G. E. and VAN NOORDEN, S. *Can. med. Ass. J.* **88**, 462 (1963).

77 RAMACHANDRAN, J., CHUNG, D. and LI, C. H. *Metabolism* **13**, 1043 (1964).

78 RASMUSSEN, H. *J. biol. Chem.* **234**, 547 (1959).

79 ROSEMBERG, L. L., EVANS, E. S. and SIMPSON, M. E. *Endocrinology* **68**, 1 (1961).

79a RUDMAN, D. *J. Lipid Res.* **4**, 119 (1963).

79b RUDMAN, D., REID, M. B., SEIDMAN, F., DI GIRHANO, M., WERTHEIM, A. R. and BERN, S. *Endocrinology* **68**, 273 (1961).

80 SAFFRAN, M. and SCHALLY, A. V. *Endocrinology* **56**, 523 (1955).

81 SAYERS, M. A., SAYERS, G. and WOODURY, L. A. *Endocrinology* **42,** 379 (1948).
82 SCHWYZER, R., COSTOPANAGIOTIS, A. and SIEBER, P. *Helv. chim. Acta* **46,** 870 (1963).
83 SCHWYZER, R., ISELIN, B., KAPPELER, H., RINIKER, B., RITTEL, W. and ZUBER, H. *Helv. chim. Acta* **46,** 1975 (1963).
84 SCHWYZER, R., RITTEL, W. and COSTOPANAGIOTIS, A. *Helv. chim. Acta* **45,** 2472 (1962).
85 SCHWYZER, R. and SIEBER, P. *Nature, Lond.* **199,** 172 (1963).
86 SHEPHERD, R. G., HOWARD, K. S., BELL, P. H., CACCIOLA, A. R., CHILD, R. G., DAVIS, M. G., ENGLISH, J. P., FINN, B. M., MEISENHELDER, J. H., MOYER, A. W. and VAN DER SCHEER, J. *J. Amer. chem. Soc.* **78,** 5051 (1956).
87 SHIZUME, K., LERNER, A. B. and FITZPATRICK, T. B. *Endocrinology* **54,** 553 (1954).
88 TANAKA, A., PICKERING, B. T. and LI, C. H. *Archs. Biochem. Biophys.* **99,** 294 (1962).
89 WALLER, J.-P. and DIXON, H. B. F. *Biochem. J.* **75,** 320 (1960).
90 WALSER, A. and KOLLER, F. *Experientia* **19,** 320 (1963).
91 WHITE, W. F. *J. Amer. chem. Soc.* **75,** 503 (1953).
92 WHITE, W. F. *J. Amer. chem. Soc.* **77,** 4691 (1955).
93 WILLIAMS, W. C., ISLAND, D., OLDFIELD, R. A. A. *J. clin. Endocr.* **21,** 426 (1961).

4

GROWTH HORMONE

Growth hormone is secreted by the anterior pituitary gland. Its site of origin is probably the acidophils, there being some direct evidence for this from studies by the fluorescent antibody technique (31, 55, 70).

In the human and in the monkey the placenta may also be a source of a growth hormone (43, 46). A substance has been extracted which cross-reacts immunologically with antisera to human growth hormone (HGH) and has lactogenic activity and slight growth activity. Its site of origin has been studied in experiments with fluorescein-labelled antiserum to growth hormone of pituitary origin; specific fluorescence was localized in the cytoplasm of the syncytiotrophoblast of the chorionic villi (85) of placentae as early as the twelfth week of gestation. It is interesting that similar experiments with anti-serum to chorionic gonadotrophin indicated that this hormone was also present in the syncytiotrophoblast (see page 125).

Biological activity

It has long been known that growth hormone has a marked effect on skeletal and visceral growth in experimental animals but the underlying metabolic changes are still incompletely understood. Its nitrogen-retaining properties and its effects on fat metabolism are well established. It probably stimulates biosynthesis of protein by regulating the rate of synthesis of RNA including messenger RNA (48). In the human and monkey, growth hormone appears to be associated also with lactogenic activity. Extensive publications on these and other effects have appeared (4, 15, 47).

Growth hormone of animal origin is active in experimental animals but has no biological activity in man. Wilhelmi demonstrated that the hormone from fish is active in fish but not in the rat, and showed that it possessed distinct physico-chemical differences when compared with the bovine hor-

76

mone which is active in both species (92). Observations such as these stimulated both research into HGH and, later, attempts to isolate the 'active core' of animal growth hormone.

Biological assay

There are several well-established procedures for the assay of growth hormone but they are not very suitable for clinical applications either because of their difficulty or their lack of sensitivity.

Thus Evans and Simpson (19) employed rats at six months of age. These animals grow very slowly and are referred to as 'plateaued' rats. Growth hormone causes these animals to resume growth but unfortunately the sensitivity of the response is low and fifteen to twenty days are required for the assay.

Other assays require the use of hypophysectomized rats which resume growth on administration of growth hormone. An end point which is commonly used is the increase in width of the proximal epiphyseal cartilage of the tibia. This assay requires four to five days to perform and is sensitive to between 5 and 120 μg of growth hormone (28).

An *in vitro* effect which has been adapted as an assay procedure depends on the incorporation of ^{35}S into cartilage taken from hypophysectomized rats, the 'sulphation factor' (14). This effect has been studied extensively and it appears that some of the ^{35}S is incorporated into chondroitin sulphate (12). It should be noted that similar effects are reported for lactogenic hormone, thyroxine and testosterone, while cortisone and hydrocortisone reduce the incorporation of ^{35}S. Almquist has improved the design of the assay and has obtained an index of precision (λ) of 0·14 with a working range of 0·1–0·6 μg HGH per ml (1). The assay is therefore suitable for clinical application.

Finally the effect of growth hormone on fat metabolism affords another means of assay. The fasting unesterified fatty acids in plasma are raised by growth hormone and also by corticotrophin and thyrotrophin while glucose and insulin suppress the effect (9, 78). This action may be duplicated *in vitro* using the epididymal fat pad of the rat (91) thus providing a useful but non-specific method for the study of growth hormone, particularly during chemical fractionations (68).

STANDARDS A number of standards of bovine and ovine growth hormone have been available in America for some years and potencies have been expressed in terms of these in early publications. Several are equipotent with the USP and international standards but variations in potency have been reported when different methods of assay are used. This suggests that there are some qualitative differences between preparations (22).

Methods of preparation

(a) FROM PITUITARY GLANDS   There was an early report on the isolation of growth hormone from bovine pituitaries in an apparently homogeneous form according to electrophoretic, diffusion and solubility studies (59). The contamination with other pituitary hormones was probably of a low order but the yield was poor. This has been improved in subsequent modifications of the method (16, 72, 73, 94) which depends initially on the extraction of the glands with calcium hydroxide at pH 11·5.

Several other methods are available for the initial extraction of ovine or bovine glands; they involve the use of salt solutions such as 0·3 M-KCl at pH 5·5 (81, 94), 0·25M-$(NH_4)_2$ SO_4 at pH 5·5 or 7·5 (18) and sodium borate at pH 5·5 (21, 90).

Subsequent purification in the earlier methods involved the careful adjustment of the pH and of the concentration of salt or ethanol. Chromatography on ion-exchange resins (e.g. Amberlite IRC-50) and countercurrent distributions in systems such as s-butanol–0·4 per cent dichloroacetic acid (72, 73) have also been used. The methods of gel filtration have been introduced into later methods; an apparently homogeneous preparation was split into two fractions by the use of Sephadex G-75 in acetate buffer at pH 4, the slower moving component containing the major activity (16). Even so it is doubtful if any of the preparations so far obtained are absolutely pure.

In an attempt to devise a simpler method using mild procedures, Ferguson and Wallace (21, 90) extracted ovine growth hormone in borate buffer at pH 8·6–8·8 and purified it by chromatography on a single column of DEAE-cellulose. The activity occurred in the first peak while all the other pituitary hormones remained adsorbed. The product was approximately equipotent with NIH-GH-B2 and in starch gel electrophoresis showed two principal components migrating towards the cathode. The yield by this method was about 0·2 per cent from fresh pituitaries or about 1·6 per cent from the acetone dried powder, which is rather less than that reported by Ellis (18) using a modification of the method of Wilhelmi (94).

A comparison of the potencies and yields by various methods is given in Table 4.1.

It was disappointing, but of great interest, when it was found that these preparations of growth hormone which were very effective in experimental animals, were totally ineffective in man or monkey. When work commenced on HGH another interesting species difference became apparent. Methods which had been successful for the extraction and purification of ovine and bovine growth hormones failed when applied to HGH. Thus the fractional extraction of pituitaries by water and ammonium sulphate used by Ellis (18) showed that HGH by contrast was distributed over several fractions and was not separated from other hormones (93). In the fractionation on DEAE-

TABLE 4.1

Methods for the extraction of growth hormone from mammalian pituitary glands

Reference	Method	Species	Potency i.u. per mg	Yield i.u. per g fresh pituitaries
21	Extraction in borate buffers; DEAE-cellulose.	Ovine	0·86–0·99	about 1·9
90	As 21	Ovine	1·0	2·0
		Bovine	0·4	2·0
		Porcine	1·9	8·0
		Cetacean	0·6	3·1
18	Extraction in water pH 5·5; fractional precipitation from ammonium sulphate	Ovine	0·9–1·2	4·5
		Bovine	0·9–1·2	4·9
16	Extraction in calcium hydroxide; fractional precipitation from ethanol and gel filtration	Bovine	1·25–2·72	about 2·2 (1·0 of purest fraction)
77	Extraction in acid-acetone (Raben method)	Porcine	0·5	7·5 (from acetone dried powder)

cellulose of Ferguson and Wallace it was found that whereas ovine growth hormone was unadsorbed, HGH was adsorbed even more firmly than the other hormones such as gonadotrophins and thyrotrophin.

Modified methods were therefore developed. The hormone is extracted under mild conditions by 0·3 M-KCl at pH 5·5 and pH 10·0 (80) or by 0·8 per cent NaCl at pH 7·4 (60). In the first method the extract was then purified by gel filtration on Sephadex G-200 and in this way the growth activity was separated from other proteins including luteinizing hormone which contaminated the initial extract. The product contained 2–2·5 i.u. per mg and 4 i.u. prolactin per mg but had no detectable luteinizing activity. Disc electrophoresis revealed a major and two minor components while in the untracentrifuge a single boundary with $S_{20,w} = 2·3$ was observed.

In the second method Li *et al.* (60) fractionated their material by precipitation with ammonium sulphate and then by chromatography on Amberlite IRC-50 (XE-97) at pH 5·1. Finally, by gel filtration on Sephadex G-50 in 0·1 N-acetic acid, they obtained a fraction which was homogeneous by countercurrent distribution in the system s-butanol–0·1 per cent dichloroacetic acid and by gel filtration on Sephadex G-75.

The method which has had the greatest impact, however, is that described by Raben (77). Its success has probably been due to the fact that under the conditions employed most of the other biologically active components are destroyed.

Acetone-dried powder of human pituitary glands is extracted in a mixture of acetic acid and acetone at 70° which is sufficient to destroy bacteria and viruses. The hormone is fractionally precipitated using acetone and ether and is freed from corticotrophin which is adsorbed on to oxycellulose. Other impurities are salted out and the hormone is finally precipitated from ethanol. The average yield of growth hormone from acetone-dried human pituitaries is about 4·4 per cent, while it is 3 per cent from simian glands and 1·5 per cent from porcine glands. These results are compared with others in Table 4.2.

TABLE 4.2

Methods for the extraction of growth hormone from human pituitary glands

Reference	Method of extraction	Potency i.u. per mg	Yield i.u. per g
77	Acetone-dried powder extracted in hot acetic acid and acetone; fractional precipitation from acetone and ether.	approximately 1	44 (from acetone-dried powder)
93	Extraction and fractional precipitation from ammonium sulphate.	0·63	10·6 (from acetone-dried powder)
80	Extraction in 0·3M-KCl, pH 5·5 and 10; gel filtration on G-200.	2–2·5	approx. 600 (from acetone-dried powder)
90	Extraction in borate buffer; DEAE-cellulose.	2	20 (from fresh glands)

Growth hormone prepared by this and other methods is not chemically pure and electrophoresis on starch gel or polyacrylamide gels reveals up to five protein bands, several of which are active (3, 11, 20, 22, 50). Some preparations have been shown to contain albumin but this may be removed by gel filtration.

All preparations of HGH to date possess lactogenic activity which follows the growth activity through gel filtration, and chromatography on DEAE-cellulose (13, but see also 86b) and carboxymethyl cellulose (37). There is an interesting observation that the secretion of growth hormone by human pituitaries *in vitro* decreases rapidly while the lactogenic activity increases; this suggests that the structures required for the two activities may not be identical (8). This observation, however, at present lacks confirmation and the growth activity was measured by an immunological method; it is well known that for other hormones, e.g. for human chorionic gonadotrophin, such estimates may not always parallel the biological activity. Further investigations of this nature will be awaited with interest.

(b) PLACENTA   A protein which cross-reacts with antiserum to HGH has been extracted from placentae (43, 86b). The tissue was extracted at pH 8·6, and precipitates which formed at pH 6·4 and at 4·5 were removed. The protein was then precipitated from half-saturated ammonium sulphate and then chromatographed on Amberlite CG-50 resin as in the method for pituitary growth hormone of Li (56). Furthermore the method of Raben has also been applied to placentae (46).

The product exhibits lactogenic activity but its growth hormone activity is somewhat uncertain. It has been reported to be inactive by the tibial method of assay, but it does increase the uptake of ^{35}S by cartilage and its action is inhibited by antiserum to HGH (46). It gives a reaction of partial identity with HGH in double diffusion experiments in agar gel and electrophoretically it moves slightly ahead of HGH and albumin.

Further work on the biological significance and characterization of this placental factor will be awaited with great interest.

(c) BLOOD   There is evidence from the use of ^{131}I-labelled HGH that in serum the hormone is bound to an α_2-macroglobulin (34). It may be extracted from blood by methods similar to those used for pituitaries. Thus when serum is treated with an equal volume of saturated ammonium sulphate the hormone is precipitated and may then be fractionated on Amberlite IRC-50 in phosphate buffer at pH 5·1. It is eluted in 0·18 M-phosphate buffer containing 0·45 M-ammonium sulphate at pH 6·0 and is precipitated by increasing the concentration of ammonium sulphate (89).

Several other methods have been described which are suitable for use in the immunoassay of HGH in plasma. Hunter and Greenwood (41) have used a modification of the method of Raben in which the HGH is extracted in the albumin fraction in a mixture of acetic acid and acetone (1:1 v/v) and is then precipitated by ether. In the method of Gemzell (26) the hormone is precipitated from trichloroacetic acid after which it is extracted with the albumin fraction by ethanol. It is then precipitated on adjusting the pH to 6·1. In a modification of this, Dominguez and Pearson (17) extracted HGH from an ammonium sulphate precipitate in trichloroacetic acid and acetone and then precipitated it by adjusting the pH to 6·1.

(d) URINE   There are conflicting reports on the occurrence of growth hormone in urine. Extraction of urine by the kaolin adsorption method and fractionation with ammonium sulphate gives material which shows some cross reaction with antiserum to HGH (10, 25, 46). However other workers

G

TABLE 4.3

Some physico-chemical constants of growth hormones

Species	Human	Simian	Bovine	Porcine	Ovine	Rat	Cetacean
Sedimentation coefficient $S_{20,w}$	2·47	1·88	3·2	3·02 (75)	2·76	2·2 (82)	2·84
Diffusion coefficient $D_{20,w}$	8·88	7·20	7·23	6·54 (75)			
Molecular weight	21,000 (58, 67) 27,100 (62) 29,000 (69, 86)	23,000 (58) 25,400 (62)	45,000 (58, 66) 30,000 (2, 96)	41,600 (58, 75) 25,000	48,000 (58) 47,800 (72)	24,000 (82) —	40,000 (58, 73)
Isoelectric point	4·9 (62)	5·5 (62)	6·9	5–5·5 6·3 (75)	6·8		6·2 (73)
pK	9·8	10·2	10·4				

These results were reported in the references given and by LI, C. H. in *Comparative Endocrinology*, Vol. 1 (edited by U. S. von Euler and H. Heller), p. 434, Academic Press, New York (1963).

have failed to confirm this; certainly the evidence for growth activity by biological assay in experiments reported so far is slight (25).

Chemical properties

Growth hormones from many species have been examined. They are all simple proteins containing no carbohydrate. There is a considerable range in molecular weights among the different species, the bovine and ovine having the highest and the primates the lowest (see Table 4.3). There are also differences in isoelectric points, the hormones from the monkey and the human being the most acidic.

A chemical property of great interest is that the ovine and bovine hormones have two N-terminal amino acids, phenylalanine and alanine, indicating the presence of two polypeptide chains. The other growth hormones however have only one N-terminal amino acid, phenylalanine, and therefore may be composed of single chains (74).

Studies with carboxypeptidase have shown that phenylalanine is at the C-terminus in all growth hormones (35, 65, 75). The bovine GH has been considered to exist as a branched chain structure with a single C-terminus (35, 44), but recently there is evidence of two C-terminal phenylalanine chains (2, 96).

All the common amino acids are present in growth hormone and the number of residues is given in Table 4.4. The sequences from the N- and C-termini are also indicated as far as they are known at present. The preparation of growth hormone from rat pituitaries is interesting in that it lacks tryptophan. Its secondary structure may well be less complex since it contains only one cystine and three methionine residues per molecule (82).

Enzymic transformations

Partial (up to 40 per cent) hydrolysis of HGH with chymotrypsin or pepsin does not reduce the activity (57, 58). Further hydrolysis however abolishes the activity. Some of the other growth hormones are not as stable but it seems clear that the whole molecule is not required for biological activity. The C-terminal phenylalanine is also not essential since it may be removed by carboxypeptidase without loss of activity.

Since only human and simian growth hormones are effective in the human, the possibility of partially digesting the readily available bovine or ovine growth hormone to reveal an active core is appealing. The early observations that an active core results after treatment with chymotrypsin (24, 63, 64) have not always been confirmed (5, 6). Laron *et al.* (52) submitted both bovine and human growth hormones to digestion with pepsin and the products were investigated by electrophoresis in agar gel. They were split up into several components, the majority of which moved to the cathode. One component of bovine growth hormone, however, moved to the anode with a

TABLE 4.4

Amino acids in various preparations of growth hormone
(number of residues to nearest whole number)

Species	Human	Simian	Bovine	Rat
Assumed molecular weight	21,500	23,000	45,700	24,000
Reference	58	58	58	82
Aspartic acid	20	21	36	17
Glutamic acid	27	27	49	24
Threonine	10	10	25	8
Serine	18	17	27	12
Proline	9	10	15	9
Glycine	9	10	23	11
Alanine	8	7	29	14
Valine	7	6	14	9
Leucine	23	23	49	18
Isoleucine	7	7	13	7
Lysine	9	9	22	11
Arginine	10	11	24	9
Histidine	3	3	7	3
Tyrosine	7	8	12	5
Tryptophan	1	1	3	—
Phenylalanine	12	13	25	9
Methionine	3	3	8	3
Half-cystine	4	6	8	2

Amino-acid sequences:

		N-terminus		C-terminus
	Reference		Reference	
Bovine	76	Phe-Ala-Thr- . . . Ala-Phe-Ala- . . .	35	. . . -Leu-Ala-Phe-Phe
Ovine	72	Phe- . . . Ala- . . .	58	. . . -Tyr-Ala-Phe
Porcine	75	Phe-Pro-Ala-Met-Pro-Leu-. . .	75	. . . -Phe-Ala-Phe
Cetacean	58, 76	Phe- . . .	65	. . . -Leu-Ala-Phe
Simian	58, 76	Phe- . . .	58	. . . -Ala-Gly-Phe
Human	60	Phe-Pro-Thr-Leu-Asp-Leu- . . .	58	. . . -Leu-Phe

mobility similar to that of undigested HGH. The immunological activities of both bovine and human hormones decreased but weak haemagglutination was found with up to 60–70 per cent digestion. The anodic component of the digested bovine hormone gave a positive haemagglutination reaction with antiserum to HGH. This gives some evidence in favour of a common immunological core with HGH.

HGH which has been treated with pepsin or chymotrypsin continues to cause nitrogen retention in man (6). However antibodies have been found within a week of giving the latter preparation, and even the pepsin-treated hormone is slightly antigenic.

A study of growth hormone by disc electrophoresis has revealed that on standing in alkali it fragments to give five protein bands (53). Since this breakdown can be prevented by the proteinase inhibitor di-iso-propyl-fluorophosphate, the indication is that the initial breakdown is caused by proteolysis. Proteinase activity is in fact found in bovine growth hormone which has been extracted by alkali; when extracted by hot acetic acid, how-ever, the proteinase is inactivated and such preparations show no loss of activity when stored in acidic buffers. Lewis (54) has studied the factors that affect the fragmentation of growth hormones prepared by different methods and it seems likely that the method of isolation determines the amount and the kind of contaminating proteinase.

Effect of heat

The biological activity of bovine growth hormone is destroyed by heating at 100° for ten minutes (59) but HGH remains active even after fifteen minutes (57). Prolonged heating affects the electrophoretic mobility of HGH and after thirty minutes at 100° it migrates as albumin (51). The heated prepara-tion reacts more slowly in double diffusion experiments with antiserum to HGH and its haemagglutination capacity decreases.

Immunological properties

The development of the haemagglutination method of Boyden (see p. 28), and the preparation of HGH in a high state of purity by Raben no doubt stimulated Read and Bryan (79) to investigate the immunoassay of HGH. Some preparations obtained by the Raben method produce antibodies in rabbits which react solely to HGH and simian growth hormone (32, 33, 39). By the use of the tanned red cell haemagglutination-inhibition reaction excellent results were obtained for purified preparations of HGH. However, when applied to the determination of HGH in serum, the end points were less clear, and falsely high readings were obtained, particularly in cases of hypopituitarism. A number of non-specific inhibitors occur in plasma and also interfere in the assay (45). The method created a great deal of interest in immunological assays which led to the development of assays for other pituitary hormones and to much work on HGH itself.

Firstly methods were investigated for the extraction of plasma prior to the immunoassay as described on page 81. Although the specificity was un-doubtedly improved by this means, it soon became clear that a more sensitive method was really required.

Quantitative precipitin reactions (61) and the complement fixation method

(88) are alternative techniques but are no more sensitive than the haemagglu-tination-inhibition reaction. The method of choice is undoubtedly by use of ^{131}I-labelled antigen where the lower limit of sensitivity is between 0·1 and 0·2 ng (27, 41).

The labelling of HGH is conveniently performed by the method of Hunter and Greenwood (29). Small amounts of carrier-free [^{131}I]iodide (2 mc) are allowed to react with small quantities of HGH (5 μg) in the presence of the oxidizing agent chloramine-T. Sodium metabisulphite is added to convert any [^{131}I]iodine into [^{131}I]iodide and the labelled HGH is then separated from the reaction mixture by gel filtration through Sephadex G-50. The efficiency of the method is high (approximately 70 per cent transfer of ^{131}I to the HGH) and the product has a high specific activity (250–590 μc per μg). The hormone is calculated to contain up to 1·2 atoms of iodine per molecule. Preparations of up to 300 μc per μg contain no detectable degradation products and are immunologically identical with the unlabelled hormone. At 500 μc per μg and above, however, there is a progressive loss of affinity of the hormone for the antiserum.

There are several methods for separating the bound and the free ^{131}I-anti-gen. Hunter and Greenwood used electrophoresis on cellulose acetate; paper (27) or polyacrylamide gel (23) have been used instead. Alternatively the ^{131}I-antigen bound to antibody may be precipitated by a second antibody such as goat antiserum to rabbit γ-globulin (36, 84, 89).

When certain preparations of HGH obtained by the method of Raben or by the method of Li and Papkoff (60, 62) have been used as antigens they have produced antibodies to albumin (7, 38, 40, 49, 71). These may be removed by suitable absorption with serum albumin before the assay but the concentra-tion is usually too low to interfere when using the ^{131}I-assay. Alternatively impurities in the HGH may be largely removed before immunization, or labelling, by gel filtration (87).

The haemagglutination and radioimmunological methods show no cross-reactions between intact non-primate growth hormones and HGH. The technique of micro-complement fixation, however, reveals significant im-munological similarities between porcine, ovine and bovine growth hormones and HGH (86a). Higher concentrations of anti-HGH antiserum are required for observing the cross-reactions than for the homologous reaction but the complement fixation obtained with HGH and its antiserum is inhibited by the non-primate growth hormones. The technique is particularly sensitive to the conformation of the antigen and has been used to measure the relatedness of several non-human primate growth hormones. It is interesting that these hormones are significantly distinguished from HGH while reactions of com-plete identity are observed by double diffusion in agar gel (86a).

CLINICAL APPLICATIONS

The radioimmunoassay of growth hormone is ideally suited to clinical investigations since it is extremely sensitive, is relatively easy to perform and large numbers of samples may be estimated together. It has proved useful as an aid to the diagnosis of abnormal pituitary function and furthermore has helped to reveal several interesting facts about the normal physiological functions of growth hormone (30, 42, 83).

The concentration of growth hormone in plasma increases gradually during fasting while it decreases if the blood sugar rises. It has been suggested that the release of growth hormone during starvation may be a mechanism whereby the stores of protein in the body are conserved while the utilization of fat is enhanced (95). The antagonistic action of growth hormone and insulin ensures that the amounts of glucose, fatty acids and amino acids in the blood remain within a restricted range, and so prevents hyper- or hypoglycaemia. Undoubtedly further applications of the method will help towards a fuller understanding of the many and varied functions of growth hormone.

REFERENCES

1 ALMQUIST, S. *Acta endocr. Copenh.* **36**, 31 (1961).

2 ANDREWS, P. and FOLLEY, S. J. *Biochem. J.* **87**, 3P (1963).

3 BARRETT, R. J., FRIESEN, H. and ASTWOOD, E. B. *J. biol. Chem.* **237**, 432 (1962).

4 BECK, J. C., GONDA, A., HAMID, M. A., MORGEN, R. O., RUBINSTEIN, D. and McGARRY, E. E. *Metabolism* **13**, 1108 (1964).

5 BERGENSTAL, D. M. and LIPSETT, M. B. *J. clin. Endocr.* **20**, 1427 (1960).

6 BIGLIERI, E. G., WATLINGTON, C. O. and FORSHAM, P. H. *J. clin. Endocr.* **21**, 361 (1961).

7 BOUCHER, B. J. *Nature, Lond.* **188**, 1025 (1960).

8 BRAUMAN, J., BRAUMAN, H. and PASTEELS, J. L. *Nature, Lond.* **202**, 1116 (1964).

9 BUCKLE, R. M., RUBINSTEIN, D., McGARRY, E. E. and BECK, J. *Endocrinology* **69**, 1009 (1961).

10 BUTT, W. R. *Ciba Fdn Colloq. Endocr.* **14**, 397 (1962).

11 CHADWICK, A., FOLLEY, S. J. and GEMZELL, C. A. *Lancet* ii, 241 (1961).

12 COLLINS, E. J. and BAKER, V. F. *Acta endocr. Copenh.* **37**, 176 (1961).

13 DAMM, H. C., DOMINGUEZ, J. M., PENSKY, J. and PEARSON, O. H. *Endocrinology* **74**, 366 (1964).

14 DAUGHADAY, W. H., SALMON, W. D. and ALEXANDER, F. *J. clin. Endocr.* **19**, 743 (1959).

15 DE BODO, R. C. and ALTZULER, M. *Physiol. Rev.* **38**, 389 (1958).

16 DELLARCHA, J. M. and SONENBERG, M. *J. biol. Chem.* **239**, 1515 (1964).

17 DOMINGUEZ, J. M. and PEARSON, O. H. *J. clin. Endocr.* **22**, 865 (1962).

18 ELLIS, S. *Endocrinology* **69,** 554 (1961).
19 EVANS, H. M. and SIMPSON, M. E. *Amer. J. Physiol.* **98,** 511 (1931).
20 FERGUSON, K. A. and WALLACE, A. L. C. *Nature, Lond.* **190,** 632 (1961).
21 FERGUSON, K. A. and WALLACE, A. L. C. *J. Endocr.* **26,** 259 (1963).
22 FERGUSON, K. A. and WALLACE, A. L. C. *Recent Prog. Horm. Res.* **19,** 1 (1963).
23 FITSCHEN, W. *Biochem. J.* **88,** 13P (1963).
24 FORSHAM, P. H., LI, C. H., DI RAIMONDO, V. C., KOLB, F. O., MITCHELL, D. and NEWMAN, S. *Metabolism* **7,** 762 (1958).
25 GELLER, J. and LOH, A. *J. clin. Endocr.* **23,** 1107 (1963).
26 GEMZELL, C. A. *J. clin. Endocr.* **19,** 1049 (1959).
27 GLICK, C. M., ROTH, J., YALOW, R. S., BERSON, S. A. *Nature, Lond.* **199,** 784 (1963).
28 GREENSPAN, F. S., LI, C. H., SIMPSON, M. E. and EVANS, H. M. *Endocrinology* **45,** 455 (1949).
29 GREENWOOD, F. C., HUNTER, W. M. and GLOVER, J. S. *Biochem. J.* **89,** 114 (1963).
30 GREENWOOD, F. C., HUNTER, W. M. and KLOPPER, A. *Br. med. J.* **1,** 22 (1964).
31 GRUMBACH, M. M. *Ciba Fdn Colloq. Endocr.* **14,** 373 (1962).
32 GRUMBACH, M. M. and KAPLAN, S. L. *Ciba Fdn Colloq. Endocr.* **14,** 63 (1962).
33 GRUMBACH, M. M., KAPLAN, S. L. and SOLOMON, S. *Nature, Lond.* **185,** 170 (1960).
34 HADDEN, D. R. and PROUT, T. E. *Nature, Lond.* **202,** 1342 (1965).
35 HARRIS, J. I., LI, C. H., CONDLIFFE, P. G. and PON, D. G. *J. biol. Chem.* **209,** 133 (1959).
36 HARTOG, M., GAAFAR, M. A. and FRASER, R. *Lancet* ii, 376 (1964).
37 HARTREE, A. S. *Biochem. J.* **85,** 7P (1962).
38 HAYASHIDA, T. and GRUNBAUM, B. W. *Endocrinology* **71,** 734 (1962).
39 HAYASHIDA, T. and LI, C. H. *Endocrinology* **65,** 944 (1959).
40 HIRSCHFIELD, J., GEMZELL, C. A. and WIDE, L. *Nature, Lond.* **187,** 64 (1960).
41 HUNTER, W. M. and GREENWOOD, F. C. *Biochem. J.* **91,** 43, 1964.
42 HUNTER, W. M. and GREENWOOD, F. C. *Br. med. J.* i, 804 (1964).
43 JASMOVICH, J. B. and MACLAREN, J. A. *Endocrinology* **71,** 209 (1962).
44 JUTISZ, M. In *Symposium on Protein Structure* (edited by A. Neuberger), p. 330, Methuen, London (1958).
45 KAPLAN, S. L. and GRUMBACH, M. M. *J. clin. Endocr.* **22,** 1153 (1962).
46 KAPLAN, S. L. and GRUMBACH, M. M. *J. clin. Endocr.* **24,** 80 (1964).
47 KNOBIL, E. and GREEP, R. O. *Recent Prog. Horm. Res.* **15,** 1 (1959).
48 KORNER, A. *Biochem. J.* **92,** 449 (1964).
49 LARON, Z. and ASSA, S. *Acta endocr. Copenh.* **40,** 311 (1962).

50 LARON, Z., ASSA, S. and MENARCHE, R. *J. clin. Endocr.* **23,** 315 (1963).
51 LARON, Z., YED-LEKACH, A., ASSA, S. and KOWADLO-SILBERGELD, A. *Acta endocr. Copenh.* **46,** 465 (1964).
52 LARON, Z., YED-LEKACH, A., ASSA, S. and KOWADLO-SILBERGELD, A. *Endocrinology* **74,** 532 (1964).
53 LEWIS, U. J. *J. biol. Chem.* **237,** 3141 (1962).
54 LEWIS, U. J. *J. biol. Chem.* **238,** 3330 (1963).
55 LEZNOFF, A., FISHMAN, J., GOODFRIEND, L., MCGARRY, E. E., BECK, J. C. and ROSE, B. *Proc. Soc. exp. Biol. Med.* **104,** 232 (1960).
56 LI, C. H. *Fedn Proc.* **16,** 775 (1957).
57 LI, C. H. *J. gen. Physiol.* **45,** Pt. 2, 169 (1962).
58 LI, C. H. *Proc. 2nd. International Congress of Endocrinology, London,* 1192 (1964).
59 LI, C. H., EVANS, H. M. and SIMPSON, M. E. *J. biol. Chem.* **159,** 353 (1945).
60 LI, C. H., LUI, W.-K. and DIXON, J. S. *Archs Biochem.* Suppl. 1, 237 (1962).
61 LI, C. H., MOUDGAL, N. R. and PAPKOFF, H. *J. biol. Chem.* **235,** 1038 (1960).
62 LI, C. H. and PAPKOFF, H. *Science,* **124,** 1293 (1956).
63 LI, C. H. PAPKOFF, H., FØNSS-BECH, P. and CONDLIFFE, P. G., *J. biol. Chem.* **218,** 41 (1956).
64 LI, C. H., PAPKOFF, H. and HAYASHIDA, T. *Archs Biochem. Biophys.* **85,** 97 (1959).
65 LI, C. H., PARCELLS, A. J. and PAPKOFF, H. *J. biol. Chem.* **233,** 1143 (1958).
66 LI, C. H. and PEDERSEN, K. O. *J. biol. Chem.* **201,** 595 (1953).
67 LI, C. H. and STARMAN, B. *Biochim. biophys. Acta* **86,** 175 (1964).
68 LI, C. H., TARNAKA, A. and PICKERING, B. T. *Acta endocr. Copenh.* Suppl. 90, **155** (1964).
69 MEISINGER, M. A. P., CIRILLO, V. J., DAVIS, G. E. and REISFELD, R. A. *Nature, Lond.* **201,** 820 (1964).
70 MENEGHELLI, V. and SCAPINELLI, R. *Acta anat.* (Basel), **51,** 198 (1962).
71 O'CONNOR, P. J. and SKINNER, L. G. *J. Endocr.* **26,** 219 (1963).
72 PAPKOFF, H. and LI, C. H. *Biochim. biophys. Acta* **29,** 145 (1958).
73 PAPKOFF, H. and LI, C. H. *J. biol. Chem.* **231,** 367 (1958).
74 PAPKOFF, H. and LI, C. H. *Metabolism* **13,** 1082 (1964).
75 PAPKOFF, H., LI, C. H. and LIU, W.-K. *Archs Biochem. Biophys.* **96,** 216 (1962).
76 PARCELLS, A. J. and LI, C. H. *J. biol. Chem.* **233,** 1140 (1958).
77 RABEN, M. S. *Recent Prog. Horm. Res.* **15,** 71 (1959).
78 RABEN, M. S. and HOLLENBERG, C. H. *J. clin. Invest.* **38,** 484 (1959).
79 READ, C. H. and BRYAN, G. T. *Recent Prog. Horm. Res.* **16,** 187 (1960).
80 REISFELD, R. A., HALLOWS, B. G., WILLIAMS, D. E., BRINK, N. G. and STEELMAN, S. L. *Nature, Lond.* **197,** 1206 (1963).

81 REISFELD, R. A., LEWIS, U. J., BRINK, N. G. and STEELMAN, S. L. *Endocrinology* **71,** 559 (1962).
82 REISFELD, R. A., MUCCILLI, A. S., WILLIAMS, D. E. and STEELMAN, S. L. *Nature, Lond.* **201,** 821 (1964).
83 ROTH, J., GLICK, S. M., YALOW, R. S. and BERSON, S. A. *Metabolism* **12,** 577 (1963).
84 SCHALCH, D. S. and PARKER, M. L. *Nature, Lond.* **203,** 1141 (1964).
85 SCIARRA, J. J., KAPLAN, S. L. and GRUMBACH, M. M. *Nature, Lond.* **199,** 1005 (1963).
86 SQUIRE, P. G. and PEDERSEN, K. O. *J. Amer. chem. soc.* **83,** 476 (1961).
86a TASHJIAN, A. H., LEVINE, L. and WILHELMI, A. E. *Endocrinology* **77,** 563 (1965).
86b TASHJIAN, A. H., LEVINE, L. and WILHELMI, A. E. *Endocrinology* **77,** 1023 (1965).
87 TOUBER, J. L. and MAINGAY, D. *Lancet* i, 1403 (1963).
88 TRENKLE, A., MOUDGAL, N. R., SADRI, K. and LI, C. H. *Nature, Lond.* **192,** 260 (1961).
89 UTIGER, R. D. *J. clin. Endocr.* **24,** 60 (1964).
90 WALLACE, A. L. C. and FERGUSON, K. A. *J. Endocr.* **30,** 387 (1964).
91 WHITE, J. E. and ENGEL, F. L. *J. clin. Invest.* **37,** 1556 (1958).
92 WILHELMI, A. E. In *Hypophyseal Growth Hormone, Nature and Actions* (edited by R. W. Smith, O. H. Gaebler and C. N. H. Long), p. 59, McGraw-Hill, New York (1955).
93 WILHELMI, A. E. *Ciba Fdn Colloq. Endocr.* **13,** 25 (1960).
94 WILHELMI, A. E., FISHMAN, J. B. and RUSSELL, J. A. *J. biol. Chem.* **176,** 735 (1948).
95 YOUNG, F. G. *Recent Prog. Horm. Res.* **8,** 471 (1953).
96 YOUNG, F. G. *Proc. Ass. clin. Biochem.* **3,** 206 (1965).

5

PROLACTIN

The terms *prolactin* and *lactogenic hormone* are synonymous and there seems little doubt that they describe also the substance known as the *luteotrophic hormone*. Usually the former terms are used for the hormone concerned with mammary development and lactation while the latter name is reserved for the hormone which prolongs the active life of the corpus luteum in some species.

Origin

It has long been known that the anterior pituitary is a source of prolactin. In contrast to some of the other hormones of this gland, its secretion is not stimulated by the hypothalamus. In fact the secretion may be depressed by the hypothalamus and it increases when the connection between the hypothalamus and the anterior pituitary is severed (40). Furthermore prolactin (and growth hormone) does not participate in the usual 'feed-back' system with the secretion of its target organs. Probably the central nervous system is the primary factor involved in regulating the secretion of prolactin.

Early evidence from the study of the pituitaries of birds, and later of mammals, indicated that the site of formation of prolactin was in the acidophils. Barrnett, Roth and Salzer (6) employed a histochemical method making use of the fact that only prolactin of all the anterior pituitary hormones was precipitated by 0·5 per cent w/v trichloroacetic acid. After the glands had been immersed in this solution, staining methods (for S—S groups) were used to locate the remaining prolactin which appeared in the granular cytoplasm of the acidophils.

Preliminary studies with the electron microscope apparently distinguishes the type of acidophil which secretes prolactin (4, 22). In the mouse and rat these cells have been called ε cells, to distinguish them from the α cells which secrete growth hormone.

91

A second source of the hormone seemed likely after early studies had demonstrated prolactin-like activity persisting after hypophysectomy in the pregnant rat, mouse and monkey. Reports of prolactin in the urine of pregnant women and in the placenta followed, culminating in the recent biological and immunological investigations of Jasmovich and Maclaren (23) and of Kaplan and Grumbach (24) which were described in the preceding chapter.

Biological activity

Prolactin is responsible for the initiation and maintenance of lactation; it also prolongs the active life of the corpus luteum in some animals, but its function in this respect in other species including the human is obscure.

These effects have been recognized for many years but another important function, concerned with metabolism, has become evident only recently. At present, human prolactin has not been separated from growth hormone, the metabolic effects of which were described in the last chapter. Highly purified prolactin from other species, although separable from growth hormone, sustains and increases the body weight of hypophysectomized pigeons, an effect also given and enhanced by growth hormone, thyroxine and prednisone (7).

There are therefore three prominent activities demonstrated by this hormone, the first concerned with growth, the second with the control of the reproductive cycle and the third which may be said to be concerned with parental behaviour. It is clear therefore that prolactin is of fundamental importance in the process of life. It was one of the first protein hormones to be purified but appears to have been neglected for many years and very little is known about its secretion in man. This is probably because of the great difficulties concerned with the methods of biological assay. Considerable advances should come from the application of immunological methods now being developed. There is an extensive and important review on the physiological significance of prolactin by Riddle (45).

Biological assay

Three distinct types of assay have been used for prolactin. These depend on:
(a) the rapid proliferation of the epithelial lining of the crop sac of pigeons;
(b) the effect on the mammary gland of rabbits or guinea-pigs;
(c) the luteotrophic effects in mice.

(a) CROP SAC METHODS   The end point may be the increase in weight of the crop gland or the changed appearance of the gland, the mucosa of which is thickened and opaque.

In the early methods systemic injections of prolactin were given, but greater sensitivity is achieved by local application (39). The material is injected in small doses intradermally directly into the skin over the gland. Only that portion of the crop sac directly under the site of injection is affected by the injection so that other areas of the gland serve as controls, or are used for other dosages. A positive response can be seen with the naked eye when the stretched membrane is held up to the light. The proliferation of the epithelial lining is associated with basophilic changes in the cytoplasm and since they are highly specific for prolactin it has been suggested that these changes, rather than the mere appearance, should be used as the end point (3).

(b) LACTATIONAL METHODS   In this type of assay, rabbits are injected with oestrogens and progesterone to make them pseudo-pregnant and then pro-lactin will stimulate the secretion of milk. The amount required when injected systemically however is prohibitive but the sensitivity is increased by using intraductal injections (38). Factors affecting the response have been investi-gated by Chadwick (9). It appears that the sensitivity of different breeds varies considerably and even in sensitive strains the precision is poor.

(c) LUTEOTROPHIC METHODS   When prolactin is injected into adult rats or mice at appropriate stages of the cycle, the reappearance of oestrus is in-hibited. This effect has been described for the rat by Astwood (2) and developed into an assay procedure using mice by Kovačić (25). The method is simple but is not specific since several other hormones affect the oestrus cycle.

The luteotrophic effect of prolactin may also be recognized by the forma-tion of deciduomata in the damaged uterine horn of adult hypophysectomized rats (15) or mice (26). An assay procedure developed by Kovačić (26) is laborious but is reasonably sensitive and precise. An advantage of the method is that the luteotrophic effect can be recognized in the presence of conta-minants such as the gonadotrophic hormones.

STANDARDS   A second international standard for prolactin is now avail-able. It was prepared from ovine glands and its potency is 22 i.u. per mg.

Methods of extraction

Most of the methods that have been described for the extraction of prolac-tin were developed for the ovine hormone but fairly extensive work has been done on the bovine and porcine hormones also.

In the method for ovine glands described by Cole and Li (13) the acetone-dried powder was extracted at pH 3 and the crude hormone precipitated by adding NaCl to 0·06 saturation. After fractional precipitation at pH 5·6 the material was submitted to countercurrent distribution in the system s-butanol–0·4 per cent dichloroacetic acid. In this way 2 g of hormone possessing 35 i.u. per mg was obtained from 1 kilogramme of fresh glands. Bovine pro-lactin has been extracted by a similar method (31); its partition coefficient in the solvent system s-butanol–0·4 per cent dichloroacetic acid, however, is higher than for ovine prolactin.

In a later modification of the method (47) iso-electric precipitation (pH 5·5–5·6) was used instead of countercurrent distribution, followed by chromatography on DEAE-cellulose in 0·01 M–tris buffer at pH 8·2. By stepwise elution with increasing concentrations of NaCl, three active fractions were obtained, all essentially with the same amino acid composition. Gel filtration on Sephadex G-75 of each showed that the fractions represented different degrees of association of the molecule (49). The monomeric form was eluted in 0·055 M-NaCl, while a highly polymerized form was eluted in 0·09 M-NaCl and aggregates of intermediate molecular weight in 0·25 M-NaCl. Starch gel electrophoresis of the unfractionated material showed six bands, the monomer containing only two of these.

Further chromatography of the monomer on DEAE-cellulose in the eluting buffer (0·055 M-NaCl in tris) effected a further separation into two components, each of which showed essentially only one band on electrophoresis. These two components had the same amino acid composition and activity.

Another preparation of ovine prolactin which was essentially pure by electrophoresis was obtained by a similar method (44). The purification consisted of chromatography on two columns of DEAE-cellulose in tris buffer at pH 9·0 with a salt gradient. It was judged to contain only one component by electrophoresis on paper, starch gel and polyacrylamide gel.

In a recent method described for porcine glands, Eppstein (14) extracted the hormone in dilute acetic acid and removed corticotrophin by adsorption on oxycellulose. The pH was then brought to 7·0 and the prolactin precipitated by adding one volume of ethanol. It was then dialysed and filtered through Sephadex G-75 in 0·1 M-sodium bicarbonate. The retarded peak contained prolactin which was purified further on DEAE-cellulose in tris buffer at pH 8·2, ionic strength 0·1 and an ionic gradient to 0·5. The final extract contained 30 i.u. per mg assayed by the local pigeon crop sac method.

A simple method has been described for the extraction of bovine, porcine and ovine prolactins by alkaline ethanol followed by precipitation of the active material at pH 5·5 with 83 per cent v/v ethanol (23a). Fractional precipitation from ammonium sulphate gives products with specific activities between 15 and 25 i.u. per mg. The ovine and bovine hormones are purified by column chromatography on DEAE-cellulose. By means of gradient elution to 0·22 M-NaCl specific activities of 35–40 i.u. per mg are attained.

The methods available for the extraction of human prolactin are the same as those for growth hormone since the two activities have not at present been separated (see p. 80). One of these methods is interesting in that a comparison has been made between the behaviours of prolactin and growth hormone from five species (51). The glands were extracted in borate buffer at pH 8·8 and submitted to fractionation on DEAE-cellulose with a changing pH and salt gradient in phosphate buffer at pH 7·2. Finally the buffer was replaced by 0·1 M-NaCl–0·12 M-Na_2CO_3 at pH 11·5. In this way up to eight fractions, A to

H, were collected from the different species. The distribution of the various activities are shown in Fig. 5.1. It is interesting to note that the prolactin activity for all species occurred in closely similar elution volumes but the growth activity occurred in various positions of the chromatogram.

The yields of prolactin and growth hormone obtained by this method varied as shown in Table 5.1. Prolactin was not definitely identified in the whale although slight crop sac proliferation was given by one of the fractions. The potencies were not as high as in some of the other methods, which is hardly surprising since no further purification was attempted; the ovine hormone possessed 12 i.u. per mg, the bovine 7·0 and the porcine only 0·1 i.u. per mg.

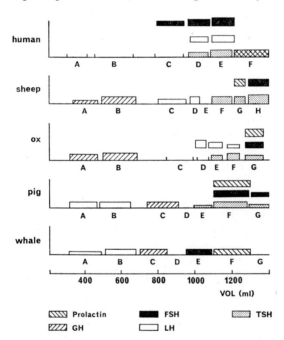

FIG. 5.1. Distribution of hormonal activities from various species eluted from DEAE-cellulose (From Reference 51, reproduced by permission)

Human growth hormone prepared by the methods of Raben (42) or of Li and Papkoff (37) possesses pigeon-crop stimulating activity (5, 16), lactogenic activity in the pseudo-pregnant rabbit (10, 19) and luteotrophic activity in the mouse (27).

The activities by the first assay are widely divergent in different laboratories, but the precision of these assays is poor and at present it is difficult to decide whether the discrepancies are due to errors in the bioassays, to differences between the strains of birds or to real differences in the preparations. Recorded figures range from negligible activity to values up to almost 5 i.u. per mg.

TABLE 5.1

*Recovery of prolactin and growth hormone
from the pituitaries of various species*

Species	Prolactin	Growth hormone
	(i.u. per g fresh gland)	
Man	83	20·0
Sheep	38	2·0
Ox	21	2·0
Pig	9	8.0
Whale	—	3·1

(From Reference 51, reprinted by permission)

Activity by the lactogenic response appears to be significantly higher. Wilhelmi (52) has reported a level of 25 i.u. per mg while Forsyth *et al.* (19) have found up to 15 i.u. per mg.

In the luteotrophic assays the activity is somewhat higher than by the pigeon crop sac method. A value of about 6 i.u. per mg has been reported by Kovačić using both the prolongation of dioestrus and the deciduoma response (27).

Similar results have been reported for simian growth hormone which is highly lactogenic in the rabbit (18).

At the time of writing an important new method for the preparation of human prolactin based on extraction with water and precipitation near the isoelectric point has been described (1). The interest in this method lies in the observation that the product contains up to 24 i.u. per mg measured by the pigeon crop method, but surprisingly little growth hormone activity (about 0·3 i.u. per mg) as measured by the tibia test. If this observation is confirmed it will strongly suggest that human prolactin and growth hormone **are** distinct entities.

Chemical properties

Although several preparations of prolactin have been shown to be homogeneous by a number of criteria, it is only recently that any appear to be pure by starch gel electrophoresis. There are three or four components in most of the purified preparations (17), each of which contains lactogenic activity.

Pierce and Carsten (41) found three components in ovine prolactin and made the interesting observation that only one of these passed a stretched membrane permeable to proteins of molecular weight 30,000 or under.

Three components were demonstrated in the ovine prolactin, NIH-P-S-3, by agar gel electrophoresis, migrating between the β- and α-globulins, with α_2-globulin and with α_1-globulin.

Reisfeld et al. (43) found that one of the three components in their preparation was highly active while the others were less potent and were considered to be altered forms of the hormone. They have recently been able to separate one component which appears to be pure (44).

Physico-chemical properties

Some of the physico-chemical properties of the ovine prolactins prepared by Sluyser and Li (47) and by Reisfeld et al. (44) are given in Table 5.2. According to Eppstein (14) the isoelectric point of porcine prolactin is 4·97 compared with 5·73 for ovine prolactin. The molecular weight of the porcine hormone is 25,000 from ultracentrifugal data.

TABLE 5.2

Some physical-chemical properties of ovine prolactin

Isoelectric point (pH)	5·74, 5·73[a]
Sedimentation coefficient, $S_{20,w}$	2·17, 2·19[31,b], 2·05 [31,c]
Diffusion constant, $D_{20,w}(cm^2/s)$	$8·62 \times 10^{-7}$, $8·44 \times 10^{-7}$ [31,d]
Molecular weight	23,400, 24,200[a], 22,720 [47]
Potency	30 i.u./mg.

These results were reported in reference 44 unless otherwise stated.
Reference (a) is DIXON, J. S. and LI, C. H. *Metabolism*, **13**, 1093 (1964).
(b) : in 0·1M-NaHCO$_3$
(c) : in borate buffer at pH 8·43.
(d) : by an electrophoretic-diffusion method.

Composition

The amino acid composition of ovine and porcine prolactins are similar but it will be noticed that whereas there are fourteen half-cysteine residues in porcine there are only six in ovine (and bovine) prolactin (Table 5.3).

The N-terminal amino acid is threonine in ovine and bovine prolactins (12) while it is alanine in porcine prolactin. The amino acid sequence at present established for ovine prolactin is Thr-Pro-Val-Thr-Pro.

The hormone is unreactive to carboxypeptidase which suggests that there

H

TABLE 5.3

Amino acid composition of ovine and porcine prolactins

	Ovine	Porcine
Molecular weight	23,300	25,000

	Number of residues to nearest whole number	
Alanine	10*, 9[44]	15†
Arginine	11*	14†
Half-cysteine	6*	14†
Aspartic acid	23*	22†
Glutamic acid	24*, 23[44]	30†
Glycine	11*, 27[47]	16†
Histidine	8*	10†
Leucine	24*, 23[44]	24†
Isoleucine	10*	12†
Lysine	10*, 9[44]	10†
Methionine	7*	4†
Phenylalanine	6*	7†
Proline	12*, 11[44]	11†
Serine	15*, 14[44]	17†
Threonine	9*	6†
Valine	10*, 11[47]	9†
Tyrosine	7*	7†
Tryptophan	2*	3†

* DIXON, J. S. and LI, C. H. *Metabolism* **13**, 1093 (1964).
† EPPSTEIN, S. *Nature, Lond.* **202**, 899 (1964).

is no *C*-terminal amino acid. It seems likely that it has a looped configuration formed by a cysteine residue. Evidence for this was obtained by reduction of the S—S bonds to SH groups with mercaptoethanol and treatment with iodo-acetamide to prevent reoxidation (33). Digestion with carboxypeptidase then revealed that cysteic acid occupied the *C*-terminus of the chain, a finding confirmed by another experiment involving hydrazinolysis of performic acid oxidized prolactin (32). Although S—S bridges are oxidized by performic acid no peptide fragments were observed suggesting that all the S—S bridges are intra-chain linkages, the protein consisting of a single polypeptide chain. The sequence from the *C*-terminus is Asp-Leu-Tyr giving the following structure:

H₂N—Thr—Pro—Val—Thr—Pro—

[————————CyS————————] —Tyr—Leu—Asp(NH₂)—CyS—COOH

Chemical modifications and biological activity

There are several early reports concerning the effects of reagents on the biological activity of prolactin which do not appear to have been repeated on the purer preparations now available.

Some of the tyrosine residues in the molecule react with iodine at the same rate as tyrosine itself, but other groups react more slowly. The activity is destroyed almost completely in the process, which suggests that the tyrosine groups are of importance (36).

The activity is not destroyed by treatment with urea (30); indeed urea has been included in the buffer used for the chromatography of ovine prolactin on the ion-exchange resin, IRC-50, in order to prevent hydrogen bonding between the protein and the resin (11).

True inactivation occurs in the presence of a 200-fold amount of cysteine (20). Less cysteine leads to inactivation due to the transformation of the hormone to a less soluble state, but if the hormone is redissolved the original activity is regained. Thioglycollic acid is about fifty times as effective as cysteine in destroying activity.

In more recent work it has been found that certain changes in the molecule occur at pH 10·5. Reisfeld *et al.* (44) found that their electrophoretically homogeneous ovine prolactin developed additional electrophoretic components at this pH but this did not occur at pH 8 or pH 9. Lewis (29) also reported electrophoretic changes at pH 7·5 after eighteen hours at 25° and presented evidence that the changes were due to the action of proteinases contaminating the hormone. Reisfeld *et al.* (44). however, could find no proteinase activity in their preparation. Moreover they found that no polymerization occurred in solution or after freeze-drying, although this occurred with the monomer isolated by Sluyser and Li (47). It was suggested that this could be explained by the presence of small amounts of EDTA in the former preparation.

ACETYLATION AND GUANIDINATION   Treatment with O-methylisourea had no effect on biological activity (31). It was shown that the lysine residues were converted to homoarginines and the N-terminal threonine was unchanged. Furthermore, acetylation of the guanidinated compound caused no loss of activity although it should be noted that when the native hormone was acetylated by keten loss of activity did occur (35).

It was concluded that the α-amino group is not essential for activity. This was confirmed by the observation that oxidation of the N-terminal threonine with periodate did not destroy activity.

OTHER REACTIONS   Esterification of the hormone with methyl alcohol in dilute hydrochloric acid progressively decreased activity as the number of methoxyl groups increased (34). In this reaction it is probable that the loss of activity is due to the esterification of the carboxyl groups.

Early observations on the digestion of the hormone with pepsin and trypsin are probably misleading since the experiments were carried out with impure preparations. It has recently been shown that following limited digestion with chymotrypsin it is possible to isolate an active 'core' from ovine prolactin. After 50 per cent digestion at 25° the bulk of the protein sedimented at approximately the same velocity as the untreated hormone and formed aggregates just as the undigested hormone. The N-terminal amino acids were alanine and leucine with glycine and aspartic acid next; leucine and phenylalanine were at the C-terminus (48, 50).

Immunological properties

It has been known for more than thirty years that prolactin can act as an antigen; when pigeons were injected with crude bovine pituitary extracts there was initially a marked stimulation of the crop sac but the birds eventually developed marked refractoriness to further injections. When purified preparations became available it was soon demonstrated that antibodies could be produced in rabbits (46, 53).

Antisera to purified ovine prolactin give a single precipitin line in double diffusion and immunoelectrophoretic experiments (21, 28, 50). A reaction of identity is given by bovine prolactin although the two proteins have slightly different electrophoretic mobilities (21). Goat prolactin is also identical immunologically but there is no cross-reaction with human or rat prolactins. Other hormones of the anterior pituitary give no precipitation with up to 250 μg whereas as little as 2 μg of ovine prolactin is effective.

Numerous other methods have been used to investigate the antigenicity of prolactin. In precipitin ring tests 0·1–0·2 μg ovine prolactin can be detected while in haemagglutination-inhibition tests as little as 0·01–0·02 μg of the purified hormone is recognized (21). The complement fixation method using ^{51}Cr-labelled red cells as the end point is also sensitive to 0·02 μg (8). Furthermore the antiserum is active *in vivo* as an inhibitor of crop sac stimulating activity.

Trenkle *et al.* (50) have shown that not all the molecule of prolactin is required for immunological activity. An active core is prepared by treating the native ovine hormone with chymotrypsin at pH 9·5 for 100 minutes at 25°. The antiserum to this core gave a single precipitin line in agar gel but again there was no cross reaction with human prolactin. Periodate-treated prolactin also reacted with this antiserum. When oxidized with performic acid however which oxidizes the disulphide bridges it no longer reacted with the antiserum to the native hormone. However it was still antigenic and its antiserum gave two precipitin lines.

REFERENCES

1 APOSTOLAKIS, M. *Acta endocr. Copenh.* **49,** 1 (1965).
2 ASTWOOD, E. B. *Ciba Fdn Colloq. Endocr.* **5,** 74 (1953).
3 BAHN, R. C. and BATES, R. W. *J. clin. Endocr.* **16,** 1337 (1956).
4 BARNES, B. G. *Endocrinology* **71,** 618 (1962).
5 BARRETT, R. J., FRIESEN, H. and ASTWOOD, E. B. *J. biol. Chem.* **237,** 432 (1962).
6 BARRNETT, R. J., ROTH, W. D. and SALZER, J. *Endocrinology* **69,** 1047 (1961).
7 BATES, R. W., MILLER, R. A. and GARRISON, M. M. *Endocrinology* **71,** 345 (1962).
8 BRAUMAN, J., BRAUMAN, H. and PASTEELS, J. L. *Nature, Lond.* **202,** 1116 (1964).
9 CHADWICK, A. *J. Endocrin.* **27,** 253 (1963).
10 CHADWICK, A., FOLLEY, S. J. and GEMZELL, C. A. *Lancet* ii, 241 (1961).
11 COLE, R. D. *J. biol. Chem.* **236,** 1369 (1961).
12 COLE, R. D., GESCHWIND, I. I. and LI, C. H. *J. biol. Chem.* **224,** 399 (1957).
13 COLE, R. D. and LI, C. H. *J. biol. Chem.* **213,** 197 (1955).
14 EPPSTEIN, S. *Nature, Lond.* **202,** 899 (1964).
15 EVANS, H. M., SIMPSON, M. E. and LYONS, W. R. *Proc. Soc. exp. Biol. Med.* **46,** 586 (1941).
16 FERGUSON, K. A. and WALLACE, A. L. C. *Nature, Lond.* **190,** 632 (1961).
17 FERGUSON, K. A. and WALLACE, A. L. C. *Recent Prog. Horm. Res.* **19,** 1 (1963).
18 FORSYTH, I. A. *J. Endocr.* **31,** xxx (1965).
19 FORSYTH, I. A., FOLLEY, S. J. and CHADWICK, A. *J. Endocr.* **31,** 115 (1965).
20 FRAENKEL-CONRAT, H. L., SIMPSON, M. E. and EVANS, H. M. *J. biol. Chem.* **142,** 107 (1942).
21 HAYASHIDA, T. *Ciba Fdn Colloq. Endocr.* **14,** 338 (1962).
22 HYMER, W. C., MCSHAN, W. H. and CHRISTIANSEN, R. G. *Endocrinology* **69,** 81 (1961).
23 JASMOVICH, J. B. and MACLAREN, J. A. *Endocrinology* **71,** 209 (1962).
23a JIANG, N.-S. and WILHELMI, A. E. *Endocrinology* **77,** 150 (1965).
24 KAPLAN, S. L. and GRUMBACH, M. M. *J. clin. Endocr.* **24,** 80 (1964).
25 KOVAČIĆ, N. *J. Endocr.* **24,** 227 (1962).
26 KOVAČIĆ, N. *J. Endocr.* **28,** 45 (1963).
27 KOVAČIĆ, N. *J. Reprod. Fert.* **8,** 165 (1964).
28 LARON, Z. and ASSA, S. *Nature, Lond.* **197,** 299 (1963).
29 LEWIS, U. J. *J. biol. Chem.* **237,** 3141 (1962).
30 LI, C. H. *J. biol. Chem.* **155,** 45 (1945).
31 LI, C. H. *Adv. Protein Chem.* **12,** 295 (1957).
32 LI, C. H. and CUMMINS, J. T. *J. biol. Chem.* **229,** 157 (1957).

33 LI, C. H. and CUMMINS, J. T. *J. biol. Chem.* **233,** 73 (1958).

34 LI, C. H. and FRAENKEL-CONRAT, H. L. *J. biol. Chem.* **167,** 495 (1947).

35 LI, C. H. and KALMAN, A. *J. Amer. chem. Soc.* **68,** 285 (1946).

36 LI, C. H., LYONS, W. R. and EVANS, H. M. *J. biol. Chem.* **139,** 43 (1941).

37 LI, C. H. and PAPKOFF, H. *Science* **124,** 1293 (1956).

38 LYONS, W. R. *Proc. Soc. exp. Biol. Med.* **51,** 308 (1942).

39 LYONS, W. R. and PAGE, E. *Proc. Soc. exp. Biol. Med.* **32,** 1049 (1935).

40 MEITES, J., NICOLL, C. S. and TALWALKER, P. K. In *Advances in Neuroendocrinology* (edited by A. V. Nalbandov), p. 238, University of Illinois Press (1963).

41 PIERCE, J. G. and CARSTEN, M. E. *J. Amer. chem. Soc.* **80,** 3482 (1958).

42 RABEN, M. S. *Recent Prog. Horm. Res.* **15,** 71 (1959).

43 REISFELD, R. A., TONG, G. L., RICKES, E. L., BRINK, N. G. and STEELMAN, S. L. *J. Amer. chem. Soc.* **83,** 2717 (1961).

44 REISFELD, R. A., WILLIAMS, D. E., CIRELLO, V. J., TONG, G. L. and BRINK, N. G. *J. biol. Chem.* **239,** 1777 (1964).

45 RIDDLE, O. *J. natn Canc. Inst.* **31,** 1039 (1963).

46 ROWLANDS, I. W. and YOUNG, F. G. *J. Physiol. Lond.* **95,** 410 (1939).

47 SLUYSER, M. and LI, C. H. *Archs Biochim. Biophys.* **104,** 50 (1964).

48 SLUYSER, M. and LI, C. H. *Biochim. biophys. Acta* **82,** 595 (1964).

49 SQUIRE, P. G., STARMAN, B. and LI, C. H. *J. biol. Chem.* **238,** 1389 (1963).

50 TRENKLE, A., LI, C. H. and MOUDGAL, N. R. *Archs Biochem. Biophys.* **100,** 255 (1963).

51 WALLACE, A. L. C. and FERGUSON, K. A. *J. Endocr.* **30,** 387 (1964).

52 WILHELMI, A. E. *Can. J. Biochem.* **39,** 1659 (1961).

53 YOUNG, F. G. *Biochem. J.* **32,** 656 (1938).

6

THE GONADOTROPHINS

The gonadotrophins are protein hormones produced by the anterior pituitary and by the placenta. Those of pituitary origin consist of *follicle stimulating hormone* (FSH), *luteinizing hormone* (LH, also referred to as *interstitial cell stimulating hormone*, ICSH) and *luteotrophic hormone* (probably identical with *prolactin* or *lactogenic hormone*). The luteotrophic hormone was considered separately in Chapter 5. The urine of postmenopausal women is a particularly rich source of gonadotrophins and extracts from such urine contain both FSH and LH activities, normally referred to as *human menopausal gonadotrophin* (HMG).

The placental hormone is *chorionic gonadotrophin* (HCG) and is found in high concentration in the blood and the urine during pregnancy, particularly between the eighth and twelfth weeks. Another rich source of gonadotrophin is the serum of pregnant mares (pregnant mare's serum, PMS) but it is interesting to note that this hormone has a very different type of activity from HCG.

Pituitary gonadotrophins

CELLULAR ORIGIN OF THE PITUITARY GONADOTROPHINS

By means of histochemical techniques it has been reasonably well established that the gonadotrophins arise from the basophilic cells of the anterior pituitary (144, 145, 175). Recent work supports the suggestion that the peripherally situated cells which are deeply stained by periodic acid-Schiff's reagent (PAS) are responsible for the production of FSH, while the centrally located basophils with less intense reaction for glycoprotein are considered to be the source of LH (63, 93, 107). An opposite view is taken by Hildebrand *et al.* (94, 157), who used a modified PAS reaction. An independent technique such as the fluorescent antibody method is required to help clarify

103

the position, but so far preparations of the gonadotrophins of sufficient purity have not been available for the production of the necessary antisera. An attempt was made by McGarry and Beck (126) with an antiserum to human pituitary FSH, but the antigen contained impurities including albumin, and uniform staining of the pituitary was obtained.

Another approach was used by Bourdel and Li (20). Antiserum to ovine LH was injected into female rats and was found to counteract endogenous LH. Histological examination of the pituitary revealed certain important changes. The basophilic cells were enlarged and stained less intensely than those in the untreated animals. The cells at the periphery showed no alteration, however, but the central basophils had undergone degenerative changes. This finding lends support to the view that the cells producing LH were centrally located and were those to which the action of the antiserum was directed.

BIOLOGICAL PROPERTIES

It is generally believed that the sequence of ovarian changes occurring during the normal menstrual cycle is governed by the release of gonadotrophin from the anterior pituitary which in turn is dependent on hypothalamic control (see Chapter 2). FSH is responsible for the growth of the follicle which produces oestrogen and stimulates endometrial growth in the uterus. Then LH, possibly in combination with FSH, induces the final stages of follicular ripening, release of the ovum and transformation of the follicular remnant to a functional corpus luteum. The corpus luteum secretes progesterone and oestrogen which induce the secretory phase of the endometrium. There is good evidence that the steroids produced during this cycle of events react by a 'feed-back' mechanism on the anterior pituitary, or hypothalamus to control the further release of gonadotrophin.

In the male, FSH causes growth of the seminiferous tubules and maintains spermatogenesis, while LH promotes the secretion of androgen by the interstitial cells (Leydig cells).

These hormones are recognized by a large number of biological assays. Some are not specific for either FSH or LH but may still be of value in routine clinical work. They are of lesser value in following the progress of chemical fractionations and will not be considered here.

ASSAYS FOR FSH   The method depending on the stimulation of ovarian growth in hypophysectomized rats (60) is highly specific but very laborious. For most purposes a test depending on the augmenting effect of LH (usually in the form of HCG) on FSH in increasing the weight of the ovaries in normal immature rats or mice is satisfactory (30, 179). It is unaffected by other pituitary hormones, is sensitive and is reasonably precise.

ASSAYS FOR LH   A highly specific test depending on the repair of interstitial tissues of the ovaries in hypophysectomized rats was described by

Evans (60), but, again, is very laborious. For several years much use has been made of a test depending on the increase in weight of the ventral prostate gland in hypophysectomized rats (86). The specificity is satisfactory (119) but it is technically difficult and time-consuming.

Another highly specific and more sensitive test was described by Parlow (138). This depends on the depletion of ovarian ascorbic acid in intact, immature, pseudo-pregnant rats (OAAD test). Some difficulty has been experienced in certain laboratories in obtaining satisfactory precision in this assay. The reason is probably because the procedure is not followed exactly as laid down by Parlow. It is particularly important to extract the ovaries immediately after dissection: they should be weighed and homogenized in metaphosphoric acid within one minute. Careful intravenous injection of the test material is also recommended although other methods of administration may be used at the expense of sensitivity rather than precision.

Other hormones of the anterior pituitary do not interfere in this assay. Lysine vasopressin is inactive but large doses of arginine vasopressin will cause depletion of ovarian ascorbic acid, as will angiotensin II, possibly due to its high pressor activity (125, 165).

A method has been described (13) in which depletion of cholesterol rather than ascorbic acid is measured. It is claimed to be remarkably sensitive but at the moment it does not appear to be as reproducible in different centres as the OAAD method.

Standard preparations

The sensitivity to gonadotrophins of different strains of animal varies considerably and it is therefore necessary to prepare standard substances so that the results obtained in different laboratories can be expressed in common units rather than as animal units.

PITUITARY GONADOTROPHINS Several preparations from ovine pituitaries have been available as standards for some years. One of the first was a preparation of FSH from Armour Laboratories identified as FSH 264-151X. Later preparations have been available from the American National Institutes of Health, NIH-FSH-S1, S2, etc. The equivalent preparations of LH are Armour LH 227-80 and NIH-LH-S1 etc. Although the preparations of LH are reasonably free of FSH, the FSH is certainly not free of LH.

At the present time international standard preparations of human pituitary FSH and LH are not available, although there are now methods available for the preparation of fractions that are purer than the ovine standards.

URINARY GONADOTROPHINS Standards prepared from the urine of post-menopausal women have been available in this country for over ten years. The first was called HMG 20 (Organon Laboratories Ltd.) and was prepared by adsorption on to kaolin, elution by alkali, precipitation by acetone and purification by treatment with calcium phosphate. An almost identical material, HMG 24, eventually became the first international reference preparation (IRP-HMG).

A new standard is now available which was prepared by Serono, Rome (Pergonal 23). It was also extracted by kaolin and was purified by chromatography on Permutit. It has now become the second 'international reference preparation for human postmenopausal gonadotrophins' (2nd IRP-HMG). One ampoule, which contains 5 mg of the standard, is equivalent to 40 i.u. of FSH and 40 i.u. of LH activity.

COMPARISON OF ACTIVITIES The biological activities of these standards have been compared in many centres by a variety of assay methods. The results of most value are those obtained by assays believed to be specific for FSH or LH and only these will be considered here. The potencies given in Table 6.1 have been collected from published work, have been obtained in

TABLE 6.1

Assays for FSH (ovarian augmentation method in mice or rats)

	Equivalent amounts	Potency as i.u. FSH per mg
2nd-IRP-HMG	1 ampoule (40 i.u.)	8[a]
1st IRP-HMG	280 mg	0·14
NIH-FSH-S1	1·56 mg	26
Armour 264-151X[b]	2·8–4·2 mg	9·6–14·2

(a) Assuming 5 mg HMG per ampoule.
(b) Armour 264–151X has been variously estimated to be 37–55% of the potency of NIH-FSH-S1 and since 1963 has shown some loss of potency.

Assays for LH by the OAAD method

	Equivalent amounts	Potency as i.u. LH per mg
2nd IRP-HMG	1 ampoule (40 i.u.)	8
1st IRP-HMG	80 mg	0·5
NIH-LH-S1	0·0264 mg	1500
Armour 227–80	0·0264 mg	1500
2nd Int.Std.HCG	approx. 50 i.u. HCG	approx. 0·8 per i.u.HCG

Note: Because of differences in the biological properties of ovine and human LH the relative potencies of NIH-LH-S1 and Armour 227–80 would be significantly different from those given if measured in terms of human LH by the ventral prostate method (see ROSEMBERG, E., SOLOD, A. and ALBERT, A. *J. clin. Endocr.* **24**, 714, 1964).

the author's laboratory, or, wherever possible, are the results of collaborative assays. By means of these results it is possible to convert potencies given in terms of any one standard into international units.

METHODS OF PREPARATION OF THE PITUITARY GONADOTROPHINS
1. *FSH*

The extraction of crude pituitary powders in mixtures of ethanol and acetate buffers has proved a most useful method for the gonadotrophins (106). The yields are high and there is virtually complete separation from growth hormone, corticotrophin and prolactin.

The purification of pituitary gonadotrophin was originally achieved by salting-out procedures, particularly with ammonium sulphate, since FSH alone of the pituitary hormones is not precipitated by 50 per cent saturated ammonium sulphate. Later, the ion-exchange celluloses have proved useful; from solutions of low ionic strength only LH is adsorbed on to carboxymethyl cellulose, while it is eluted before FSH from columns of DEAE-cellulose (181).

Other methods used with success are electrophoresis on starch, polyacrylamide gels (40, 115, 162) or ethanolized cellulose (116), gel filtration (15, 150) and chromatography on calcium phosphate (37).

According to early reports equine pituitaries are particularly rich in FSH, since they contain much more than either ovine or porcine pituitaries (64). This has not always been confirmed by later work, probably because of the different methods of extraction used. Ovine FSH has been the most readily available, but in recent years there has been a steady increase in demands for human FSH for clinical use.

(a) OVINE FSH   A preparation of high purity was obtained by a method which involves extraction in calcium hydroxide and fractional precipitation using ammonium sulphate (114). The product was homogeneous in free electrophoresis at six different pH values and in the ultracentrifuge, but it was later shown to be heterogeneous by zone electrophoresis in starch (147) and the main protein peak did not correspond to the major activity. It was refractionated two or three times and appeared almost homogeneous but still contained traces of LH activity.

Fractional precipitation with ammonium sulphate has also been used by Woods *et al.* (201), Reichert and Parlow (149), Steelman and Segaloff (180) and by Courrier (50). The product has been further purified by chromatography on DEAE-cellulose and other ion-exchange materials, by gel filtration on Sephadex G-100, by chromatography on hydroxyl apatite and by starch gel electrophoresis.

It is somewhat difficult to compare the biological potencies of the different preparations, since a variety of standards and several assay methods have been used. Nevertheless it is clear that preparations with the greatest potency have been shown to be heterogeneous by physico-chemical criteria, while less potent ones are apparently homogeneous. Potencies of several of these have been recalculated in terms of the international units and are given in Table 6.2.

TABLE 6.2

Potencies of ovine FSH

| Method of extraction | FSH Potency | | LH Con-tamination | Reference |
	As reported	Converted to i.u. FSH per mg	Converted to i.u. LH per mg	
40% v/v ethanol: fractional precipitation from $(NH_4)_2SO_4$: DEAE-chromatography.	32–45 × NIH-FSH-S1	830–1,170	Detectable	201, 202
DEAE-chromatography: zone electrophoresis.	30–40 × Armour Standard 264-151X	360–480	10	180, (a)
Extraction with and fractional precipitation from $(NH_4)_2SO_4$: gel filtration on Sephadex G-100.	22–23 × NIH-FSH-S1	570–600	not reported	50
Extraction at pH 5·5: fractional precipitation from $(NH_4)_2SO_4$.	1·4 × NIH-FSH-S1	36	0·3	149
Zone electrophoresis: Sephadex G-25: DEAE-chromatography in urea buffers: starch gel electrophoresis.	9·7 × NIH-FSH-S1	250	Detectable	54

(a) ELLIS, S. *J. biol. Chem.* **233**, 63 (1958).

The LH contamination in some of these preparations cannot be compared directly since different methods of bioassay were used. Although the potency of the preparation in Reference 149 is relatively low, the contamination with LH appears to be the least.

It has been reported that by use of a chloroform-butanol extraction procedure in combination with DEAE-cellulose chromatography and gel filtration on Sephadex G-100 that ovine FSH with a potency of 50× NIH-FSH-S1 (i.e. 1290 i.u. per mg) has been obtained (148d). The same method has been used to prepare *bovine* FSH of potency 3·1 × NIH-FSH-S1 (80 i.u. per mg).

(b) PORCINE FSH Preparations of high potency may be obtained by first removing the corticotrophin in acid–acetone and then extracting the gonadotrophin at an alkaline pH, followed by fractional precipitation from ammonium sulphate (180). The Armour Standard 264-151X was prepared in this way.

The potency of such preparations was reported to be increased following treatment with pancreatin and fractionation in alcohol (178). The product was then fractionated by chromatography on DEAE-cellulose in a gradient system to $0.25M$-NaCl-$0.05M$-Na$_2$HPO$_4$; the preparation obtained was essentially homogeneous both in the ultracentrifuge and in paper electrophoresis (180). When a similar method was tried on the undigested hormone the product was found to be unstable. Fractionation on hydroxyl apatite was investigated instead of DEAE-cellulose but the recoveries were poor.

Steelman and Segaloff (180) report that their preparation is between thirty and forty times as active as the Armour Standard 264-151X in assays for FSH. In international units it therefore contains about 400 units per mg. The LH contamination is probably less than 0.0075 mg NIH-LH-S1 per mg, i.e. 10 i.u./mg.

(c) HUMAN FSH　Gonadotrophins are extracted efficiently from human glands by mixtures of acetate buffer of ionic strength 0.5 at pH 5.0 and ethanol (15, 37, 171) as originally described by Koenig and King (106). Other satisfactory methods make use of calcium hydroxide (115) or aqueous solutions at various pH values (56, 57, 181, 200).

The separation of FSH from LH and other contaminants is then possible by methods similar to those used for ovine gonadotrophins. Fractional precipitation from ammonium sulphate is described in some methods (162) while chromatography on DEAE-cellulose is used in nearly all. Good yields are obtained by stepwise elution in phosphate or acetate buffers, and by elution in salt gradients (8). Amir et al. (8) employ DEAE-Sephadex which is equilibrated in 5-mM-phosphate at pH 7.0. Gradient elution to 0.8 M-NaCl separates FSH from most of the LH but the main peak is still contaminated with albumin. The latter is not completely removed by gel filtration on Sephadex G-100 but by using the side fractions from the DEAE column followed by gel filtration a preparation essentially free of albumin is obtained.

Preparations of extremely high potency have been obtained by stepwise elution from DEAE-cellulose and gel filtration on Sephadex G-100 by Reichert and Parlow (139, 151, 155) and by Roos and Gemzell (162). In the latter method, the final product was purified by electrophoresis on a column of acrylamide gel (Table 6.3) and was homogeneous in the ultracentrifuge and in zone-electrophoresis. Before the electrophoresis on acrylamide gel, three components were demonstrated in the ultracentrifuge but although these were separated on acrylamide there was no increase in activity.

It is clear from these latter studies that as purification proceeds the stability of the hormone decreases. Crude FSH may be precipitated from acetone or alcohol, or be freeze-dried without appreciable loss of activity, but when highly purified the safest method appears to be concentration by ultrafiltration. Neither of the extremely potent preparations of FSH (8, 155, 162) were obtained as solids and the protein concentration was calculated from the ultraviolet absorptions.

TABLE 6.3

Potencies of purified human FSH

Method of preparation	FSH potency as reported	FSH potency as i.u.FSH per mg	LH i.u. per mg	Reference
(a) Preparations obtained as dry powders				
Extraction in ammonium acetate: ethanol; CM- and DEAE-cellulose.	55 × Armour 264-151X	660	not reported	181
Extraction in ammonium acetate: ethanol; CM- and DEAE-cellulose; calcium phosphate; urea-ammonium sulphate-cellosolve partition.	1,036 i.u.	1,036	180 i.u.	42
Extraction in aqueous salts: CM- and DEAE-cellulose; gel filtration on Sephadex G-100.	47 × NIH-FSH-S1	1,210	not reported	139
(b) Preparations obtained only in solution				
Reference 139	75–94 × NIH-FSH-S1 (based on u.v. absorption at 215–225 mμ)	1,930–2,440	not reported	139, 155
Extraction of frozen pituitaries in aqueous salts; fractional precipitation from ammonium sulphate; DEAE-cellulose; Sephadex G-100; electrophoresis on polyacrylamide gel.	150–200 × NIH-FSH-S1	3,900–5,200	—	162
	428 × NIH-FSH-S2 (based on u.v. absorption at 230 mμ)	11,000	present	(a)

(a) ROOS, P. and GEMZELL, C.A. *Ciba Foundation Study Group on Physicochemical and Immunological Properties of the Gonadotrophins*, p. 11 (1965). The LH potency of this preparation was determined by the seminal vesicle method in rats and was expressed as i.u. HCG. The result of less than 6 i.u. HCG per estimated mg cannot at present be converted to i.u. LH.

A method which has been found to give good yields of FSH of high potency and biological purity is shown in Figure 6.1. The product contains between 450 and 600 i.u. FSH per mg and 250–500 i.u. LH per mg. It is stable almost indefinitely at room temperature if kept dry. In solution (1 mg per ml physiological saline) at −15° it retains its potency for at least a year. The preparation is active in the human and has been widely used in clinical trials (51).

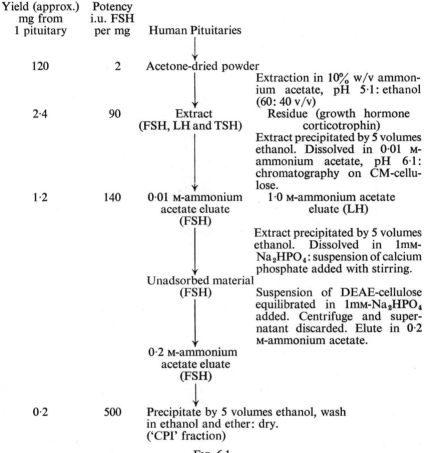

Yield (approx.) mg from 1 pituitary	Potency i.u. FSH per mg	
		Human Pituitaries
120	2	Acetone-dried powder
		Extraction in 10% w/v ammonium acetate, pH 5·1: ethanol (60: 40 v/v)
2·4	90	Extract (FSH, LH and TSH) — Residue (growth hormone corticotrophin)
		Extract precipitated by 5 volumes ethanol. Dissolved in 0·01 M-ammonium acetate, pH 6·1: chromatography on CM-cellulose.
1·2	140	0·01 M-ammonium acetate eluate (FSH) — 1·0 M-ammonium acetate eluate (LH)
		Extract precipitated by 5 volumes ethanol. Dissolved in 1mM-Na₂HPO₄: suspension of calcium phosphate added with stirring.
		Unadsorbed material (FSH) — Suspension of DEAE-cellulose equilibrated in 1mM-Na₂HPO₄ added. Centrifuge and supernatant discarded. Elute in 0·2 M-ammonium acetate.
		0·2 M-ammonium acetate eluate (FSH)
0·2	500	Precipitate by 5 volumes ethanol, wash in ethanol and ether: dry. ('CPI' fraction)

Fig. 6.1

Electrophoresis in starch gel demonstrates that it is heterogeneous (Fig. 6.2). Elution of the FSH region, however, gives a preparation virtually free of LH. An interesting synergistic effect of such a preparation with purified LH has been reported (43), the potency of these hormones when combined in optimal proportions being increased by more than threefold. The preparation of FSH is not free of albumin, however. In order to overcome this difficulty treatment with urea, or fractionation in cellosolve-salt systems prior to electrophoresis has been proposed (32, 42). The cellosolve-salt systems consist of mixtures of ethyl or butyl cellosolves and strong solutions of ammonium sulphate or sodium and potassium phosphates which may also contain urea. They are interesting systems in that the FSH may be preferentially soluble in the organic layers (see Table 6.3).

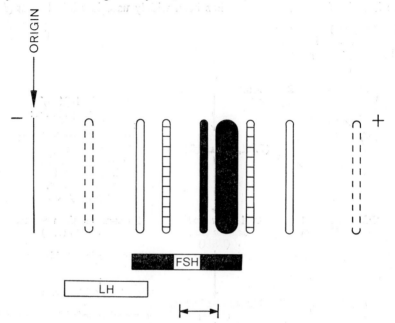

FIG. 6.2. A typical starch gel electrophoretic pattern obtained with human FSH (CPI fraction, References 37 and 40)

The gel buffer consisted of a mixture of 0·0033 M-citric acid–0·016 M-tris and 0·02 M-lithium hydroxide–0·076 M-boric acid (9:1 v/v, pH 8·1) and the electrode vessels contained 0·1 M-lithium hydroxide–0.38 M-boric acid (pH 8·5), (as FERGUSON, K. A. and WALLACE, A. L. C. *Recent Prog. Horm. Res.* **19**, 1 (1963)).

The voltage gradient was 20 V/cm for 5 hours and the gel was stained with nigrosine.

The portion of gel indicated (←→) contained, in a typical experiment, approximately 120 i.u. FSH and less than 3 i.u. LH, but was not free of albumin.

2. *LH*

Early reports suggested that the pituitaries of sheep were richest in LH, followed by those of the pig, horse and man (64, 190). However, according to Steelman and Segaloff (180) equine pituitaries are much more active than was first suggested. Equine LH however has a longer biological half-life in plasma than ovine, bovine or porcine LH so that the relative potencies may vary with the method of assay. In a recent study (155a) in which the OAAD method was used the yield of purified material was similar to that from ovine, bovine or porcine glands, but it varied somewhat according to the age of the glands initially extracted.

TABLE 6.4

Potencies of purified preparations of ovine LH

Method of preparation	LH potency		FSH potency			Reference
	as reported	i.u. per mg	as reported	i.u. per mg		
Aqueous extraction: ammonium sulphate precipitation: DEAE-cellulose.	1·6 × NIH-LH-S1 (Ref. 150)	2,400	Not detected at 6,000 × MED for LH			202
Ethanol-acetate extraction: CM-cellulose	1·93 × Armour 227-80	2,900	1 mg < 0·1 × Armour 264-151-X	< 1·2		187 188 189
NaCl extraction, pH 4·55: sulphosalicylic acid and ammonium sulphate precipitation: IRC-50: zone electrophoresis on starch	2·4 × NIH-LH-S1 (Ref. 150)	3,600	—	—		176
Aqueous extraction, pH 5·5: ammonium sulphate precipitation: metaphosphoric acid precipitation: ethanol fractionation: IRC-50: gel filtration on Sephadex G-100	4·2–4·5 × NIH-LH-S1	6,300–6,800	< 0·012 × NIH-FSH-S1 (also contains < 0·1 unit TSH per mg)	< 0·3		150

(a) OVINE LH   Preparations of high potency were obtained over twenty years ago by fractionation with ammonium sulphate, and although they satisfied the current criteria of homogeneity they would probably now be shown to be impure. Later methods have employed ion exchange resins and celluloses as in the purification of FSH. Thus Squire and Li (176) used the carboxylic acid resin IRC-50 and Woods and Simpson (202) used in addition DEAE-cellulose. Steelman and Segaloff (180) separated FSH and LH on carboxymethyl cellulose as before mentioned and then refractionated the LH on a second column (181, 187, 188).

Reichert and Parlow (150) succeeded in purifying ovine LH by precipitating impurities by metaphosphoric acid and submitting the extract to gel filtration of Sephadex G-100.

Where possible the potencies of these preparations have been converted to i.u. and are shown in the Table 6.4. The best preparations are essentially free of FSH; it appears to be easier to separate FSH from LH, than to remove LH from FSH.

(b) PORCINE AND BOVINE LH   Methods used for porcine and bovine LH follow much the same pattern as those for ovine LH and range from the early method using ammonium sulphate fractionation (174) to the recent method of Reichert (148 a and b) using metaphosphoric acid precipitation and gel filtration of Sephadex G-100.

(c) HUMAN LH   Three recent methods for the preparation of human LH differ in the conditions for extraction, but in each, ion-exchange celluloses are employed for subsequent purification.

Squire, Li and Andersen (177) extracted pituitaries in calcium hydroxide and precipitated the active material by ammonium sulphate. Next, the LH was adsorbed on to CM-cellulose and eluted by stepwise increases in concentration of ammonium acetate at pH 6·1. Active fractions were eluted with 0·04, 0·08 and 0·2 M-ammonium acetate and electrophoretic examinations of each suggested that LH is partly complexed with inactive protein, one complex being dissociated at pH 3·6 while the other is not. A product of high potency was obtained from the 0·08 M-eluate by electrophoresis on a column of Pevikon (polyvinylchloride-polyvinyl acetate polymer) at pH 3·6 (see Table 6.5).

Hartree, Butt and Kirkham (92) used the ammonium acetate–ethanol and CM-cellulose fractionation of Steelman, Segaloff and Andersen (181). They obtained a twofold concentration of activity by chromatography on IRC-50 at pH 7·5 using a gradient to 1M-NaCl. Further purification was achieved by use of DEAE-cellulose equilibrated in glycine buffer at pH 9·5. The active material was eluted by application of a gradient to 0·25 M-ammonium acetate at pH 6·1, the main contaminant, TSH, being retained slightly more firmly on this ion-exchanger.

Reichert and Parlow (153, 155) extracted their material in ammonium

TABLE 6.5

Potencies of purified human LH

Method of preparation	LH potency		FSH Potency		TSH potency	Reference
	as reported	i.u. per mg	as reported	i.u. per mg	i.u. per mg	
Extraction in ammonium acetate: ethanol; CM-cellulose; IRC-50; DEAE-cellulose	6,400 mg 1st IRP-HMG per mg	3,200	<1 mg 1st IRP-HMG per mg	<0·14	6×10^{-3}	92
Ammonium sulphate; DEAE-cellulose; IRC-50	$3 \cdot 2 \times$ NIH-LH-S1	4,800	$0 \cdot 11 \times$ NIH-FSH-S1	2·8	0·18	153 155
Ammonium sulphate; CM- and DEAE-cellulose; gel filtration on Sephadex G-100	$3 \times$ NIH-LH-S1	4,500	$0 \cdot 14 \times$ NIH-FSH-S1	3·6	<0·1	139
Extraction in ammonium acetate: ethanol; CM-cellulose*	$6–10 \times$ Armour 227–80*		$<1 \cdot 0 \times$ Armour 264-151-X	<6	—	171 181

A method of extraction in calcium hydroxide followed by fractionation with ammonium sulphate, IRC-50, CM-cellulose and electrophoresis has been reported (177). The only potency reported was in terms of HCG by the ventral prostate method: it was 500 i.u. per mg.

* Assayed by the ventral prostate method: a later assay by the OAAD method gave a potency of only $0 \cdot 35 \times$ Armour 227–80 (i.e. 525 i.u. per mg, see Reference 151).

sulphate at pH 4 and separated the LH from FSH by chromatography on DEAE-cellulose, the LH being unadsorbed. Subsequent purification was achieved on IRC-50 in 0·007 M-phosphate–0·003 M-borate buffer at pH 8·0. This latter procedure was found to remove pH 4 proteinase activity which was found to contaminate the cruder preparations.

A comparison of the activities of these preparations is given in Table 6.5. Unfortunately a different method of assay was used for the preparation of Squire *et al.* (177) so that a direct comparison of activities is not possible. No details of possible TSH contamination are given for this preparation; the other two are not completely free of TSH.

CHEMICAL PROPERTIES

The exact composition of FSH and LH is at present unknown since neither has been obtained completely pure. They appear to be proteins containing carbohydrate which seems to be essential for the biological activity. The hexose consists of galactose and mannose and has been variously estimated in FSH to be between 2·1 and 5·0 per cent and in LH to be between 2·1 and 5·5 per cent (87, 180, 186). Recent work in the author's laboratory, however, suggest that human FSH and LH contain a much higher proportion of hexose (8a). The total carbohydrate accounts for about 22 per cent of the FSH molecule and consists of 10·7 per cent mannose, 1·18 per cent galactose, 1·7 per cent fucose, 4·5 per cent glucosamine and 3·37 per cent *N*-acetylneuraminic acid. In porcine FSH the two hexoses are in approximately equal amounts, while in the ovine there is more galactose than mannose. There is more mannose than galactose in both human and ovine LH.

Ovine FSH contains at least twice as much sialic acid as ovine LH but in human FSH and LH the amount in each is about the same (8a). All the common amino acids are detected in FSH and LH except methionine in FSH (8a) and tryptophan in LH (8a, 143). In this respect LH resembles TSH; there are other similarities. Both contain about nine cysteine residues per molecule, the highest number reported for any pituitary hormone. LH contains more proline than TSH however.

The nature of the carbohydrate-protein linkages is at present unknown. Partial hydrolysis of ovine LH with pronase (a proteolytic enzyme of *Streptomyces griseus*) gave a glycopeptide of molecular weight about 3,000, but all the amino acids commonly found to take part in carbohydrate-protein covalent linkages are present in the peptide, i.e. aspartic acid, glutamic acid, threonine and serine (137, 186). Reaction with carboxypeptidase did not help since no amino acids were liberated.

In a more recent study on LH of several species, however, the amino acids were investigated by dinitrophenylation, digestion with carboxypeptidase A and hydrazinolysis (148c). Dinitrophenylation revealed serine, threonine and phenylalanine as the principal amino acids in ovine, bovine and porcine LH at the N-terminus while serine was found in human LH along with valine and aspartic acid. Carboxypeptidase A also released serine from these preparations with leucine from ovine and bovine and leucine and glycine from human and porcine LH. A surprising number of amino acids were therefore detected and the possibility of heterogeneity in the preparations must be entertained.

It has been observed that LH has a rather high cysteine content and there is reported to be a high degree of disulphide cross-linking along the peptide chain (189). In a study of the optical rotatory dispersion of pituitary hormones it was found that LH possessed a very low dispersion constant $(\lambda_0 = 213)$ and neither this nor the specific rotation was altered by treatment with 7 M-urea or 4 M-guanidine at 50-60° although there was almost complete loss of biological activity (97). Jorgensens concluded that LH was a globular protein locked in a non-helical, rigid conformation by the disulphide cross-linkages. The dispersion constant for FSH is also rather low $(\lambda_0 = 233)$ and it appears to possess only slight helical conformation.

TABLE 6.6

Some physico-chemical constants of different preparations of FSH and LH

	FSH			LH		
	Ovine	Porcine*	Human	Ovine	Porcine	Human
Molecular weight	67,000[134]	29,000[180]		28,000–30,000[177, 188] monomer 16,300[a]	45,000[c] 25,000–33,000[d]	26,000[177]
$S_{20,w}$	4·7[134]	2·49[180]	1·64[37] 1·67[116] 2·9[b]	2·32[188] 2·47[176] 2·7[177]		2·14[116] 2·71[177]
Isoelectric point	4·5[134]	5·1–5·2[180]		7·3[177] 7·7[187, 189]	7·45	5·4[177]

* digested with pancreatin.

(*a*) LI, C. H. and STARMAN, B. *Nature, Lond.* **202,** 291 (1964).

(*b*) ROOS, P. and GEMZELL, C. A. Ciba Foundation Study Group on Physicochemical and Immunological Properties of the Gonadotropins, p. 11 (1965).

(*c*) REICHERT, L. Ciba Foundation Study Group on Physicochemical and Immunological Properties of the Gonadotropins, p. 30 (1965). This result was obtained by the method of gel filtration: the molecular weight has probably been overestimated.

(*d*) REICHERT, L. E. and JIANG, N. S. *Endocrinology* **77,** 78 (1965). This result was obtained by the sucrose density gradient centrifugation method. Preparations of LH from several other species were compared and found to have similar molecular weights by this method.

Physical constants

The above mentioned and other physical constants are given in Table 6.6.

Ovine LH has been reported in two forms, one associated with an acidic protein (187, 188). The isoelectric point of this 'combining' protein is 5·2.

Stability

Crude preparations of both FSH and LH are stable when dry for several years and pituitary glands retain their gonadotrophic activity when stored in acetone at −5° for many months. The only evidence of deterioration in national standards concerns NIH-FSH-S1, some ampoules of which have suffered loss of activity since 1961. The purest preparations, particularly of FSH, are difficult to obtain in a stable, dry form. Losses may occur during freeze-drying and when kept in solution the initial high activity soon falls (8, 139, 151, 162, 180). FSH which was 74·5 times NIH-FSH-S1 dropped in potency to 47 times NIH-FSH-S1 within eight days of freeze-drying and five weeks later was only 38 times NIH-FSH-S1.

In contrast LH is more stable in highly purified form and no losses appear to occur on freeze-drying. It has been reported that in the dry state it may be heated to 100° for twenty-four hours with only about 30 per cent loss of activity (152). However it is completely inactivated within six minutes when in solution at pH 7·4 at this temperature. It is also very unstable in 0·01 N-HCl even at −20°; it is more stable at neutral pH values and activity is retained for some time even at pH 11 (55, 152).

Effect of various reagents on biological activity

Much of the work reported on the effects of reagents on activity was done with preparations that are now recognized as impure. Results that have been misleading in view of subsequent work are therefore omitted but in many cases the early conclusions still hold.

FSH   Digestion to 60–75 per cent with trypsin, chymotrypsin (131) or pronase (8) destroys biological activity. However, it should be noted that highly potent porcine FSH has been prepared after digestion with pancreatin (178). Moreover it is suggested that whereas highly active FSH which has not been treated with pancreatin is unstable in the freeze-dried state, preparations of comparable activity but treated in the early stages of fractionation with pancreatin seem to be exceedingly stable. According to Reichert and Parlow (152) most preparations of FSH contain proteinase but there is no correlation between the stability of the preparation and the amount of enzyme.

Ptyaline and takadiastase destroy activity, suggesting that the carbohydrate is essential for biological activity (129). This conclusion is supported by the finding that the terminal sialic acid is essential in NIH-FSH S1 (85) and in purified human FSH (8) which are inactivated by treatment with neuraminidase. Oxidation with periodic acid (8, 38, 72) or with hydrogen peroxide (38) also reduces activity.

Terminal amino groups and S—S linkages seem to be important since treatment with keten (112) or reduction with cysteine (38, 66, 67, 178) leads to inactivation.

LH   Early reports of the inactivation of LH by enzymes (47) have been confirmed recently when it was shown that trypsin, acetylated trypsin and chymotrypsin appreciably reduce the activity (2). Carboxypeptidase A reduces the activity by half with the liberation of serine and lysine, the *C*-terminal amino acid. A more rapid inactivation occurs with the proteolytic enzyme from *clostridium histolytium*, clostripaine, which cleaves peptides on the carboxyl side of arginine at a much greater rate than it cleaves lysine residues.

In contrast no inactivation of ovine LH occurs following treatment for six to sixteen hours at 37° with neuraminidase. This is probably accounted for by the very low sialic acid content of this hormone. Periodate oxidation, however, destroys the biological activity but apparently not the immunological properties (184). Performic acid oxidation for thirty minutes destroys both types of activity (2, 184). Oxidation with H_2O_2 has also been studied and found to lead to inactivation (148).

Reaction with keten or reduction with cysteine (66) destroys LH, as it does FSH, activity. It has been reported that LH is more susceptible to reduction with borohydride than is FSH (38) but unfortunately the experiments were done on rather crude preparations and do not appear to have been repeated on highly purified materials.

Sodium in liquid ammonia completely inactivates LH; almost 70 per cent is destroyed by dimercaptopropanol while sodium thioglycollate (50 min) causes slight loss of activity (2).

The active material may be precipitated by picrolinic, flavianic, picric and trichloroacetic acids (65, 113).

Treatment with urea leads to inactivation of LH (55, 166). Thus after twenty-four hours at 25–40° in 6 M-urea over 95 per cent of the activity is lost, but at 5° only 75 per cent inactivation occurs. Ovine LH is virtually destroyed within the first hour at 24° and after removal of urea by dialysis there is no regeneration of activity (47). Since FSH is more stable to urea than is LH this affords a method of removing traces of LH from FSH preparations (42, 54).

Urinary gonadotrophins

(*a*) HUMAN MENOPAUSAL GONADOTROPHIN (HMG)

Initial extraction from urine

Many methods have been proposed for the extraction of gonadotrophins from urine, chiefly for subsequent assays in clinical studies. Precipitation from alcohol or acetone was used in the earlier methods, but clearly these are impractical for dealing with large volumes of urine since up to five volumes of solvent are required for one of urine for efficient precipitation.

Ultrafiltration through collodion membranes has been used (75, 100, 159), but undoubtedly the most popular methods have been those depending on adsorption, usually on to kaolin (170). The adsorption is most efficiently carried out at pH 4·0 and the gonadotrophin is eluted at about pH 11·0. It may then be precipitated by ethanol or acetone at pH 5·5.

In the method of Loraine and Brown (118), HCl is used for the acidification of the urine and dilute NaOH at pH 11·3 for elution. The reagents described earlier by Bradbury, Brown and Brown (27) and subsequently adopted by Albert et al. (6) were acetic acid and ammonia. An advantage in the latter method is that only two volumes instead of five volumes of acetone are required for the final precipitation.

Other adsorbents are aluminium hydroxide (124), attapulgite (163) and ion exchange materials (98).

Methods depending on precipitation are preferred in some laboratories. The reagents include tannic acid (99) which gives very satisfactory recoveries, a mixture of benzoic and tungstic acids (31) and zinc acetate (50).

The efficiencies of several of these methods have been compared, and although some differences were found they can probably be explained by variations in local conditions, by the errors involved in biological assays and by qualitative differences in the products (19, 120).

Purification of HMG

Early attempts to purify HMG were designed to separate the FSH and LH components and to remove toxic impurities from the crude extracts. Methods which showed promise were fractional precipitation from ammonium sulphate (98) and chromatography on calcium phosphate (34). Some separation of FSH and LH was claimed for the latter method but it eventually proved of use chiefly for the removal of toxic material and was subsequently adopted for the preparation of the first reference preparation, HMG 24.

A major improvement in the specific activity of HMG was obtained in the method of Johnsen (98). Urine at pH 4·5 was passed through a column of ion exchange material (a sodium aluminium silicate) and after careful washing of the column, active material was eluted in a mixture of ammonium acetate and ethanol. It was subsequently fractionated by precipitation from ammonium sulphate yielding a product 60–80 times the potency of 1st IRP-HMG (8·5–11·5 i.u. per mg). A large batch of this material, HMG J5, was distributed to several laboratories and its potency was confirmed. It contained LH as well as FSH but relatively more of the latter than IRP-HMG. After fractionation on calcium phosphate its potency was increased to 345 times 1st IRP-HMG (50 i.u. per mg) but it was still not homogeneous, showing in the ultracentrifuge a major component (90·9 per cent) with sedimentation coefficient, $S_{20, w}$, of 2·0 and a minor component with a higher constant (37).

Another preparation of high potency was obtained by precipitation with ethanol, adsorption on kaolin and chromatography on the ion exchange material, Decalso (synthetic sodium aluminium silicate) and finally electrophoresis on starch (26). This preparation was homogeneous by free electrophoresis with a mobility of $-4·76 \times 10^{-5}$ at pH 8·6.

There are two factors in particular which have contributed to later progress in the purification of HMG. Firstly there is the improvement in specific activity of the initial extracts achieved by using the kaolin method of Albert (4, 6). In this method the active material is eluted from the kaolin and precipitated with only two volumes of acetone. It is then re-extracted in a mixture of ammonium acetate and ethanol to yield material already ten times as active as 1st IRP-HMG (1·5 i.u. per mg). This technique has served for the preparation of the starting material in nearly all later methods.

Secondly the use of the ion-exchange cellulose materials (142) has greatly facilitated the subsequent purification. Butt and Round (44) investigated stepwise elution from DEAE-cellulose and found some improvement in potency. Segaloff et al. (172) used gradient elution to 0·5 M-NaCl in 0·1 M-NaH$_2$PO$_4$. The active material was eluted early and was then fractionated on a second column. The material appeared homogeneous on DEAE-cellulose and by paper electrophoresis at pH 6·8 and 8·5. Its activity was equal to that of the Armour standard 264-151-X in assays for FSH (about 12 i.u. per mg).

Albert et al. (7) showed subsequently that for large-scale preparations the fractionation on DEAE could be achieved by a batch technique. Impurities were adsorbed on to the DEAE-cellulose while the FSH activity remained in the solution of 0·05 M-phosphate.*

This step was used in two recent methods. Donini, Puzzuoli and Montezemolo (53) passed the fraction they obtained through Permutit at pH 5·4 and then eluted the active material in a solution of 10 per cent ammonium acetate and 45 per cent ethanol and then reprecipitated it by increasing the concentration of ethanol. The activity varied from batch to batch between 138 and 467 times 1st IRP-HMG (18–66 i.u. per mg). The potency increased to 621 times 1st IRP-HMG (88 i.u. per mg) after filtration through Sephadex G-200 but it still contained some LH. There was immunological evidence that other common impurities such as albumin had been removed, however.

Reichert and Parlow (154) obtained material which was over 90 times as

---

* Although suitable for the purification of HMG it should be noted that some loss of efficiency is encountered when this method is applied to extracts of pituitary FSH since all the LH as well as FSH remains unadsorbed. If a weaker solution is used the FSH is preferentially adsorbed leaving LH in solution. See also Ref. 154 below.

TABLE 6.7

Potencies of various preparations of HMG

Method of preparation	FSH potency as assayed	FSH potency i.u. per mg	LH potency as assayed	LH potency i.u. per mg	Reference
Adsorption on ion-exchange resin: fractional precipitation from ammonium sulphate ('HMG J5'): chromatography on calcium phosphate	345 × 1st IRP-HMG	50	not assayed	—	37
Kaolin: DEAE-cellulose: Sephadex G-100	1·9 × NIH-FSH-S1	50	0·0035 × NIH-LH-S1	5·3	154
Kaolin: DEAE-cellulose: Permutit: Sephadex G-200: followed by column electrophoresis	621 × 1st IRP-HMG	88	116 × 1st IRP-HMG	58	53,(a)
	1,325 × 1st IRP-HMG	190	27 × 1st IRP-HMG	14	(b)

(a) DONINI, P., PUZZUOLI, D. and D'ALESSIO, I. *Acta endocr. Copenh.* **45**, 329 (1964).
(b) DONINI, P. *Ciba Foundation Study Group on Physicochemical and Immunological Properties of the Gonadotropins*, p. 98 (1965). ROOS, P. and GEMZELL, C. A., *Ciba Foundation Study Group on Physicochemical and Immunological Properties of the Gonadotropins*, p. 11 (1965) have reported the preparation of HMG using DEAE-cellulose, Sephadex G-100 and electrophoresis on polyacrylamide gel. It was not isolated from solution however: the potency estimated from the ultraviolet absorption was 12 × NIH-FSH-S1 (i.e. 310 i.u. per mg) and LH activity was present.

active as 1st IRP-HMG by this technique but found that when the step was repeated some FSH activity was lost by adsorption to the DEAE-cellulose. Subsequent chromatography on DEAE-cellulose in 0·0213 M-borate–0·035 M-phosphate buffer at pH 8·0 gave a material over 350 times as potent as 1st IRP-HMG (50 i.u. per mg).

The potencies of these various preparations are given in the table with the amount of LH included where possible.

(b) Gonadotrophins from the urine of males

Relatively little work has been done on the purification of gonadotrophins from the urine of normal males, but the assay of these gonadotrophins is often of clinical value.

They may be extracted by the kaolin, tannic acid or benzoic acid-tungstic acid methods, although in the hands of Borth the latter gave poor results (19). Hamburger and Johnsen (90) showed that the Permutit adsorption method could be used for male as well as for post-menopausal urine. They did extensive biological investigations of their product but did not attempt to purify it. Albert et al. (7) used the kaolin method followed by reprecipitation from ammonium acetate-ethanol and then removed impurities by adsorption on DEAE-cellulose. Active material was then precipitated by tannic acid at pH 5·0 and the gonadotrophin was then eluted from the precipitate by borate buffer. Although this method was devised essentially for clinical assays it is a useful preliminary procedure for further purification.

Gonadotrophin of high activity may be obtained by similar methods from the urine of eunuchs. It contains both FSH and LH and the ratio of FSH to LH is reported to be rather higher than in HMG (3, 5, 154). By purification of the gonadotrophin with DEAE-cellulose it has been possible to obtain a potency of 41 i.u. per mg as FSH and 15 i.u. per mg as LH. Partial separation of these factors is achieved by chromatography on a column of DEAE-cellulose; LH is not retained by the exchanger from a solution of 0·01 M-phosphate-borate buffer, pH 8·0, and its potency is increased to 20 i.u. per mg. The FSH retained on the column is eluted by increase of salt concentration to 0·1 M-NaCl. It contained 106 i.u. per mg as FSH and only 3·2 i.u. per mg as LH (154).

(c) Gonadotrophins from other sources

The tannic acid (182) and the kaolin (123) methods have been used to extract gonadotrophin from the urine of sheep. The gonadotrophin behaves similarly to human gonadotrophin on DEAE-cellulose but requires rather more ethanol (86 per cent by volume) for complete precipitation.

Chemical properties of HMG

When prepared as a dry powder HMG is stable indefinitely: in solution its potency soon falls unless kept deep frozen. HMG is less stable in acid than in

neutral or alkaline solutions. Full activity is retained after twenty minutes at
room temperature at pH 11·5 (38).

Oxidation with periodic acid or with hydrogen peroxide causes considerable loss of biological activity. Slight loss of activity occurs after treatment
with ascorbic acid, thioglycollic acid or methionine and rather more with
cysteine. Sodium borohydride causes some qualitative changes, since the
LH activity falls rather more than FSH activity.

Incubation of HMG with 6 M-urea at 40° leads to almost complete loss of
both FSH and LH activities within twenty-four hours (166). 4 M-urea under
the same conditions causes less destruction, while after six hours FSH
activity is much less affected than LH (14). It is likely that with the weaker
solution of urea the cyanate produced (at pH 7) is responsible for the effect
on biological activity rather than the urea.

Since it is unlikely that any HMG so far prepared is homogeneous the
physicochemical properties are unknown. The best preparations are glycoproteins containing about 15 per cent hexose, 11 per cent hexosamine and
up to 10 per cent neuraminic acid (22). All the common amino acids have
been detected and the carbohydrate moiety contains mannose, galactose,
glucose and glucosamine. During electrophoresis the active material migrates
in the region of α_1-glycoprotein (7).

IMMUNOLOGICAL PROPERTIES OF GONADOTROPHINS

It has been shown repeatedly that antisera may be raised to both urinary
and pituitary gonadotrophins. They are effective in neutralizing the biological
activity of the homologous antigens but antisera to FSH and HMG are not
yet sufficiently specific for use in immunoassays. Methods for assaying HCG
and LH have been developed, however, and are widely used; they are discussed on pp. 132–133).

FSH

The main contaminants in purified human FSH which interfere in immunological investigations are LH and proteins related to albumin (32). Most of
the LH is removed by electrophoresis in starch gel but the albumin remains
(42). Much of this can be removed by fractionation before electrophoresis
in the partition system consisting of urea-ammonium sulphate-ethyl cellosolve described on pp. 111–112.

Preparations obtained by this method give a single precipitin line in the
α_2-globulin region with antiserum to pituitary FSH, but some albumin is
usually detected by the more sensitive haemagglutination-inhibition method.
There is also a slight cross-reaction between the antiserum and LH or HCG in
spite of the lack of LH in the antigen.

Promising results have also been reported by Saxena and Henneman (164)
who used a similar method for the initial extraction of FSH and then purified

the antigen by two electrophoreses in starch gel. A single precipitin line was obtained in double diffusion and immuno-electrophoretic experiments.

Antisera to human pituitary FSH cross-react in double diffusion experiments and neutralize the biological activity of HMG. There is some evidence that they also cross-react with equine FSH but not with ovine FSH.

Preliminary observations by the haemagglutination-inhibition method are sufficiently encouraging to suggest that before very long an immunological assay for this hormone will be possible (42).

Antisera to ovine NIH-FSH-S1 show as many as six precipitin lines in agar gel and starch gel immuno-electrophoresis (58). The antisera inhibit the effect of FSH in normal and hypophysectomized rats; this property is retained after absorption of the antisera with various tissues from sheep and with NIH-LH-S1 while the number of precipitin lines is reduced to two.

HMG

The purest preparations of HMG which contain a high proportion of FSH give multiple precipitin lines in immuno-electrophoresis (53, 77, 96). Some of these may be removed by pre-absorption of the antisera with extracts of urine from hypophysectomized patients or from children (76, 77).

Donini *et al.* (53) worked with HMG of high potency which had been purified on columns of the ion exchange material, Permutit. It gave two lines in the α_1–α_2 globulin region and one or two in the β region in immuno-electrophoresis. It is interesting to note that there were no lines in the albumin region.

Antisera to HMG neutralize the biological activity of HMG and of pituitary FSH (37, 198). There is some evidence that they are less efficient against LH or HCG (37, 122) but this is not a universal finding (198).

Human chorionic Gonadotrophin (HCG)

Human chorionic gonadotrophin (HCG) was first recognized in the blood and urine of pregnant women by Aschheim and Zondek in 1927 (10). They believed originally that it was produced from the anterior pituitary but it is now known to arise from the chorionic tissue of the placenta (52) and its detection in urine forms the basis of most tests for the early diagnosis of pregnancy. The major site of production in the placenta is probably the cytotrophoblast but as yet no definite conclusion can be made as to the specific types of cells which are responsible (52). More information should soon be forthcoming from investigations which have commenced with fluorescein- and ferritin-labelled antibodies to HCG (110, 130, 169). At present the evidence is contradictory, since staining with fluorescein appears only in the syncytiotrophoblast and not the cytotrophoblast.

HCG is also produced by certain tumours of the uterus and testes. At present there is no good evidence for any biological or chemical differences between the hormones produced from these different sources.

Biological properties of HCG

(a) FUNCTION   In early pregnancy HCG prolongs the active life of the corpus luteum which in the human produces progesterone and oestrogen. Eventually the placenta itself takes over the production of these steroids but HCG is observed throughout pregnancy; so it may possess other functions yet unknown.

(b) BIOASSAY   There are numerous biological tests for HCG, the first of which was developed by Aschheim and Zondek (10) and depends on the formation of haemorrhagic follicles and corpora lutea in the ovaries of intact immature mice. It has probably been the most widely used of all tests for the diagnosis of pregnancy and is only now being replaced by immunological tests.

Amphibia have been used, HCG causing ovulation in the female (e.g. *Xenopus laevis*) and the expulsion of spermatozoa in the male (e.g. *Bufo arenarum, Bufo bufo, Rana pipiens* and *Xenopus laevis*). These responses are extremely rapid but the sensitivity varies considerably.

The test depending on the increase in prostatic weight in normal rats, a secondary effect of the hormone, is suitable for quantitative assay (117). The ovarian ascorbic acid depletion assay (OAAD) described for pituitary LH may also be used for HCG. It may be noted at this stage that there are no recognized differences in the biological activities of LH and HCG.

HCG has been used successfully in the human as a luteinizing hormone. When infertile women are treated with human FSH followed by HCG they may ovulate as indicated by the changes in the excretion of steroids and in many cases by the ensuing pregnancies (9, 51, 71, 121).

Standards

The first international standard was established in 1938 when 0·1 mg of a preparation of HCG containing lactose was defined as the unit. The second international standard has recently been set up. Like the first international standard, it is only of medium potency and certainly not pure. It is claimed, however, that the cruder material is more stable than the highly purified preparations and therefore is more suitable. It was prepared from urine by adsorption on Permutit from which it was eluted in a mixture of ammonium acetate and ethanol (158). It was then precipitated by the addition of more ethanol, and pyrogens were removed by calcium phosphate. Lactose was added and the preparation was freeze-dried in ampoules.

Collaborative assays showed that each ampoule (approximately 6·8 mg) contained 5,300 i.u.

METHODS OF EXTRACTION FROM URINE

Most of the methods used for extracting the pituitary gonadotrophins from urine are equally suitable for HCG. The first methods used depended on direct precipitation with acetone or ethanol, but a more economical method which depends on adsorption on to benzoic acid has been described by Katzman and Doisy (103). A saturated solution of benzoic acid in acetone is added to urine which is then slowly acidified to about pH 3·5. The benzoic acid is precipitated as fine crystals on to which HCG and other proteins are adsorbed. Alternatively a solution of sodium benzoate may be added to the urine and on acidification to pH 3·5 the benzoic acid is precipitated as before. The precipitate is separated and mixed with acetone or ethanol which dissolves the benzoic acid and simultaneously precipitates the proteins. These are separated, washed with acetone and ether and dried.

It is interesting to note that the benzoic acid method is unsuitable for the extraction of pituitary gonadotrophins, e.g. from the urine of postmenopausal women (102, 185). Thus Butt and Crooke (41) were able to extract HCG from the urine of pregnant women by use of the benzoic acid method and then the gonadotrophins of pituitary origin by the kaolin method from the residual urine.

The hormone may be adsorbed from acidified urine on to a column of Permutit (synthetic aluminium silicate) (104). After washing with water and mixtures of ammonium acetate and ethanol, the active material is eluted in 38 per cent (by volume) ethanol in 10 per cent (w/v) ammonium acetate and is then precipitated by increasing the concentration of ethanol. The synthetic ion-exchanger, Decalso (Permutit Ltd), may be used as the adsorbent and a product of very high potency (12,000 i.u. per mg) was thus obtained by Morris (134).

Methods of purification

The crude material extracted by benzoic acid is seldom more potent than about 500 i.u. per mg. Claesson *et al.* (48) improved the potency of their extract by precipitating non-specific material with protamine at pH 7·4 and eventually they obtained a product containing 6–8,000 i.u. per mg.

Got and Bourrillon (83) purified their benzoic acid extract by a lengthy procedure but they achieved extremely high potency. They reprecipitated the material several times, from acetate buffer at pH 4·5, and from a solution containing calcium chloride. It was also re-adsorbed on kaolin as in the method for HMG and was finally fractionally eluted from a column of Permutit by a mixture of ammonium acetate and ethanol (60:40 v/v). The product contained 13,000 i.u. per mg and was reported to be homogeneous by electrophoretic, sedimentation, solubility, diffusion and immunoelectrophoretic studies (82).

Reisfeld and Hertz (156) used a much shorter method. After initial extraction by kaolin the product was fractionated on a column of DEAE-cellulose in tris buffer at pH 8·6. The pH was kept constant and the salt concentration was increased by the addition of NaCl. The main activity was eluted early with 0·01–0·12 M-NaCl and the product contained 1,500 i.u. per mg. It was then fractionated again on DEAE-cellulose prepared in phosphate buffer at pH 6·0. The active material was eluted by a salt gradient to 0·3 M-NaCl and it now contained 15,000 i.u. per mg. These workers also investigated the method used by Legault-Démare (108) for the purification of PMS. Here non-specific proteins were precipitated with barium and HCG remained in solution. The product contained 13,000 i.u. per mg but three components were demonstrated by electrophoresis whereas in the chromatographic method the material behaved as a single component for over 200 minutes, showing some heterogeneity only after 240 minutes.

CHEMICAL PROPERTIES OF HCG

Although much of the information available on the chemical properties of HCG has been obtained from preparations which are now known to have been impure, it is clear that the hormone is a glycoprotein with a high carbohydrate content, and that the whole molecule is required for full hormonal activity.

Zilliacus and Roos (203) showed that the sugars in their preparation (6–8,000 i.u. per mg) included galactose, mannose and glucosamine. Later work has shown that HCG also contains fucose (1·2 per cent) and sialic acid (8·5 per cent) consisting of N-acetyl- and N-glycollyl-neuraminic acids (82). The ratio of hexose to hexosamine has been found to vary in different preparations between 1·2 and 2·5 (Table 6.8). The amino acids, glycine, leucine, alanine, valine, aspartic acid, glutamic acid, serine, threonine, cystine, lysine, phenylalanine, proline, isoleucine and methionine were identified in the preparation of Morris (134).

HCG is reported to be stable at 0° in 0·2 per cent aqueous solution at pH 1·0–13·0 for 18 hours and at pH 3·0–11·0 for 8 days (134). The activity drops with increasing temperature, particularly above 37°, and with decrease of pH below 4·6 (11).

Several of the common protein precipitants (picric, flavianic, trichloroacetic and sulphosalicylic acids) do not precipitate HCG, but tungstic, phosphotungstic and phosphomolybdic do.

Effect of various reagents on biological activity

Many reagents destroy the biological activity of HCG. Among these are benzoyl chloride, phenylisocyanate, 2:4-dinitro-fluorobenzene, sodium hypobromite, Folin's phenol reagent, diazobenzene sulphonate (134), silver nitrate, mercuric chloride, sodium lauryl sulphate, sodium bisulphite and m-dinitrobenzene (12).

TABLE 6.8

Some properties of HCG

Hexose (galactose and mannose)%	11·0 (10·7[a], 12·2[134])
Hexosamine (glucosamine and galactosamine)%	8·7 (5·2[a], 4·9[134])
Fucose %	1·2
Sialic acid (N-acetyl and N-glycollyl neuraminic acid)%	8·5
Isoelectric point	2·95 (3·2–3·3[a], 3·5–3·6[b])
Diffusion constant $D_{20, w}$ cm^2/s	8·2 × 10^{-7}
$S_{20, w}$	2·7
Molecular weight	30,000

These results are taken from References 82 and 83; others as indicated. The C-terminal residue is glycine (82).

(a) LUNDGREN, H. P., GURIN, S., BACHMAN, C. and WILSON, D. W. *J. biol. Chem.* **142,** 367 (1942).

(b) RAACKE, I. D., LI, C. H. and LOSTROH, A. *Acta endocr. Copenh.* **17,** 366 (1954).

Formaldehyde reduces the activity slowly as also does keten, probably due to the acetylation of the phenolic groups of tyrosine (112). The hormone appears to be stable in 0·1 N-nitrous acid at 2°.

The behaviour of HCG in solutions of urea resembles that of LH. When incubated with 40 per cent urea at pH 7·2 at 37·5°, 80 per cent of the activity is lost within 60 minutes.

Although periodate is known to destroy other gonadotrophic activity it is less effective against HCG (194). This important claim clearly requires further investigation. The oxidized hormone differs from the original in being resistant to influenza virus.

Fraenkel-Conrat *et al.* (68) found that a solution containing 1 mg per ml was almost completely inactivated when a 40-fold amount of cysteine was added at pH 7·8, but that there was no inactivation when the concentration was 0·1 mg per ml. They concluded that the integrity of some disulphide bonds which are not easily reduced is essential for hormonal activity. Similar findings were reported by Bischoff (16). The hormonal activity is also reduced by ascorbic acid at pH 4·6 at 22° (12) and the potency is partly restored by subsequent treatment with 1 per cent hydrogen peroxide.

Effect of enzymes on biological activity

Abramonitz and Hisaw (1) found that the activity was rapidly reduced by hydrolysis with trypsin or chymotrypsin and slowly with ptyalin. Bourrillon *et al.* (25) examined their highly purified preparation in the presence of various enzymes and found that it could not be split further without loss of biological activity. Thus the proteolytic enzymes trypsin, chymotrypsin and papain partially destroyed the activity so that by 24 hours only 20 per cent of

K

the initial activity remained. Inactivation with carboxypeptidase was even more rapid and there was also a very rapid reaction with pepsin but this was probably due to the low pH employed. There was appreciable reduction in activity with the salivary enzyme ptyalin and some reduction with glucosidase and lysozyme. However, hyaluronidase was without effect.

MOLECULAR WEIGHT   The molecular weight of the hormone has been variously estimated at between 30,000 and 120,000. The most reliable figure is probably 30,000 obtained by Got (82) by the methods of light-scattering and ultracentrifugation. This agrees with the estimate from the method of radiation inactivation of biological activity (136, 140). This method is less affected by impurities than many others.

HCG and pituitary LH

The similarity between the biological properties of these two hormones is well known. Comparatively little is known of the chemical properties of the highly purified preparations of either, but particularly of LH. The sedimentation coefficients are similar ($S_{20, \text{w}} = 2.7$) and the molecular weights are in the region of 30,000. However the isoelectric points are widely different, LH is 5.4 but HCG is about 3.0. These results are consistent with the finding of a sialic acid content in HCG higher than in LH. It is interesting that the sialic acid appears to be important with regard to the activity of HCG since hydrolysis with neuraminidase reduces the activity (29, 167) whereas, not surprisingly, it has no effect on LH (2). Thus, in spite of the similar biological activities, the chemical structure of the active centres appears to be different in each hormone.

IMMUNOCHEMISTRY OF HCG

In the short time since the immunological assay for HCG was described, numerous publications have appeared, chiefly because of the application of the method to the diagnosis of pregnancy. As usually performed it is certainly not specific for HCG and probably estimates in addition inactivated forms of HCG and other proteins characteristic of pregnancy. In the last two trimesters of pregnancy the immunological results are usually higher than the biological results and immunologically active material has been found to remain unextracted by kaolin from pregnancy urine while all HCG is removed (95).

It is well established that antisera raised to HCG will block the biological activity of HCG in experimental animals (36, 89, 109, 122, 127, 131, 133, 168, 183, 196); these antisera are not necessarily specific for HCG, however, since they affect other gonadotrophins such as HMG and pituitary LH (28, 36, 133, 183).

The antisera are usually produced in rabbits by the administration of HCG with adjuvants such as Freund's (28, 45, 70, 89, 101, 105, 109, 122, 127, 131,

168, 173, 193) or adsorbed on bentonite (36, 133). It has seldom been possible to use the purest HCG, and since it is known that secondary antibodies tend to continue to rise in titre relative to the main component if immunization is prolonged, a short course of injections is advisable. A course extending over six to eight weeks is often sufficient but animals vary considerably in responsiveness, and some require much longer. Wide (195) showed that in a series of sixteen rabbits injections were extended from six to thirty weeks and the total amount of HCG required per rabbit varied from 9,000 i.u. to 120,000 i.u. Even then two rabbits failed to produce satisfactory antibodies.

Studies in double diffusion and immunoelectrophoresis

The presence of three to five components is found in antisera raised to most commercial preparations of HCG. Some of these cross-react to components in the urine of non-pregnant females, males, children and to normal human serum (28, 45, 101, 173). It has been repeatedly observed that the number of precipitins may be reduced, sometimes to only one, by absorbing the antiserum with concentrates from the urine of males, or of hypophysectomized patients or by human serum. There is some evidence that the remaining precipitin line is due to the specific HCG–anti-HCG reaction.

This evidence is:

(a) The position of the precipitin line in immuno-electrophoretic experiments (in the β-globulin position) is in the region of the biologically active component of HCG (109, 122).

(b) Highly purified preparations of HCG give a single precipitin line in the same electrophoretic position (84).

(c) The absorbed antiserum will still neutralize the biological activity of HCG.

(d) The absorbed antiserum may be used in the haemagglutination-inhibition or complement fixation tests for the diagnosis of pregnancy; quantitative estimations by these methods give results in reasonable agreement with bioassay.

Although antisera to HCG are purified considerably by such absorption they continue to react with pituitary LH. At the moment it seems unlikely that the reaction to LH is one of complete identity with HCG. It is usually observed that the precipitin line between LH and anti-HCG forms as a spur on the HCG–anti-HCG line (33, 78, 141). Immunoelectrophoretic investigations show that the LH–anti-HCG line is more extended to the anode than the HCG line. These results suggest that some of the antigenic properties of LH and HCG are alike, but not all.

No immunological differences have been detected between HCG extracted from the urine of pregnant women and that obtained from the urine of patients with chorio-epithelioma (109) or with testicular tumours secreting chorionic gonadotrophin (131). Although some chemical differences between HCG from different tissues has been suggested (78) there seems to be no evidence for this on immunological grounds. It is possible of course that differences in the molecular structure could exist which are not related to their biological activity or antigenic sites.

Haemagglutination methods

These are the most widely used methods for clinical work. Usually formalinized sheep cells are treated with tannic acid and sensitized with purified HCG (e.g. 196). Red cells treated with pyruvic aldehyde have also been used and they do not require prior treatment with tannic acid (36). Alternatively the cells may be washed in buffer containing hydroquinone and then formalinized and sensitized directly with HCG (70). The bis-diazotized benzidine method has also been used for HCG (89).

Other particles including latex (74, 79, 183), barium sulphate (73) and bentonite have been examined as substitutes for red cells but none appear to offer any great advantages.

The haemagglutination-inhibition reaction has proved most useful for measurements in both urine and serum. Non-specific agglutination of the cells occurs with some specimens of urine. Salts, particularly phosphates, may be the cause and these can be removed by refrigerating the urine and removing the insoluble material. In other cases the HCG is best extracted by precipitation with acetone or benzoic acid.

The sensitivity of the method can be adjusted by varying the concentrations of the antiserum and of the sensitized red cells. For the routine diagnosis of pregnancy a sensitivity of 0·5–1·0 i.u. of HCG per ml is adequate.

Determinations in serum are preferably carried out on extracted material so that interference from serum proteins is minimized. A completely satisfactory method has not been described; precipitation with acetone gives reasonable results (132) but the extracts are still rather crude. Fractional precipitation from ethanol is suggested as an alternative. Non-specific protein is removed by precipitation from ammonium acetate–ethanol (40:60 v/v) and then the HCG is precipitated by increasing the concentration of ethanol to 80 per cent by volume. This gives cleaner extracts than the acetone method.

Very satisfactory results have been obtained for serum by using the alternative technique of complement fixation. This compares in sensitivity and specificity with the haemagglutination-inhibition method and as performed by Brody and Carlström no extraction is required (28).

SPECIFICITY   The only other hormone likely to interfere in the determination of HCG is pituitary LH (35, 197). There is evidence that with some antisera the reaction may not be complete, since the immunological estimates are lower than the biological estimates of potency (39). However these same antisera give results in agreement with bioassay for LH as it occurs in urine, which suggests that the antigenic groups in the LH extracted from pituitaries and from urine may not be identical.

Radioimmunological methods for HCG

Methods for the assay of HCG using ^{131}I-labelled antigen have been described (140, 199). The method of Hunter and Greenwood (p. 86) is suitable for labelling HCG and the separation of free and bound antigen is achieved by precipitation of the bound with anti γ-globulin.

The advantage of the radioimmunoassay is its high sensitivity; it is possible to detect less than 0·01 i.u. HCG per ml. It should therefore be of great use in the determination of HCG in serum and will probably be applicable to the determination of LH in serum or urine.

Immunological and biological activity

In view of the apparent lack of purity in the antigen usually employed, it is surprising that the immunological test for HCG has been so successful. The shapes of the curves for the excretion of HCG throughout pregnancy are similar by immunological and biological methods and the results by both methods fall sharply after labour or abortion.

In the second and third trimesters of pregnancy, however, the immunological results are rather higher than the biological results. Furthermore if HCG is heated to 100° its biological activity is rapidly destroyed but its immunological potency is not (196). Thus it is probable that the antigenic groups are not those that are essential for biological activity.

In a very careful study the loss of hormonal activity of HCG on exposure to a 2·0 MeV electron beam was compared with the loss of immunological activity (140). The rate of inactivation was consistently greater when assayed biologically than when measured immunologically. The molecular weight calculated from the biological results was 27,000 which agreed well with other physical measurements. The molecular weight from the immunological data, however, was only 11,200. These findings were interpreted as demonstrating that the structural unit required for immunological activity is considerably smaller than that required for biological activity.

Pregnant mare's serum gonadotrophin

Pregnant mare's serum gonadotrophin (PMS) was first recognized by Cole and Hart (49) and by Zondek (204). It is produced chiefly between about the 40th and 150th days of gestation, its origin being the structures known as the 'endometrial cups'. The sticky secretion from these cups is an extremely rich source of gonadotrophin.

PMS appears to behave as a mixture of FSH and LH although until now there is no confirmation of claims in the past for the separation of these factors.

Methods of assay include those depending on the increase in ovarian or uterine weights in immature mice or rats, vaginal cornification, formation of corpora lutea and ovulation in rabbits. The method of choice is probably the ovarian weight test as it is satisfactory from the criteria of simplicity, precision, sensitivity and practicability (91, 158).

International standard

This was set up in 1939 and the unit was defined as the activity of 0·25 mg of the reference standard (158). This standard contains PMS contributed from five different centres and is in the form of 25 mg tablets containing lactose.

EXTRACTION AND PURIFICATION

PMS is a glycoprotein and methods for its extraction and purification include fractional precipitation from salts (80) or from ethanol or acetone (46, 81) and adsorption on to aluminium hydroxide (59, 88) or benzoic acid (160).

(a) *From serum*

In the method of Goss and Cole (81) the serum is brought to pH 9 and is mixed with 90–95 per cent of its volume of acetone. After standing for 12–18 hours, the precipitate is separated by filtration and washed with 50 per cent acetone. The combined filtrates are acidified to pH 6 with HCl and left at 2°. The inactive precipitate which forms is removed and gonadotrophin is then precipitated by increasing the concentration of acetone to 70 per cent.

The specific activity is increased by fractional precipitation from acetone. The extract is dissolved in 40 per cent acetone and the pH is adjusted to 5·5. After increasing the acetone concentration to 50 per cent, an inactive precipitate forms and is removed. Finally the active material is precipitated by adjusting the pH to 4·5. Li *et al.* (111) used this method and obtained a high degree of purity, as judged by the electrophoretic pattern.

One of the most active of the early preparations was obtained by Rimington and Rowlands (160, 161). They first removed inert proteins from the serum by precipitation with metaphosphoric acid and then adsorbed the active material on to benzoic acid at pH 4·6. The benzoic acid was removed from the precipitate by acetone and the protein was dissolved in water adjusted to pH 7 with NaOH. An inert precipitate formed on adding an equal volume of ethanol and sufficient acetic acid to bring the pH to between 4·7 and 4·8. Active material precipitated on increasing the concentration of ethanol to 66 per cent. It was finally purified by fractional precipitation from ethanol and its potency was 12,500 i.u. per mg.

More recently Bourrillon and Got (21, 24) and Legault-Démare et al. (108) have made notable contributions to the purification of PMS. In the first method, fractional precipitation with ethanol at various pH values between 4·8 and 8·5 gave a product of 5–6,000 i.u. per mg. This was heterogeneous, but after electrophoresis on starch, a fraction was obtained which was homogeneous in electrophoresis between pH 1·95 and 8·6, in the ultracentrifuge and by solubility studies, and contained between 8,000 and 10,000 i.u. per mg.

Legault-Démare used precipitation from ethanol and then adsorbed the product on Permutit ion exchange resin. After elution, impurities were removed by adsorption on barium carbonate and a surprising increase in activity to between 10,000 and 13,000 i.u. per mg was obtained.

Frahm and Schneider (69) reported the fractionation of purified PMS by paper electrophoresis into three zones which they considered may represent different biological activities. This interesting finding was not confirmed, however, by the work of Raacke et al. (146), who submitted PMS to zone electrophoresis on starch at different pH values, but FSH and LH activities were retained in similar proportions throughout. It was claimed that the best fraction had the remarkable potency of 30,000 i.u. per mg.

(b) From endometrial cups

The secretion from the endometrial cups taken from mares in early pregnancy may be freeze-dried to give material containing about 100 i.u. per mg (135). It may also be extracted in 10 per cent ammonium acetate, pH 5·1, and ethanol (60:40 v/v) and when precipitated from ethanol contains between 300 and 800 i.u. per mg (33). The total amount of gonadotrophin obtained in this way from individual mares is between 200,000 and 500,000 i.u. between the 50th and 70th days of pregnancy.

The gonadotrophin may be purified by methods similar to those described for human gonadotrophin. The active material is not retained by carboxymethyl cellulose from 0·01 M-ammonium acetate (pH 6·1) but is adsorbed from weak buffers at pH 7 on to DEAE-cellulose. When eluted in 0·2 M-ammonium acetate the potency is increased to about 5,000 i.u. per mg. This material shows three components in starch gel electrophoresis.

Material of the same potency was obtained by chromatography on DEAE-cellulose at pH 4·6 followed by chromatography on ECTEOLA-cellulose at pH 4·0. A threefold enhancement of specific activity was obtained by subsequent gel filtration on Sephadex G-200 (135).

Gonadotrophin which resembles PMS may be obtained by similar methods from endometrial cups of the zebra, but the total amount of active material appears to be less than from the mare (33).

PHYSICOCHEMICAL PROPERTIES

Some of the properties of purified PMS are given in Table 6.9. It will be seen that PMS is an acidic protein with an isoelectric point of 1·8. It contains a high proportion of carbohydrate, including 10·4 per cent sialic acid. Both *N*-acetyl and *N*-glycolloyl neuraminic acids have been detected (24). The hexose consists of galactose (13 per cent), mannose (4 per cent) and glucose (1·6 per cent) and the hexosamines are acetyl glucosamine (14·6 per cent) and acetyl galactosamine (2·9 per cent).

The molecular weight of about 70,000 was obtained from a consideration of the diffusion coefficient and the sedimentation coefficient in 0·1 M-NaCl (23) and is consistent with the chromatographic behaviour on Sephadex gels. Morris (135) has discussed reasons for the different estimates reported in earlier papers.

TABLE 6.9

Some properties of PMS

Hexose %	18·6
Hexosamine %	17·5
Fucose %	1·4
L-Rhamnose %	0·7
Sialic acid %	10·4
$S_{20, w}$	3·7, 3·2[135]
Molecular weight	75,000, 68,500[135]
Isoelectric point	1·8, 2·4[146]

These results are taken from Reference 24 unless otherwise indicated.

Stability

Early workers reported somewhat capricious behaviour for PMS, some preparations showing a rapid decline in activity while others showed little change after months. It may be that some of these preparations were contaminated with proteolytic enzymes, bacteria or other impurities which would explain these observations. There are reports that even the dry powder loses activity fairly rapidly (111, 161). In general it seems that PMS is fairly stable in neutral or slightly alkaline solutions. No inactivation occurs in solution at pH 7·5 over the course of thirty-five days at 1·5°, but fairly rapid loss of activity occurs in alkali, even at room temperature (111). As the temperature is increased the loss of activity is more rapid; at 37° the activity decreases somewhat at pH 5·25 over thirty hours, while at pH 3·63 it decreases by 50 per cent within ten hours (61). At 60°, 50 per cent of the potency is lost within two days at pH 5·9 and 85 per cent is lost within four days (161).

Effect of reagents on activity

Loss of activity has been reported after treatment with keten, nitrous acid and formaldehyde (17, 18, 46, 111, 161). It thus seems that free amino groups play an important role in the activity of the hormone.

A large excess of cysteine results in complete inactivation and some loss has been noted with HCN at pH 8·0 (62, 67). Whitten (193) claimed that periodate preferentially destroyed the FSH component but Raacke *et al.* (147) could not confirm this and found that both types of activity were partly reduced.

Loss of potency occurs after incubation with trypsin, pepsin, chymotrypsin, papain and carboxypeptidase (46, 59, 61, 80, 161). Biological activity is rapidly abolished by carbohydrate-splitting enzymes such as ptyalin and takadiastase which suggests that the intact carbohydrate residue is essential for activity (61, 128). Morris (134) is cautious about drawing too many conclusions from these experiments since the commercial takadiastase used sometimes contains an enzyme which is effective in inactivating PMS but is not identical with diastase or *N*-acetyl glucosaminidase and is not a proteolytic enzyme. Whitten (191) confirmed that diastase (from saliva) rapidly inactivated PMS but found that two other sources of α-amylase—malted barley and parotid salivary glands—did not. Thus the actions of saliva and takadiastase may not be due to amylase. It is clear that results of significance can be obtained only by the action of highly purified enzymes on highly purified hormones and such experiments have not yet been reported.

Whitten (192) found that the receptor destroying enzyme of *Vibrio cholerae* cultures rapidly inactivated PMS, as did the allantoic fluid from chicken embryos which had been infected with adapted LEE-B strain of influenza virus. In this respect its behaviour is similar to HCG which is also inactivated under these conditions. Similar loss of activity occurs after hydrolysis with neuraminidase, which demonstrates the importance of the sialic acids with respect to activity.

References

1 ABRAMOWITZ, A. A. and HISAW, F. L. *Endocrinology* **25,** 633 (1939).

2 ADAMS-MAYNE, M. and WARD, D. N. *Endocrinology* **75,** 333 (1964).

3 ALBERT, A., DERNER, I., LEIFERMAN, J., STELLMACHER, V. and BARNUM, J. *J. clin. Endocr.* **21,** 839 (1961).

4 ALBERT, A., DERNER, I., STELLMACHER, V., LEIFERMAN, J. and BARNUM, J. *J. clin. Endocr.* **21,** 1260 (1961).

5 ALBERT, A., DERNER, I., STELLMACHER, V., LEIFERMAN, J. and BARNUM, J. *J. clin. Endocr.* **22,** 996 (1962).

6 ALBERT, A., KELLY, S., SILVER, L. and KOBI, J. *J. clin. Endocr.* **18,** 600 (1958).

7 ALBERT, A., KOBI, J., LEIFERMAN, J. and DERNER, I. *J. clin. Endocr.* **21,** 1 (1961).

8 AMIR, S. M., BARKER, S. A., BUTT, W. R. and CROOKE, A. C. *Nature, Lond.* **209,** 1092 (1966).

8a AMIR, S. M., BUTT, W. R., JENKINS, J. and SOMER, P. J. *Biochim. biophys. Acta* (in the press), 1967.

9 APOSTOLAKIS, M., BETTENDORF, G. and VOIGT, K. D. *Acta endocr. Copenh.* **41,** 14 (1962).

10 ASCHHEIM, S. and ZONDEK, B. *Klin. Wschr.* **6,** 1322 (1927).

11 BANIK, U. K. *Ann. Biochem. exp. Med.* **19,** 5 (1959).

12 BANIK, U. K. *Ann. Biochem. exp. Med.* **19,** 29 (1959).

13 BELL, E. T., MUKERJI, S. and LORAINE, J. A. *J. Endocr.* **28,** 321 (1964).

14 BELL, E. T. and LORAINE, J. A. *Ciba Fdn Study Grp. No.* **22** (edited by G. E. W. Wolstenholme and Julie Knight) p. 29, Churchill, London (1965).

15 BETTENDORF, G., APOSTOLAKIS, M. and VOIGT, K. D. *Acta endocr. Copenh.* **41,** 1 (1962).

16 BISCHOFF, F. *J. biol. Chem.* **134,** 641 (1940).

17 BISCHOFF, F. *Endocrinology,* **29,** 520 (1941).

18 BISCHOFF, F. *Endocrinology* **30,** 525 (1942).

19 BORTH, R. and MENZI, A. *Acta endocr. Copenh.* Suppl. 90, 17 (1964).

20 BOURDEL, G. and LI, C. H. *Acta endocr. Copenh.* **42,** 473 (1963).

21 BOURRILLON, R. and GOT, R. *Acta endocr. Copenh.* **24,** 82 (1957).

22 BOURRILLON, R. and GOT, R. *Acta endocr. Copenh.* Suppl. 51, 201 (1960).

23 BOURRILLON, R. and GOT, R. *Acta endocr. Copenh.* **35,** 221 (1960).

24 BOURRILLON, R. and GOT, R. *Acta endocr. Copenh.* Suppl. 51, 683 (1960).

25 BOURRILLON, R., GOT, R. and MARCY, R. *Acta endocr. Copenh.* **31,** 553 (1959).

26 BOURRILLON, R., GOT, R. and MARCY, R. *Acta endocr. Copenh.* **35,** 225 (1960).

27 BRADBURY, J. T., BROWN, E. S. and BROWN, W. E. *Proc. Soc. exp. Biol. Med.* **71,** 228 (1949).

28 BRODY, S. and CARLSTRÖM, G. *J. clin. Endocr.* **22,** 564 (1962).

29 BROSSMER, R. and WALTER, K. *Klin. Wschr.* **36,** 925 (1958).

30 BROWN, P. S. *J. Endocrin.* **13,** 59 (1955).

31 BUTT, W. R. *J. Endocrin.* **17,** 143 (1958).

32 BUTT, W. R. In *Immunological Properties of Protein Hormones* (edited by F. Polvani and P. Crosignani) p. 57, Academic Press, New York (1966).

33 BUTT, W. R. *Ciba Fdn Study Grp No.* **22** (edited by G. E. W. Wolstenholme and Julie Knight) p. 64, Churchill, London (1965).

34 BUTT, W. R. and CROOKE, A. C. *Ciba Fdn Colloq. Endocr.* **5,** 44 (1953).

35 BUTT, W. R., CROOKE, A. C. and CUNNINGHAM, F. J. *Proc. R. Soc. Med.* **64,** 647 (1961).

36 BUTT, W. R., CROOKE, A. C. and CUNNINGHAM, F. J. *Ciba Fdn Colloq. Endocr.* **14,** 310, 1962.

37 BUTT, W. R., CROOKE, A. C. and CUNNINGHAM, F. J. *Biochem. J.* **81,** 596, 1961.

38 BUTT, W. R., CROOKE, A. C., CUNNINGHAM, F. J. and EVANS, A. J. *Biochem. J.* **79,** 64, 1961.

39 BUTT, W. R., CROOKE, A. C., CUNNINGHAM, F. J. and INGRASSIA, F. *Proc. R. Soc. Med.* **57,** 851 (1964).

40 BUTT, W. R., CROOKE, A. C., CUNNINGHAM, F. J. and WOLF, A. *J. Endocr.* **25,** 541, 1963.

41 BUTT, W. R., CROOKE, A. C., INGRAM, J. and ROUND, B. P. *J. Endocr.* **16,** 107 (1957).

42 BUTT, W. R., CROOKE, A. C. and WOLF, A. *Ciba Fdn Study Grp No. 22* (edited by G. E. W. Wolstenholme and Julie Knight) p. 85, Churchill, London (1965).

43 BUTT, W. R., CUNNINGHAM, F. J. and HARTREE, A. S. *Proc. R. Soc. Med.* **57,** 107 (1964).

44 BUTT, W. R. and ROUND, B. P. *J. Endocr.* **17,** 75 (1958).

45 CARLSSON, M. G. *Acta endocrin. Copenh.* **46,** 142 (1964).

46 CARTLAND, F. G. and NELSON, J. W. *J. biol. Chem.* **119,** 59 (1937).

47 CHOW, B. F., GREEP, R. O. and VAN DYKE, H. B. *J. Endocr.* **1,** 440 (1939).

48 CLAESSON, L., HÖGBERG, B., ROSENBERG, T. and WESTMAN, A. *Acta endocr. Copenh.* **1,** 1 (1948).

49 COLE, H. H. and HART, G. H. *Amer. J. Physiol.* **93,** 57 (1930).

50 COURRIER, R. *Acta endocr. Copenh.* Suppl. 90, 29 (1964).

51 CROOKE, A. C., BUTT, W. R., PALMER, R. F., MORRIS, R., EDWARDS, E. L. and ANSON, C. J. *J. Obstet. Gynaec. Br. Commonw.* **70,** 604 (1963).

52 DICZFALUSY, E. and TROEN, P. *Vitams Horm.* **19,** 230 (1961).

53 DONINI, P., PUZZUOLI, D. and MONTEZEMOLO, R. *Acta endocr. Copenh.* **45,** 321 (1964).

54 DURAISWAMI, S., MCSHAN, W. H. and MEYER, R. K. *Biochim. biophys. Acta* **86,** 156 (1964).

55 ELLIS, S. *Endocrinology* **68,** 334 (1961).

56 ELLIS, S. *Endocrinology,* **69,** 554 (1961).

57 ELRICK, H., YEARWOOD-DRAYTON, V., ARAI, Y., LEAVER, F. and MORRIS, H. G. *J. clin. Endocr.* **23,** 694 (1963).

58 ELY, C. A. and TALLBERG, T. *Endocrinology* **74,** 314 (1964).

59 EVANS, H. M., GUSTUS, E. L. and SIMPSON, M. E. *J. exp. Med.* **58,** 569 (1933).

60 EVANS, H. M., SIMPSON, M. E., TOLKSDORF, S. and JENSEN, H. *Endocrinology* **25,** 529 (1939).

61 EVANS, J. S. and HAUSCHILDT, J. D. *J. biol. Chem.* **145,** 335 (1942).

62 EVANS, J. S., NELSON, J. W. and CARTLAND, G. F. *Endocrinology* **30,** 387 (1942).

63 FARQUHAR, M. G. and RINEHART, J. F. *Endocrinology* **55,** 857 (1954).

64 FEVOLD, H. L. *Endocrinology* **24,** 435 (1939).

65 FEVOLD, H. L. *J. biol. Chem.* **128,** 83 (1939).

66 FRAENKEL-CONRAT, H. L., SIMPSON, M. E. and EVANS, H. M. *J. biol. Chem.* **130,** 247 (1939).

67 FRAENKEL-CONRAT, H. L., SIMPSON, M. E. and EVANS, H. M. *Proc. Soc. exp. Biol. Med.* **45,** 627 (1940).

68 FRAENKEL-CONRAT, H. L., SIMPSON, M. E. and EVANS, H. M. *Science* **91,** 363 (1940).

69 FRAHM, H. and SCHNEIDER, W. G. *Acta endocr. Copenh.* **24,** 106 (1957).

70 FULTHORPE, A. J., PARKE, J. A. C., TOVEY, J. E. and MONCKTON, J. C. *Br. med. J.* i, 1049 (1963).

71 GEMZELL, C. A., DICZFALUSY, E. and TILLINGER, G. *J. clin. Endocr.* **18,** 1333 (1958).

72 GESCHWIND, I. I. and LI, C. H. *Endocrinology* **63,** 449 (1958).

73 GILBOA-GARBER, N. and NELKEN, D. *Nature, Lond.* **197,** 158 (1963).

74 GOLDIN, M. *Amer. J. clin. Path.* **38,** 335 (1962).

75 GORBMAN, A. *Endocrinology* **37,** 177 (1945).

76 GOSS, D. A. *J. clin. Endocr.* **24,** 408 (1964).

77 GOSS, D. A. and LEWIS, J. *J. clin. Endocr.* **23,** 986 (1963).

78 GOSS, D. A. and LEWIS, J. *Endocrinology* **74,** 83 (1964).

79 GOSS, D. A. and TAYMOR, M. L. *Endocrinology* **71,** 321 (1962).

80 GOSS, H. and COLE, H. H. *Endocrinology,* **15,** 214 (1931).

81 GOSS, H. and COLE, H. H. *Endocrinology* **26,** 244 (1940).

82 GOT, R. and BOURRILLON, R. *Acta endocr. Copenh.* Suppl. 51, 1091 (1960).

83 GOT, R. and BOURRILLON, R. *Biochim. biophys. Acta* **39,** 241 (1960).

84 GOT, R., LEVY, G. and BOURRILLON, R. *Experientia* **15,** 480 (1959).

85 GOTTSCHALK, A., WHITTEN, W. K. and GRAHAM, E. R. B. *Biochim. biophys. Acta* **37,** 375 (1960).

86 GREEP, R. O., VAN DYKE, H. B. and CHOW, B. F. *Endocrinology* **30,** 635 (1942).

87 GRÖSCHEL, U. and LI, C. H. *Biochim. biophys. Acta* **37,** 375 (1960).

88 GUSTUS, E. L., MEYER, R. K. and WOODS, O. R. *J. biol. Chem.* **114,** 59 (1936).

89 HAMASHIGE, S. and ARQUILLA, E. R. *J. clin. Invest.* **42,** 546 (1963).

90 HAMBURGER, C. and JOHNSEN, S. G. *Acta endocr. Copenh.* **26,** 1 (1957).

91 HAMBURGER, C. and PEDERSEN-BJERGAARD, K. *Q. Jl. Pharm. Pharmac.* **10,** 662 (1937).

92 HARTREE, A. S., BUTT, W. R. and KIRKHAM, K. E. *J. Endocr.* **29,** 61 (1964).

93 HELLBAUM, A. A., MCARTHUR, L. G., CAMPBELL, D. L. and FINERTY, J. C. *Endocrinology* **68**, 144 (1961).

94 HILDEBRAND, J. E., RENNELLS, E. G. and FINERTY, J. C. *Z. Zellforsch. mikrosk. Anat.* **46**, 400 (1957).

95 HOBSON, B. M. and WIDE, L. *Acta endocr. Copenh.* **46**, 632 (1964).

96 ILLEI, G. and MORITZ, P. *J. Endocr.* **29**, 263 (1964).

97 JIRGENSONS, B. *Arch. Biochem. Biophys.* **91**, 123 (1960).

98 JOHNSEN, S. G. *Acta endocr. Copenh.* **20**, 101 (1955).

99 JOHNSEN, S. G. *Acta endocr. Copenh.* **28**, 69 (1958).

100 JUNGCK, E. G., MADDOCK, W. O. and HELLER, C. G. *J. clin. Endocr.* **7**, 1 (1947).

101 KAIVOLA, S., KIISTALA, U. and AXELSON, E. *Acta endocr. Copenh.* **42**, 395 (1963).

102 KATZMAN, P. A. *Endocrinology* **21**, 89 (1937).

103 KATZMAN, P. A. and DOISY, E. A. *J. biol. Chem.* **106**, 125 (1934).

104 KATZMAN, P. A., GODFRID, M., CAIN, C. K. and DOISY, E. A. *J. biol. Chem.* **148**, 501 (1943).

105 KEELE, D. K., REMPLE, J., BEAN, J. and WEBSTER, J. *J. clin. Endocr.* **22**, 287 (1962).

106 KOENIG, V. L. and KING, E. *Archs. Biochem.* **26**, 219 (1950).

107 KRAICER, J. and LOGOTHETOPOLOUS, J. *Endocrinology* **69**, 381 (1961).

108 LEGAULT-DÉMARE, J., CLAUSER, H. and JUTISZ, M. *Biochim. biophys. Acta* **30**, 169, (1958).

109 LEWIS, J., DRAY, S., GENUTH, S. and SCHWARTZ, H. S. *J. clin. Endocr.* **24**, 197 (1964).

110 LEZNOFF, A. and DAVIS, B. A. *Can. J. Biochem. Physiol.* **41**, 2517 (1963).

111 LI, C. H., EVANS, H. M. and WONDER, D. H. *J. gen. Physiol.* **23**, 733 (1940).

112 LI, C. H., SIMPSON, M. E. and EVANS, H. M. *J. biol. Chem.* **131**, 259 (1939).

113 LI, C. H., SIMPSON, M. E. and EVANS, H. M. *Endocrinology* **27**, 803 (1940).

114 LI, C. H., SIMPSON, M. E. and EVANS, H. M. *Science* **109**, 445 (1949).

115 LI, C. H., SQUIRE, P. G. and GRÖSCHEL, V. *Proc. Soc. exp. Biol. Med.* **98**, 839 (1958).

116 LI, C. H., SQUIRE, P. G. and GRÖSCHEL, V. *Arch. Biochem. Biophys.* **86**, 110 (1960).

117 LORAINE, J. A. *J. Endocr.* **6**, 613 (1950).

118 LORAINE, J. A. and BROWN, J. B. *Acta endocr. Copenh.* **17**, 250 (1954).

119 LORAINE, J. A. and DICZFALUSY, E. *J. Endocr.* **17**, 425 (1958).

120 LORAINE, J. A. and MACKAY, M. A. *J. Endocr.* **22**, 277 (1961).

121 LUNENFELD, B. *J. Int. Fed. Gynaec. Obst.* **1**, 153 (1963).

122 LUNENFELD, B., ISERSKY, C. and SHELESNYAK, M. C. *J. clin. Endocr.* **22,** 555 (1962).

123 MACGILLIVRAY, A. J. and ROBERTSON, H. A. *J. Endocr.* **26,** 125 (1963).

124 MALBERG, R. F. and GOODMAN, J. R. *J. clin. Endocr.* **14,** 666 (1954).

125 MCCANN, S. M. and TALEISNIK, S. *Amer. J. Physiol.* **199,** 847 (1960).

126 MCGARRY, E. E. and BECK, J. C. *Fert. Steril.* **14,** 558, 1963.

127 MCKEAN, C. M. *Amer. J. Obst. Gynaec.* **86,** 596 (1960).

128 MCSHAN, W. M. and MEYER, R. K. *J. biol. Chem.* **120,** 361 (1938).

129 MCSHAN, W. M. and MEYER, R. K. *J. biol. Chem.* **135,** 473 (1940).

130 MIDGLEY, A. R. and PIERCE, G. B. *J. exp. Med.* **115,** 289 (1962).

131 MIDGLEY, A. R., PIERCE, G. B. and WEIGHE, W. O. *Proc. Soc. exp. Biol. Med.* **108,** 85 (1961).

132 MISHELL, D. R., WIDE, L. and GEMZELL, C. A. *J. clin. Endocr.* **23,** 125 (1963).

133 MORITZ, P. and ILLEI, G. *J. Endocr.* **26,** xxx (1963).

134 MORRIS, C. J. O. R. *Br. med. Bull.* **11**(2), 101 (1955).

135 MORRIS, C. J. O. R. *Acta endocr. Copenh.* Suppl. 90, 163 (1964).

136 NYDICK, M., BERRY, R. J. and ODELL, W. D. *J. clin. Endocr.* **24,** 1049 (1964).

137 PAPKOFF, H. *Biochim. biophys. Acta* **78,** 384 (1964).

138 PARLOW, A. F. In *Human Pituitary Gonadotrophins* (edited by A. Albert), p. 300, C. C. Thomas, Springfield, Ill. (1961).

139 PARLOW, A. F., CONDLIFFE, P. G., REICHERT, L. E. and WILHELMI, A. E. *Endocrinology* **76,** 27 (1965).

140 PAUL, W. E. and ODELL, W. D. *Nature, Lond.* **203,** 979 (1964).

141 PAUL, W. E. and ROSS, G. T. *Endocrinology* **75,** 352 (1964).

142 PETERSON, E. A. and SOBER, A. A. *J. Amer. chem. Soc.* **78,** 751 (1956).

143 PIERCE, G. B. and WYNSTON, L. K. *Biochim. biophys. Acta* **43,** 538 (1960).

144 PURVES, H. D. and GRIESBACH, W. E. *Endocrinology* **49,** 244 (1951).

145 PURVES, H. D. and GRIESBACH, W. E. *Endocrinology* **55,** 785 (1954).

146 RAACKE, I. D., LOSTROH, A. J., BODA, J. M. and LI, C. H. *Acta endocr. Copenh.* **26,** 377 (1957).

147 RAACKE, I. D., LOSTROH, A. J. and LI, C. H. *Archs Biochem. Biophys.* **77,** 138 (1958).

148 REICHERT, L. E. *Endocrinology* **69,** 398 (1961).

148a REICHERT, L. E. *Endocrinology* **71,** 729 (1962).

148b REICHERT, L. E. *Endocrinology* **75,** 970 (1964).

148c REICHERT, L. E. *Endocrinology* **78,** 186 (1966).

148d REICHERT, L. E. and JIANG, N. S. *Endocrinology* **77,** 124 (1965).

149 REICHERT, L. E. and PARLOW, A. F. *Endocrinology* **73,** 224 (1963).

150 REICHERT, L. E. and PARLOW, A. F. *Endocrinology* **73,** 285 (1963).

151 REICHERT, L. E. and PARLOW, A. F. *Endocrinology* **74,** 236 (1964).

152 REICHERT, L. E. and PARLOW, A. F. *Endocrinology* **74,** 809 (1964).

153 REICHERT, L. E. and PARLOW, A. F. *Endocrinology* **75**, 815 (1964).

154 REICHERT, L. E. and PARLOW, A. F. *J. clin. Endocr.* **24**, 1040 (1964).

155 REICHERT, L. E. and PARLOW, A. F. *Proc. Soc. exp. Biol. Med.* **115**, 286 (1964).

155a REICHERT, L. E. and WILHELMI, A. E. *Endocrinology* **76**, 762 (1965).

156 REISFELD, R. A. and HERTZ, R. *Biochim. biophys. Acta* **43**, 540 (1960).

157 RENNELLS, E. G. *Z. Zellforsch. mikrosk. Anat.* **45**, 464 (1957).

158 Report of the Third International Conference on Standardization of Hormones, *Bull. W. H. O.*, L. of N. **8**, 887 (1939).

159 RIGAS, D. A., PAULSON, S. A. and HELLER, C. G. *Endocrinology* **62**, 738 (1958).

160 RIMINGTON, C. and ROWLANDS, I. W. *Biochem. J.* **35**, 736 (1941).

161 RIMINGTON, C. and ROWLANDS, I. W. *Biochem. J.* **38**, 54 (1944).

162 ROOS, P. and GEMZELL, C. A. *Biochim. biophys. Acta* **82**, 218 (1964).

163 SALHANICK, H. A. In *Human Pituitary Gonadotrophins* (edited by A. Albert) p. 37, C. C. Thomas, Springfield, Ill. (1961).

164 SAXENA, B. B. and HENNEMAN, P. H. *J. clin. Endocr.* **24**, 1271 (1964).

165 SCHALLY, A. V. and BOWERS, C. Y. *Endocrinology* **75**, 312 (1964).

166 SCHMIDT-ELMENDORFF, H., LORAINE, J. A. and Bell, E. T. *J. Endocr.* **24**, 153 (1962).

167 SCHUMACHER, G., UHLING, R., BLOBEL, R., MOHR, E. and SCHUMAGER, M. D. *Naturwissenschaften* **47**, 517 (1960).

168 SCHWARTZ, H. S. and MANTEL, N. *J. clin. Endocr.* **22**, 393 (1962).

169 SCIARRA, J. J., KAPLAN, S. L. and GRUMBACH, M. M. *Nature, Lond.* **199**, 1005 (1963).

170 SCOTT, L. D. *Br. J. exp. Path.* **21**, 320 (1941).

171 SEGALOFF, A. and STEELMAN, S. L. *Recent Prog. Horm. Res.* **15**, 127 (1959).

172 SEGALOFF, A., STEELMAN, S. L., EVERETT, C. and FLORES, A. *J. clin. Endocr.* **19**, 827 (1959).

173 SHAHANI, S. K. and RAO, S. S. *Acta endocr. Copenh.* **46**, 317 (1964).

174 SHEDLOVSKY, T., ROTHEN, A., GREEP, R. O., VAN DYKE, H. B. and CHOW, B. F. *Science* **92**, 178 (1940).

175 SIPERSTEIN, E., NICHOLS, C. W., GRIESBACH, W. E. and CHEIKOFF, I. L. *Anat. Rec.* **118**, 593 (1954).

176 SQUIRE, P. G. and LI, C. H. *J. biol. Chem.* **234**, 520 (1959).

177 SQUIRE, P. G., LI, C. H. and ANDERSEN, R. N. *Biochemistry*, **1**, 412 (1962).

178 STEELMAN, S. L., LAMONT, W. A. and BALTES, B. J. *Acta endocr. Copenh.* **22**, 186 (1956).

179 STEELMAN, S. L. and POHLEY, F. M. *Endocrinology* **53**, 604 (1953).

180 STEELMAN, S. L. and SEGALOFF, A. *Recent Prog. Horm. Res.* **15**, 115 (1959).

181 STEELMAN, S. L., SEGALOFF, A. and ANDERSEN, R. N. *Proc. Soc. exp. Biol. Med.* **101,** 452 (1959).

182 SYMINGTON, R. B. *J. Endocr.* **29,** 215 (1964).

183 TAYMOR, M. L., GOSS, D. A. and BUYTENDORP. A. *Fert. Steril.* **14,** 603, 1963.

184 TRENKLE, A., LI, C. H., SADRI, K. and ROBERTSON, H. A. *Archs. Biochem. Biophys.* **99,** 288 (1962).

185 VARNEY, R. F. and KOCH, F. C. *Endocrinology,* **30,** 399 (1942).

186 WALBORG, E. F. and WARD, D. *Biochim. biophys. Acta* **78,** 304 (1963).

187 WARD, D. N., ADAMS-MAYNE, M. and WADE, J. *Acta endocr. Copenh.* **36,** 73 (1961).

188 WARD, D. N., MCGREGOR, R. F. and GRIFFIN, A. C. *Biochim. biophys. Acta* **32,** 305 (1959).

189 WARD, D. N., WALBORG, E. F. and ADAMS-MAYNE, M. *Biochim. biophys. Acta* **50,** 224 (1961).

190 WEST, E. and FEVOLD, H. L. *Proc. Soc. exp. Biol. Med.* **44,** 446 (1940).

191 WHITTEN, W. K. *Aust. J. Sci.* **10,** 49 (1947).

192 WHITTEN, W. K. *Aust. J. scient. Res.* Series B **1,** 271 (1948).

193 WHITTEN, W. K. *Aust. J. scient. Res.* Series B **3,** 346 (1950).

194 WHITTEN, W. K. *Aust. J. scient. Res.* Series B **6,** 300 (1953).

195 WIDE, L. *Acta endocr. Copenh.* Suppl. 70, 18 (1962).

196 WIDE, L. and GEMZELL, C. A. *Ciba Fdn Colloq. Endocr.* **14,** 296 (1962).

197 WIDE, L., ROOS, P. and GEMZELL, C. A. *Acta endocr. Copenh.* **37,** 445 (1961).

198 WILDE, C. E., BAGSHAWE, K. D., DREWE, A. and PALLAS, W. *J. Endocr.* **32,** 117 (1965).

199 WILDE, C. E., ORR, H. and BAGSHAWE, K. D. *Nature, Lond.* **205,** 191 (1965).

200 WILHELMI, A. E. *Can. J. Biochem. Physiol.* **39,** 1659 (1961).

201 WOODS, M. C. and SIMPSON, M. E. *Endocrinology* **66,** 575 (1960).

202 WOODS, M. C. and SIMPSON, M. E. *Endocrinology* **68,** 647 (1961).

203 ZILLIACUS, H. and ROOS, B.-E. *Acta endocr. Copenh.* **6,** 147 (1951).

204 ZONDEK, B. *Klin. Wschr.* **9,** 2285 (1930).

7

THYROID STIMULATING AND THYROID HORMONES

Thyroid stimulating hormone (TSH)

The thyroid stimulating hormone (thyrotrophin, TSH) is a protein produced in the anterior pituitary, and its function is to control the activity of the thyroid gland.

CELLULAR SOURCE

A good deal of evidence has accumulated from early biological and histochemical studies to suggest that the basophils are the source of TSH. By the use of the performic acid–alcian blue technique it seems probable that the S^2 type of cell which stains a deep purplish blue is responsible (116). Studies with antisera to TSH which have been labelled with rhodamine showed fluorescence localized in the cytoplasm of certain basophils (98). These, however, appeared to be the same cells that stained with antisera to corticotrophin labelled with fluorescein. Whether these results are due to the presence of a common antigenic determinant in the two hormones, to a contaminant or to the fact that they have a common cellular origin, will only be decided when purer preparations become available.

BIOLOGICAL ACTIVITY

It has been known for more than a hundred years that there is some relationship between the anterior pituitary and the thyroid gland. Thus it was noted that patients with diseases of the thyroid gland had abnormal pituitaries and this was soon confirmed by work on experimental animals.

The active principle was first extracted from bovine pituitary glands over thirty years ago, and considerable progress has been made since then in the purification of the hormone. However, progress has been slower than with some of the other pituitary hormones, probably because of difficulties with bioassays and the relative instability of the purified hormone.

The primary effects of TSH on the thyroid are essentially those related to the growth and function of the gland. The first effect is probably the activation of a proteolytic enzyme which promotes the hydrolysis of colloid and the liberation of thyroid hormones. Changes in the appearance of the colloid droplets can be detected within thirty minutes of administering TSH to experimental guinea-pigs or rats. An increase in the mean height of the acinar cells of the thyroid of chicks is noted after about eighteen hours and an increase in the actual weight of the gland in about twenty-four hours (79).

The uptake and turnover of iodine by the thyroid gland is increased by TSH. In the human, studies with ^{131}I demonstrate that protein-bound iodine (PBI) of the blood increases within four hours of the injection of TSH and there is increased thyroidal uptake of ^{131}I within eight hours. Eventually increased activity of the thyroid gland is reflected by an elevated basal metabolic rate.

Some interesting observations have been made regarding the nature of circulating TSH in patients with thyrotoxicosis. Adams (1) showed that the TSH principle in the blood of these patients acted on the thyroids of experimental animals over a more prolonged period than did TSH itself. This observation has been confirmed repeatedly and the response has been attributed to the existence of a 'long-acting thyroid stimulator' (LATS).

This substance has not yet been shown conclusively to be a separate compound. McKenzie (100) examined the pituitaries of six patients who suffered from thyrotoxicosis (Graves' Disease) and found TSH but no LATS. The latter, however, appeared in the sera of these patients. This immediately suggests an extra-pituitary origin for LATS, but there are other explanations, including the possibility that LATS may be TSH bound to another pituitary component or to some factor in plasma (107, 108, 171).

Another biological action noted with preparations of TSH is the exophthalmogenic effect. At one time this was considered to be due to a separate component in TSH. It now seems that the two activities run parallel during purification and that the thyrotrophic and exophthalmogenic activities are probably present in the same molecule (105).

Biological assays

Many of these effects have been employed for the biological assay of TSH. In addition to rats, mice and guinea-pigs, chicks and tadpoles are often employed as they permit assays of greater sensitivity.

The method of Gilliland and Strudwick (60) depends on the discharge of ^{131}I from the thyroid gland of one-day old chicks which have been pre-treated with thyroxine to inhibit the secretion of endogenous TSH. The accuracy and sensitivity of the method is increased by giving thyroxine and pro-pylthiouracil with the TSH (12). The index of precision (λ) of the assay as performed by Bates and Cornfield (12) is 0·2 and the working range is be-tween 4 and 30 i.u. $\times 10^{-3}$. It is interesting that even greater sensitivity has been obtained by using mice whose thyroids were labelled with ^{131}I (96, 99). TSH then caused an increase in circulating radioactivity which was maximal within two hours and permitted measurements in the range of 0·05-2 i.u. $\times 10^{-3}$. A simple, but less sensitive assay is obtained by measuring the uptake of ^{32}P by the thyroid gland of baby chicks (33). The uptake of ^{131}I in the thyroids of rats fed on an iodine-rich diet is another assay of comparable sensitivity (129). These methods are suitable for the assay of relatively active fractions from pituitary glands, but it should be noted that there has been some suggestion that growth hormone may interfere in the ^{32}P assay (105).

Extremely sensitive assays have been devised by D'Angelo et al. (34) using tadpoles. These are starved to produce atrophy of the thyroid and cessation of metamorphosis. Administration of TSH leads to the resumption of develop-ment which may be observed by the specific end-point of the measurement of thyroid cell height, or by the measurement of hind limb extrusion which may be produced by a combination of TSH and thyroid hormones.

In vitro METHODS. It is doubtful if any of the above assays is suitable for routine clinical work since those using the common laboratory animals lack the necessary sensitivity. The development of immunological methods is therefore awaited with interest. However, the need for a routine assay with the necessary sensitivity, reliability and practicability has stimulated some workers to investigate *in vitro* effects of TSH.

Bovine thyroid slices when incubated with TSH for 21 hours at 37° increase in weight due to the entry of fluid from the incubation medium. An assay based on this effect which is sensitive to 0·01 i.u. $\times 10^{-3}$ has been reported (3). It is, however, an effect which has no counterpart *in vivo*, an undesirable feature of an *in vitro* assay.

The depletion by TSH of stored labelled iodine in thyroid slices is the basis of the *in vitro* assay of Bottari and Donovan (19). The sensitivity is approx-imately 0·1 i.u. $\times 10^{-3}$ per 100 ml, the λ is satisfactory (0·13) and the method has been applied to estimations in blood (18). In another *in vitro* method depending on the use of ^{131}I, thyroid tissue is taken from male guinea-pigs which have been treated with methyl thiouracil (82). The tissue is incubated with the ^{131}I and TSH for 44 hours at 25°. A measurement of ^{131}I is made at 40 hours and potassium thiocyanate is then added and a second measurement is made after a further 4 hours. The difference in radioactivity in the two samples is inversely related to the amount of TSH. The measurement in this assay probably depends upon the rate of ^{131}I turnover in the tissue and the extent to which ^{131}I is organically bound. The sensitivity is good, the working range being between 0·007 and 0·028 i.u. $\times$ 10^{-3}, it is reasonably specific and it has been applied to estimations in human blood. As with other *in vitro* techniques, however, the method requires extreme care, particularly in the preparation and allocation of the thyroid tissue, and the λ is sometimes rather high.

STANDARDS. An international standard has been established for TSH, one i.u. being defined as the activity contained in 13·5 mg of the standard (109). The collaborative assays to determine the potency of this standard were made in comparison with the USP thyrotrophin reference substance. The units used in early literature usually refer to USP units and Junkmann-Schoeller units, one unit of the latter being equivalent to 0·1 USP unit, i.e. 0·1 i.u.

METHODS OF PREPARATION

An early method described by Ciereszko (28) for the extraction of TSH from acetone-dried bovine pituitary glands has proved useful as the initial stage in many of the later methods. It involves extraction in 2 per cent (w/v) sodium chloride solution at about pH 7·5, followed by isoelectric and acetone precipitation. A stable product with a specific activity of 0·6–1·0 i.u. per mg is obtained. The specific activity may be improved by precipitation from 3·6 M-ammonium sulphate (72) or by distribution in the system n-butanol–0·075 M-*p*-toluene sulphonic acid (23) when the active material is precipitated at the interface.

An alternative method, which depends on percolation of powdered pituitary powder with mixtures of ethanol and sodium chloride with decreasing concentrations of ethanol, gives a rather similar product (13).

Further purification is most efficiently obtained by chromatography on ion-exchange materials. The hormone is retained on the carboxylic acid, cation exchange resin, Amberlite IRC-50 (4, 36, 73), while 70–75 per cent of the inert protein passes through in 0·01 M-phosphate buffer at pH 6·5 containing 0·1 M-sodium chloride and then the TSH is recovered almost quantitatively by elution with 1 M-sodium chloride. At this stage the product contains 4–6 i.u. per mg.

The potency is increased to between 15 and 25 i.u. per mg by chromatography on carboxymethyl cellulose. The column is equilibrated in 0·05 M-formate buffer at pH 3·5 containing 0·11 M-sodium chloride. About 70 per cent of the protein passes straight through and the TSH fraction can be eluted by 0·2 M-sodium chloride in 0·05 M-formate buffer at pH 3–4.

Limanova (88) has described a batchwise technique with carboxymethyl cellulose followed by chromatography and elution in 0·2–0·3 M-sodium chloride which is suitable for both bovine and human TSH. The removal of LH from human TSH is difficult. Both IRC-50 and DEAE-cellulose were used by Hartree *et al.* (69) but the fraction richest in TSH still contained LH.

A chromatographic method using DEAE-cellulose has been described by

Carsten and Pierce (23, 24, 175). They employed a gradient of 0·05 to 0·15 M-glycine buffer at pH 9·5 and the active fraction was then submitted to a second fractionation on a similar column. Starch gel electrophoresis of the fractions obtained showed the presence of several bands which were labelled *a–j*. The biological activity was confined to fractions *a–f* and it was possible to remove the inert fractions, *h, i* and *j* by chromatography on carboxymethyl cellulose. Although these proteins were believed to be of the same molecular weight as TSH, it is interesting that they were separated also by gel filtration on Sephadex G-25 and except for the most accurate work the fractionation on carboxymethyl cellulose was not required (24). In this way a fraction was obtained that was essentially homogeneous, containing only fraction *c*, with a potency of between 30 and 60 i.u. per mg. Ovine, bovine and cetacean TSH behaved identically on these ion-exchange materials, but there was some difference in electrophoretic mobilities (175).

Gel filtration on Sephadex G-50 was used by Condliffe (30) for the purification of human TSH. After fractionation on carboxymethyl cellulose, a second gel filtration on Sephadex G-100 and chromatography on DEAE-cellulose, the product contained 20 i.u. per mg.

The final purification is difficult since, in addition to the instability of the hormone, it appears to form complexes readily with inert protein. Since urea may break down protein-protein complexes it was employed by Dedman *et al.* (36) in the final chromatography on Amberlite IRC-50. The material was applied in 0·2 M-formic acid–0·028 M-HCl–1·0 M-urea at pH 2 and development was continued in the same solvent. It was possible to prepare material of specific activity up to 60 i.u. per mg in this way, but it was extremely unstable, particularly to freeze-drying (see also 115). It is possible that the true biological activity is even higher since the same workers have obtained preparations showing transient biological activity of up to 200 i.u. per mg.

The concentration of TSH in the pituitary glands of different species varies considerably. The human pituitary has a relatively low content compared with bovine, ovine, porcine and particularly rat and mouse pituitaries (11). In an extensive investigation of human glands it was found that values ranged from 10^{-3} to 1100^{-3} i.u. per gland, and decreased with increasing age as in other species (4).

Extraction from biological fluids

(a) BLOOD Fractions obtained by precipitation with ethanol and salt at different pH values have been shown to possess TSH activity (5, 84). The active material is confined to the β-globulin fraction. Plasma is cooled to 4°, acidified to pH 1·2 with HCl, and inert protein is precipitated on adding sodium chloride to 1M. The supernatant fluid is adjusted to pH 0·5, and half as much again sodium chloride is added to precipitate further inert protein.

The supernatant is then dialysed and may be freeze-dried ready for assay. Trichloroacetic acid has also been used to remove inert proteins but gives rather variable yields.

Extracts prepared by this method when examined by the assay depending on the increase in weight of surviving bovine thyroid slices (3) gave parallel dose response lines with bovine pituitary TSH used as standard.

(b) URINE   Many of the techniques proposed for the extraction of TSH from urine are similar to those used for gonadotrophins. Thus TSH may be precipitated from ethanol or acetone or adsorbed on to benzoic acid, calcium phosphate (147) or kaolin (6). The acid-salt method described above for plasma has also been used for urine.

It has been reported that an inhibitor to TSH may be extracted from urine by the benzoic acid method (87).

CHEMICAL PROPERTIES

Since it has been impossible to obtain stable highly-purified preparations of TSH, our knowledge of the chemistry of the hormone is incomplete, and will have to be revised as better preparations become available.

The best preparations of TSH are glycoproteins of molecular weight between 28,000 and 30,000. By an electro-dialysis technique it was shown that no biological activity passed through a membrane at pH 5·0 or pH 9·5 (117). This indicated that the activity does not reside in a small peptide which is bound by electrostatic forces to a larger protein. The active material, however, passed a stretched membrane, permeable to proteins of molecular weight of the order of 26,000–30,000.

This result is in agreement with the molecular weight calculated for bovine TSH by the method of ultracentrifugation in a sucrose density gradient (51). The molecular weight was between 26,000 and 30,000 although there was some evidence of heterogeneity from the sedimentation patterns.

Composition

The composition of bovine TSH obtained by the method of Carsten and Pierce (24, 118) is given in Table 7.1. The carbohydrate consists of mannose, fucose, glucosamine and galactosamine with traces of glucose and galactose but no uronic acid. Studies by enzymic digestion gave evidence that the carbohydrate residues are in a single oligosaccharide unit which is linked to the protein by a covalent bond.

The cystine content is high, but there are no disulphide groups as measured by N-ethyl maleimide (24). Reduction and alkylation does not alter the molecular size as indicated by electro-dialysis. This suggests that the molecule does not consist of several peptide chains held together by disulphide linkages. The protein appears homogeneous with respect to its primary structure since the peptide maps of tryptic digests contain the expected number of spots judged by the calculated number of lysine and arginine residues.

TABLE 7.1

Amino acid composition of bovine TSH

Aspartic acid	13·0	Leucine	6·9
Threonine	14·3	Tyrosine	8·9
Serine	8·6	Phenylalanine	6·1
Proline	12·3	Lysine	4·6
Glutamic acid	14·3	Histidine	14·0
Glycine	8·0	Arginine	6·5
Alanine	11·1	Glucosamine	6.6
Valine	8·7	Galactosamine	4·1
Cystine (half)	13·7	Hexose	9·4
Methionine	5·1	Fucose	1·3
Isoleucine	6·2		

This table gives the calculated number of residues per arbitrary molecular weight of 28,000 (Reference 24).

Effects of reagents on biological activity

The lack of a strongly ionic character is indicated by the ease with which TSH is eluted from DEAE-cellulose. This suggests the absence of neuraminic acid and, like LH, it does in fact appear to be free of significant amounts of this acid (24, 70) and is not inactivated by treatment with neuraminidase.

The carbohydrate moiety, however, appears to be necessary for biological activity and almost complete loss of activity occurs following treatment with periodic acid (59, 70).

Reagents which affect amino groups are found to destroy activity. Examples of these are phenyl isocyanate, dinitrofluorobenzene and nitrous acid (148). However, treatment with guanidine has no effect: reaction occurs only with the ε-amino groups of lysine which therefore does not appear to be essential for activity. Acetylation of the guanidinated derivative results in loss of activity, which suggests that it is the α-amino groups that are important.

Acetylation of the native hormone is also followed by loss of activity (70) and the product has, in fact, been shown to be an inhibitor of TSH (148).

The biological activity of TSH is not consistently reduced by methylation, using methanol in HCl (70). Moreover, treatment with carboxypeptidase has no effect. These observations suggest that free carboxyl groups are not essential for biological activity.

Treatment with bromine completely inactivates TSH and the derivative may even be an inhibitor of TSH (148). This reagent could both oxidize the disulphide groups and brominate the tyrosine residues. Other reagents known to oxidize the disulphide groups such as *p*-chloromercuribenzoate and

iodoacetic acid do not inactivate the hormone, but treatment with diazobenzene sulphonic acid, affecting the tyrosine residues, does.

Iodoacetamide, which also reacts with disulphide groups, inactivates TSH
(148). In order to explain this difference in behaviour from that of other
disulphide reagents, it has been suggested that the latter act reversibly on
proteins. Undoubtedly disulphide groups play an important role in the action
of TSH and the early suggestion that cysteine reduces activity needs to be
re-investigated with purer preparations.

ENZYMIC HYDROLYSIS   Complete destruction of TSH occurs within three
hours of treatment with pepsin or trypsin (148). However, only 25 per cent
loss of activity occurs in this time with chymotrypsin, and none at all with
carboxypeptidase.

IMMUNOLOGICAL STUDIES WITH TSH

The presence of luteinizing hormone and certain serum proteins in most
preparations of TSH presents some difficulties in the preparation of specific
antisera. Purified preparations of bovine TSH are antigenic in rabbits (2, 15,
140, 168), the antisera being capable of inhibiting the biological activity of
bovine TSH. A degree of cross-reaction with human TSH has been reported
although antibodies have been demonstrated in human subjects given injections of bovine TSH over a period of several weeks (71). It has been reported that antisera to human TSH do not neutralize LATS (41, 101).

For haemagglutination reactions TSH may be attached to red cells by
the tannic acid or bis-diazotized benzidine methods. It is unlikely, however,
that the haemagglutination inhibition reaction is sufficiently sensitive for the
estimation of the small amounts of circulating TSH, and the radioimmunoassay will probably be the method of choice. The iodination of TSH has been
demonstrated by the chloramine-T method (110a, 166) and by an interesting
method of iodine distillation (74). The latter avoids the potentially destructive
influence of oxidants or organic solvents and causes no loss of biological
activity. This study clearly demonstrated another source of loss when
working with purified TSH, i.e. that through adsorption on glass or poly-
ethylene surfaces. In the method of Odell et al. (110a) the free and bound
^{131}I-TSH is separated by use of a mixture of 55 per cent v/v ethanol containing
5 per cent w/v NaCl in which free, but not bound, TSH is soluble. Serum of
hypophysectomized patients contained less than the equivalent of 3 mU per
100 ml while sera from patients with primary myxoedema contained between
7 and 156 mU per 100 ml.

Research into the development of an immunoassay for TSH in biological
fluids has now reached the stage when it is possible to demonstrate immuno-
logically-active material; the specificity of such reactions must await studies
on the biological activity of such material done in parallel.

Thyroid hormones

The isolation and chemical identification of the major thyroid hormone, *thyroxine*, was accomplished more than thirty years ago by Harington (68). Since then, a vast amount of research has been directed to the investigation of the biosynthesis and mode of action of this and other thyroid hormones, and several excellent reviews are available (75, 130, 155, 163). Much use has been made of chromatographic methods for the study of the iodinated compounds and of ^{131}I, employed as a tracer and therapeutically.

FORMATION

Iodine enters the body by the digestive tract and is quickly taken up by the thyroid gland which synthesizes and stores the thyroid hormones. Studies with ^{131}I show that the concentration in the gland rises to a maximum within 12–24 hours and then declines; such measurements are often used to measure thyroid activity. The amount taken up is increased by TSH and is inhibited by such ions as thiocyanate and perchlorate.

Although TSH controls the function of the thyroid gland, a little activity persists after hypophysectomy and furthermore it has been shown that thyroid slices are capable of synthesizing some thyroid hormones *in vitro* (106). Parenchymal cells from the follicles of ovine thyroid glands also retain their ability to concentrate and incorporate iodine into thyroid hormones. To demonstrate this, they are dispersed by trypsin and cultured as monolayers; the incorporation of iodine is increased by the addition of TSH as *in vivo* (81).

The iodide is rapidly oxidized by a peroxidase and becomes attached to tyrosine at positions 3 and 5 (Formula 1). Coupling of the iodinated tyrosines then occurs under the influence of specific enzymes, two di-iodo-tyrosines forming tetra-iodothyronine or thyroxine (T4, Formula 2), and di-iodo- and a mono-iodo-tyrosine producing tri-iodothyronine (T3, Formula 3).

$$\text{HO}-\underset{I}{\overset{I}{\bigcirc}}-CH_2 \cdot CH(NH_2) \cdot CO_2H \qquad 1$$

$$\text{HO}-\underset{I}{\overset{I}{\bigcirc}}-O-\underset{I}{\overset{I}{\bigcirc}}-CH_2 \cdot CH(NH_2) \cdot CO_2H \qquad 2$$

$$\text{HO}-\underset{I}{\overset{}{\bigcirc}}-O-\underset{I}{\overset{I}{\bigcirc}}-CH_2 \cdot CH(NH_2) \cdot CO_2H \qquad 3$$

The synthesis occurs within the thyroid follicles, or acini, which are bound together by connective tissue in groups of between twenty and forty to form a lobule. The follicles are spherical and vary in size, which increases by stimulation with TSH. Their functional capacity seems to be linked with their size, the turnover of iodine being more rapid in the smaller follicles. By the use of the two isotopes, ^{125}I and ^{131}I, it has been shown that recently formed organic iodine may be degraded and secreted before that formed earlier (139).

The walls of the follicles are made up of a single layer of lining cells. They are filled with a colloid consisting chiefly of *thyroglobulin* to which the iodinated compounds are bound. In order that the thyroid hormones may be secreted into the blood stream the globulin complex must be broken down. This is done by a proteinase and a peptidase in the gland; these, too, are stimulated by TSH. The thyroid gland is unique among the endocrine glands in storing its product in this way in an extracellular site.

It is still not clear whether the iodination in thyroid tissue occurs in the cells or in the colloid. From the results of numerous experiments on the uptake of ^{131}I, it seems likely that it occurs in the colloid, but observations on foetal tissue show that the uptake and probably the binding takes place before the formation of follicles in many species. Both ^{131}I and ^{125}I were used to locate the binding sites in rat thyroid tissue (122) and in a number of follicles much or most of the protein-bound radio-iodine was found in the epithelial cells. In an extensive review, Maloof and Soodak (97) consider that most evidence favours the concept that iodination occurs intracellularly; if this is so, it is probable that the iodinated protein is secreted so rapidly that it is very difficult to detect in the epithelium.

The iodine in the thyroid consists not only of that which enters from the circulation (called the 'first iodide pool') but that which arises from break-down products within the gland by the proteolysis of thyroglobulin—the 'second iodide pool'. Iodine from the former source may be discharged by perchlorate or thiocyanate but iodine from the latter may not.

THYROGLOBULIN

Thyroglobulin was one of the first proteins to be purified and studied by electrophoretic and ultracentrifugal methods. It was originally considered to be the only iodoprotein in the thyroid gland, but several others are now known.

Methods of extraction

The protein can be extracted in aqueous solvents, usually 0.1–0.15 M-sodium chloride (38). It is soluble in 37 per cent saturated ammonium sulphate and is insoluble in 41 per cent saturated ammonium sulphate; it may also be precipitated from 48 per cent saturated potassium phosphate at pH 6.6 (38, 43, 93, 132). When the precipitation is repeated twice from extracts of normal thyroid tissue, the product contains 85–90 per cent of a component sedimenting with $S_{20,w} = 19.4$ (111).

Several components can be identified by chromatography on DEAE-cellulose, by means of phosphate buffer at pH 6·5 with increasing concentrations of sodium chloride for elution (20, 40, 165). These components were labelled *a* to *e* by Ui *et al.* (165) in the order in which they were eluted. The proportion of iodine in these fractions showed a progressive increase from *a* to *e*: fractions, *a, b* and *c* showed single boundaries in the ultracentrifuge ($S_{20,w} = 19$) and corresponded to the main component in the original material. The other fractions, however, were not pure and sedimented with $S_{20,w} = 28$.

Independently, three distinct ultracentrifugal peaks were observed by De Groot and Carvalho (37) working with human thyroid tissue. The main component, ($S_{20,w} = 19$), made up 70–79 per cent of the protein while the other components sedimented with $S_{20,w} = 28$ and 42. Two other proteins were found in porcine thyroid glands with $S_{20,w} = 11·3$ and 6·5 (142).

The amino acid composition of several of the fractions obtained by chromatography on DEAE-cellulose is similar; it has been suggested therefore that some of the heavy components may be aggregates (165).

In view of the existence of other iodoproteins in the thyroid and the heterogeneity of most preparations, Robbins and Rall (133), in their excellent review of these hormones, suggest that the term thyroglobulin should be reserved for the soluble iodoprotein of thyroid origin which has:

1. A sedimentation coefficient, $S_{20,w} = 19$ approximately;
2. An electrophoretic mobility of approximately $-5·1^{-5}$ cm²/v/sec in barbitone buffer at pH 8·6;

and

3. A sharp range of insolubility at about 38 per cent saturated ammonium sulphate.

Composition

Thyroglobulin is a glycoprotein containing about 4 per cent glucosamine and 4·3 per cent hexose, largely galactose and mannose, and a little fucose (135). It also contains about 1·2 per cent sialic acid (61). End-group analysis by the phenylisothiocyanate technique shows that the *N*-terminal amino acids are aspartic acid, asparagine and glycine (40).

The amino acid composition of a preparation obtained as a fraction from DEAE-cellulose is given in Table 7.2. It will be seen that the acidic amino acids, aspartic and glutamic, are in high concentration. Cysteine is present but there is no information on disulphide cross-linkages.

OTHER PROPERTIES   The molecular weight is of the order of 650,000. The value of 669,000 obtained for the bovine hormone (114) by sedimentation, diffusion and light-scattering techniques agrees well with that of 655,000 obtained for the hog hormone (111). The diffusion constants are also quite

TABLE 7.2

Amino acid composition of thyroglobulin

Aspartic acid	387	Isoleucine	133
Threonine	235	Leucine	490
Serine	493	Tyrosine	129
Proline	368	Phenylalanine	268
Glutamic acid	708	Lysine	124
Glycine	427	Histidine	63
Alanine	437	Arginine	359
Valine	318	Tryptophan	69
Cystine (half)	153	Ammonia	357
Methionine	66		

This table gives the calculated number of residues per mole assuming a molecular weight of 650,000 (protein 578,000, carbohydrate 65,000, iodoamino acids 7,000). Reference 165.

similar: $2\cdot49 \times 10^{-7}$ for the former and $2\cdot60 \times 10^{-7}$ for the latter. The isoelectric point is pH $4\cdot6$, consistent with the high proportion of aspartic and glutamic acids.

The protein is stable between about pH $5\cdot0$ to pH $11\cdot3$ provided that salt is present. It is irreversibly denatured at pH $3\cdot5$. In solutions of low ionic concentration a reversible change occurs which appears to be a disaggregation of thyroglobulin. A slower sedimenting component ($S_{20,w}$ approximately 11) appears, termed the α form. Complete conversion to this form is not found even in distilled water. A similar change is noted with several other reagents, notably detergents (45, 122). The protein is split into two subunits with low concentrations of sodium dodecyl sulphate at neutral or alkaline pH. Higher concentrations completely dissociate the molecule and by observing the changes in viscosity it appears that thyroglobulin behaves as a randomly-coiled polyelectrolyte (122).

The molecule is disorganized at alkaline pH in the presence of 8 M-urea. A number of tyrosyl radicals are exposed that cannot be iodinated in the absence of urea (44, 149).

Thyroglobulin as an antigen

Thyroglobulin is not normally released into the bloodstream, but when the thyroid follicle is injured by disease or radiation, thyroglobulin may escape and then it behaves as an autoantigen. In the same way rabbits injected with extracts of their own thyroglobulin develop autoantibodies (172).

The presence of such antibodies may be demonstrated in the blood of patients suffering from chronic thyroiditis (Hashimoto's disease). The usual immunological techniques of gel diffusion, haemagglutination with tanned cells coated with thyroglobulin and complement fixation may be used (137).

IODOTHYRONINES

L-THYROXINE, the major active substance in thyroid tissue, was isolated in crystalline form as long ago as 1915 by Kendall (80); its chemical structure and synthesis was described by Harington (68). Later a second iodinated compound, 3,5,3'-L-triiodothyronine (triiodothyronine), was isolated (64, 134) and two further compounds, 3,3'-diiodothyronine and 3,3',5'-triiodothyronine, were found in the rat (136). The precursors of thyroxine, 3-monoiodotyrosine and 3,5-diiodotyrosine, have been reported to occur in extracts of normal human and rat serum (14, 39, 169). Other workers have failed to confirm this (119), and it seems possible that, in the course of preparation for chromatography, they may be formed from other compounds by the splitting of bonds that are unstable at pH 3-4 (170).

Synthesis

Since the original synthesis of thyroxine, several others have been described. Interest has centred not only on thyroxine but on analogues, because of their potential biological activities, and on the production of labelled thyronines for experimental work.

In the original method, the diphenyl ether (I, Fig. 7.1) was produced by reaction of p-methoxyphenol and 3,4,5-triiodonitrobenzene. The nitro group was then successively transformed into $-NH_2$, $-N_2Cl$ and $-CN$ from which the alanine side chain was then gradually built up.

Several other syntheses have depended on the use of 2,6-dinitro-diphenyl ethers (10, 25, 29, 46). In a synthesis from L-tyrosine, the amino group was protected by a hydantoin ring and, after nitration to give II (Fig. 7.1), was converted into the 2,6-dinitro-diphenyl ether III (Fig. 7.1) by reaction with toluene p-sulphonyl chloride in pyridine (25). Catalytic hydrogenation followed by tetrazotization with nitrosyl sulphuric acid under anhydrous conditions and reaction with iodide gave the diiodo compound IV (Fig. 7.1).

Alkaline hydrolysis yielded 3,5-diodothyronine from which DL-thyroxine was obtained by treatment with iodine in aqueous ethylamine. The appreciable racemization that may occur when the alanine side chain is protected by conversion into the hydantoin ring is prevented when the amino- and carboxy- groups are protected by acetylation and esterification respectively (25).

A synthesis of D-thyroxine has been described, starting with 3,5-dinitro-L-tyrosine and nitrosyl bromide (46). The resulting L-α-bromo-β(4-hydroxy-3, 5-dinitrophenyl) propionic acid, V, (Fig. 7.1) undergoes inversion in the presence of ammonia to give 3,5-dinitro-D-tyrosine. Then the synthesis is similar to that for L-thyroxine (25).

Methods are available for the labelling of the thyroid hormones with radioactive iodine at the 3,5 (102, 124) or the 3',5' (66) positions. 3,5-diamino-4-(4'-methoxyphenoxy)-N-acetyl phenylalanine ethyl ester is tetrazotized and added in H_2SO_4–acetic acid (1:2 v/v) to a mixture of sodium iodide, iodine

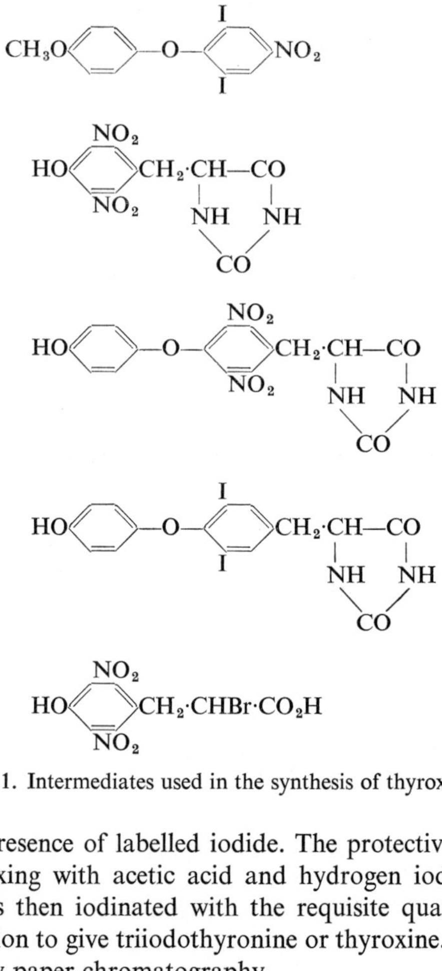

I

II

III

IV

V

FIG. 7.1. Intermediates used in the synthesis of thyroxine.

and urea in the presence of labelled iodide. The protective groups are then removed by refluxing with acetic acid and hydrogen iodide. The labelled diiodothyronine is then iodinated with the requisite quantity of iodine in ammoniacal solution to give triiodothyronine or thyroxine. The products are usually purified by paper chromatography.

The thyronines have a stereochemical structure as shown in Figure 7.2. The angle of $111°$ for the diphenyl ether oxygen prevents certain substitutions in the molecule and affects the interaction between the hormones and enzymes. A mode of interaction with protein molecules at cellular receptor sites has been proposed (77, 78). According to this theory the binding properties are conferred by the benzene ring adjacent to the alanine side chain while the second phenolic ring interacts with an adjacent functional group on the protein.

EXTRACTION AND PURIFICATION OF THE HORMONES FROM THYROID TISSUE

The thyroid hormones are released from the proteins in thyroid tissue by hydrolysis with pancreatin and trypsin in buffer at pH 8·4 (164). There is a

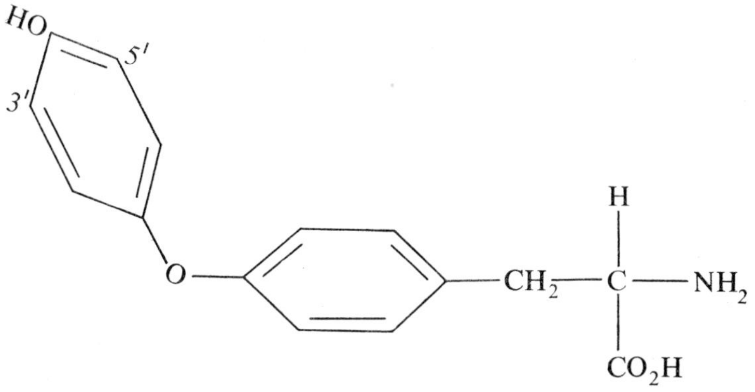

FIG. 7.2

danger that some thyroxine may be lost if the hydrolysis is too prolonged: usually 24 hours is sufficient at 37°. A bacterial enzyme, pronase, has also been used and its action compared with that of pancreatin (138). It releases thyroxine more quickly but it also de-iodinates the hormone more rapidly than pancreatin; the optimum time for hydrolysis is between four and eight hours.

After hydrolysis the iodinated compounds are extractable in n-butanol saturated with N-HCl (93) or in a mixture of methanol and ammonia (1:1 v/v) (126). They may be separated from one another by chromatography on paper or ion-exchange resins.

Numerous solvent systems have been described for paper chromatography, many containing n-butanol or ammonia (Table 7.3). Separations may not be complete after development in one direction; thus thyroxine and triiodo-thyronine are not separated adequately by n-butanol-acetic acid (138) or by n-butanol-dioxan (48). Therefore two-dimensional systems are often employed (48, 49) such as the n-butanol–dioxan system followed by n-butanol–9N-NH$_4$OH.

TABLE 7.3

Typical solvent systems used for separating the iodo-amino acids

	Reference
n-butanol–acetic acid–water (78 : 5 : 17 by vol.)	91, 92
n-butanol–acetic acid–water (85 : 10 : 75 by vol.)	42
n-butanol–9N-NH$_4$OH (1 : 1 v/v)	128
n-butanol–dioxan–2N-NH$_4$OH (4 : 1 : 5 by vol.)	48
n-butanol–n-pentanol–2N-HN$_4$OH (1 : 1 : 2 by vol.)	128
Collidine–2N-NH$_4$OH (3 : 1 v/v)	138
t-pentanol–2N-NH$_4$OH (1 : 1 v/v)	128
t-amyl alcohol–1·5N-NH$_4$OH–water (5 : 1 : 4 by vol.)	42, 91, 92
s-butanol–3·3% NH$_4$OH (3 : 1 v/v)	42

Trace amounts of thyroxine (e.g. [^{131}I]thyroxine) may be de-iodinated on paper when exposed to light and air (103) which introduces serious experimental errors. These may be avoided by working in darkness and by adding reducing agents to the paper.

The analytical grade resin, Dowex A.G.1, in the acetate form is useful for column chromatography (119, 123). At pH 4·0 the thyroid hormones are retained on the column. Mono-iodotyrosine is eluted by decreasing the pH to 3·6, diiodotyrosine to pH 2·2 and thyroxine to pH 1·4. Thyroxine and triiodothyronine are not separated completely in this system.

They are separated by partition chromatography, however. Gross and Pitt-Rivers (65) used columns of Kieselguhr with 0·5 N-sodium hydroxide as the stationary phase and 20 per cent v/v chloroform in n-butanol as the mobile phase.

METHODS OF DETECTION AND ESTIMATION

Many experiments are conducted with labelled thyroid hormones when their positions on chromatograms are readily detected by the radioactive iodine. In other instances there are several sensitive chemical reactions that can be used.

The amino group can be detected by reaction with ninhydrin when greyish-blue colours are given on paper chromatograms. The phenolic group is also readily identified. Diazotized sulphanilic acid gives a red or purple colour with thyroxine but the corresponding tetrabromothyronine does not react (8). Many diazotized amines have been investigated for use in this reaction; one of the best is the N',N'-diethyl sulphanilamide derivative. The phenolic function also reacts with nitrous acid in acid-ethanol and gives a yellow colour which turns red with ammonia.

Probably the best method for quantitative estimation is based on the decolorization of the ceric sulphate–arsenious acid reagent. This may be conveniently performed on filter paper (21).

Serial dilutions (0·01–10 μg organic I) are applied to the paper which is placed on another paper sprayed first with arsenite and the ceric sulphate reagent in acid. The papers are then placed between glass plates for fifteen minutes when the reaction is stopped by spraying with 5 per cent w/v o-phenylene diamine in acetone or methanol. The average diameter of each spot is then measured and is quantitatively related to the concentration of iodine.

The reactions of a number of analogues of thyroxine were compared by this method (9). By comparison with potassium iodide, only one tenth of the iodine in the iodinated thyronines were liberated in this reaction. Modification of the alanine side chain by acetylation or by replacement with C_1, C_2 or C_3 fatty acid residues did not alter the reaction. It was reduced, however, when the phenolic group in the molecule was replaced by H, I or was methylated, but it was unaffected when replaced by an amino group. When 4′-hydroxy-naphthyl-1′-yl was substituted for the phenolic ring the reaction was not altered but when the hydroxyl group was absent, or shifted, deiodination dropped to less than one per cent. Removal of the oxygen bridge reduced the reaction appreciably.

Thyroxine and triiodothyronine in alkali give maximum absorption in the ultra-violet at 231 and 227 mμ respectively. The extinction coefficients are about five times those at 325 mμ where absorption measurements are usually made (156).

Cathodic waves are given by thyroxine in 20 per cent v/v isopropyl alcohol in 0·5 N-sodium carbonate containing one per cent tetramethyl ammonium iodide (17, 143). Three waves are present with half-wave potentials at $-1·12$, $-1·4$ and $-1·7$ volts. Diiodothyronine gives only the last two waves. Borrows et al. (17) investigated twenty-three analogues by this polarographic method.

Immunological methods

It is possible to employ thyroxine as a hapten group for immunological studies. The coupling of thyroxine itself to protein is difficult, however, and to avoid a laborious procedure the propionic acid analogue can be used instead (27).

Tetraiodothyropropionic acid is coupled to bovine serum albumin (BSA) by the mixed anhydride procedure (27). It is mixed in tetrahydrofuran with tri-n-butylamine and isobutylchlor carbamate and is added to the BSA in aqueous tetrahydrofuran at pH 10·6. After reaction for 40 minutes followed by dialysis the conjugate is precipitated by adjusting the pH to 4·5.

Between 11 and 16 residues are conjugated to each molecule of BSA. The number of free lysine groups decreases by 16, which suggests that substitution is probably on the ε-amino groups. This assumption is supported by the fact that the conjugate migrates more rapidly than BSA towards the anode during paper electrophoresis.

Antiserum to the conjugated protein is obtained by inoculations in Freund's adjuvant. The precipitin reaction between the antiserum and the antigen is inhibited by thyroxine and various analogues (27). Concentrations of $6·5 \times 10^{-5}$ M of the hapten, tetraiodothyropropionic acid, of tetraiodothyroacetic acid, thyroxine, triiodothyropropionic acid, triiodothyroacetic acid or triiodothyronine inhibit the precipitation by about 40 per cent. In contrast, compounds without iodine substitution (e.g. thyronine or tyrosine) and those with iodine substitution but with only one aromatic ring (e.g. mono- or diiodotyrosine) produce no hapten inhibition when used in concentrations six times greater. It appears that both iodine substitutions and the diphenyl ether structure are important determinants of the specificity of the antiserum.

M

BIOSYNTHESIS

The iodination of tyrosine to mono- and diiodotyrosine and the coupling of two molecules of the latter to give thyroxine takes place within the thyroglobulin. Mono- and diiodotyrosines do not leave the thyroid but are de-iodinated and the iodine reacts again with thyroglobulin. The rates of formation of the iodotyrosines with respect to one another have been studied carefully.

It seems most likely that triiodothyronine arises from coupling between one molecule of monoiodotyrosine and one of diiodotyrosine rather than by de-iodination of thyroxine (121, 127, 128). When [^{131}I]-iodide is given to rats, initially the specific radioactivity of the monoiodotyrosine is considerably higher than that of diiodotyrosine. The specific activities become increasingly similar, however, until at 24 hours they are the same. Now if a second isotope, ^{125}I, is given 24 hours before the death of the rat, and the ^{131}I is given only 30 minutes before, it is found that monoiodotyrosine contains a slightly higher proportion of the ^{131}I than the ^{125}I, while diiodotyrosine contains relatively more of the ^{125}I than the ^{131}I. Thus monoiodotyrosine is rapidly labelled while the diiodotyrosine is labelled more slowly. This finding makes it possible to investigate the biosynthetic pathway to triiodothyronine. If this occurs by coupling of one molecule of each, at 30 minutes after injection of ^{131}I, the two rings of triiodothyronine will be labelled unequally. The β-ring iodine atom (3') is in fact labelled more heavily than the iodine at the 3 and 5 positions. This is consistent with the view that the β-ring originates from monoiodotyrosine and the α-ring from diiodotyrosine. Now thyroxine arises solely from diiodotyrosine so that the two rings are equally labelled. If triiodothyronine arose from thyroxine therefore its iodine atoms would be equally labelled also.

The method of detecting the distribution of labelled iodine is interesting (125). During reaction of thyroxine with *m*-nitrobenzene-diazonium chloride coupling occurs *ortho* to the phenol group and so iodine from the β-ring is displaced. The inorganic iodide may then be separated and the radioactivity determined separately. The same method may be applied to triiodothyronine since the diazonium salt preferentially couples in the position occupied by the iodine atom rather than at the unoccupied 5' position.

TRANSPORT OF THYROID HORMONES

After the proteolysis of the thyroglobulin complex, the next stage in the utilization of the thyroid hormones is their transport in the blood to the various tissues of the body. The majority (about 90 per cent) of the iodine in the circulation is in an organic form of which about 90 per cent is thyroxine.

Thyroglobulin itself is not normally secreted in the blood but the thyroid hormones become largely bound to other proteins. At least three binding proteins are known.

(1) an α-glycoprotein usually called 'thyroxine-binding globulin' (TBG);
(2) pre-albumin, 'thyroxine-binding pre-albumin' (TBPA);
and
(3) albumin.

The binding is of a simple, reversible nature and is probably governed by electrostatic forces. From the results of equilibrium-dialysis experiments at several pH values it has been suggested that the ionized phenolic hydroxyl groups of thyroxine interact with the ε-amino groups of lysine in albumin (152). The binding is reduced considerably when these groups are acetylated. D-thyroxine is bound as firmly to albumin as the L-isomer. The binding of triiodothyronine is reduced at pH 7·4 to one fifth of that at higher pH values; its phenolic group is less dissociated at pH 7·4. The nature of the binding sites to TBG and TBPA is at present unknown.

Purification of TBG

Fraction IV-9 obtained by the Cohn fractionation of serum proteins is a good starting material for the purification of TBG. In the method of Tata (157) a trace amount of [^{131}I]thyroxine is added to this fraction which is then submitted to starch gel electrophoresis in barbitone buffer at pH 8·6 in columns of starch gel. The electrophoresis is repeated three times, and the fraction with the highest ratio of ^{131}I to protein is collected from each experiment. Other impurities are now removed by filtration through Sephadex G-75 and then the material is fractionated on DEAE-cellulose in 0·05 M-NaH$_2$PO$_4$ with gradient elution to 0·1 M-NaCl–0·05 M-NaH$_2$PO$_4$. Finally starch gel electrophoresis is repeated, this time in glycine buffer at pH 9·0.

Ultracentrifugal studies show that TBG sediments with $S_{20,w} = 3·5$ and its molecular weight is calculated to be between 40,000 and 50,000. Its concentration in normal serum is 1–2 mg per 100 ml.

Purification of TBPA

TBPA is best purified by electrophoresis (157). In buffers other than barbitone, 20–30 per cent of thyroxine is bound to the prealbumin; however, this binding is inhibited by barbitone buffer (26, 31, 162).

Binding capacity and affinity

Distinction must be made between these two attributes of the binding proteins. TBG has a high affinity for thyroxine but a relatively low capacity, whereas albumin has a low affinity but a high capacity. Albumin may therefore be quantitatively important as a binding protein because of its higher concentration in serum. The affinity of TBG for triiodothyronine is low and it has a slight or no interaction with tetraiodothyroacetic acid (162). The binding is not affected by barbitone buffers.

There are two types of binding site of TBPA. The first is inhibited by barbitone buffers. It has a high affinity for thyroxine and for tetraiodothyroacetic acid but none for triiodothyronine. The second is unaffected by barbitone and has maximum affinity for tetraiodothyroacetic acid and none for thyroxine or triiodothyronine.

Some interesting alterations in binding capacity occur in different conditions such as in pregnancy. The thyroxine-binding protein in adult rabbit serum moves between albumin and α_1-globulin during electrophoresis: in foetal serum it is between α_2 and β-globulin (114). The distribution of thyroxine between mother and foetus can therefore be studied. It has been found that very little goes into the foetus in early pregnancy, but the amount increases as time goes on and as the binding power of foetal TBG increases.

Some thyroxine is present in the free state in the circulation and although its concentration is very small, it is important, because it is probably the fraction responsible for the biological activity. Thus only the free hormone diffuses into tissues and is exchanged from the extracellular to intracellular sites. Methods are now available for its measurement in serum (85, 91, 92, 112, 150, 151). When [^{131}I]thyroxine is added to serum, equilibration with bound thyroxine is rapidly achieved; consequently, the specific activity of the free is then the same as that of the protein-bound. The serum is passed through Sephadex G-25 when the protein-bound comes straight through the column while the free thyroxine is retarded. It is interesting that the separation is not due to the gel filtration mechanism but to the fact that phenolic compounds such as thyroxine undergo an association with the gel and the process is one of adsorption (57). The amount of thyroxine in the free state can then be calculated from the ratio of bound ^{131}I to total ^{131}I. It is found to be about 4×10^{-11}M. In an alternative method in which [^{131}I]thyroxine is added to diluted serum, which is then dialysed for 20 hours at $37°$, the range of values was found to be from 3×10^{-11}M to 1.2×10^{-10}M (113)

The total protein-bound iodine (PBI) is often used as a clinical index of thyroid function (8, 16, 47, 52). The thyroid hormones are precipitated with serum proteins by zinc hydroxide or trichloroacetic acid but inorganic iodide is not. The precipitate is then incinerated with alkali (dry ash method) or with strongly acidic reagents (wet method) in preparation for the measurement of the iodide.

Metabolism of the thyroid hormones

The liver withdraws thyroid hormones from the blood and secretes them into the bile as glucuronides and sulphates. In this way the circulating levels of the hormones are regulated. The conjugates may be hydrolysed by β-glucuronidase and sulphatase.

Oxidative de-amination, transamination and de-iodination of the hormones also occur in the liver and kidney. In skeletal muscle, however, only deiodination occurs, and this muscle is therefore a most suitable tissue for the purification of de-iodinating enzymes. However, the concentration of enzyme is much higher in liver and kidney, and some work has been done on its purification. The best preparations, however, contain up to five protein zones in starch gel electrophoresis (90, 158). The de-iodination of thyroid hormones is the most important metabolic pathway and occurs in all tissues. It has been discussed at length by Tata (159).

BIOLOGICAL ACTIVITY OF THE THYROID HORMONES

There are several distinctive biological effects of the thyroid hormones. Firstly, they increase the metabolic rate and oxygen consumption—the *calorigenic effect*; secondly, they accelerate growth and metamorphosis; thirdly, they play a part in the regulation of the synthesis of protein.

Probably the best known and most carefully studied action is the stimulation of oxygen consumption. The action may be indirect; there is a delay (latent period) after injection before the increase in respiration. Although thyroxine does not increase oxygen consumption when added to tissues *in vitro*, it prevents the decrease in respiration of rat kidney slices for several days (7, 89).

The effects of thyroid hormones on growth in animals and on metamorphosis in amphibia form the basis of many biological assay methods. Thyroxine is essential for the development of the foetus after the fifteenth to sixteenth week of pregnancy in the human, and a deficiency of the hormone leads to varying degrees of cretinism.

Small amounts of thyroxine accelerate the rate of synthesis of protein in both normal and thyroidectomized subjects (32). Thyroxine also stimulates the synthesis of microsomal protein *in vitro* (145, 146). The observations of Bronk (22) suggest that these proteins possibly include those associated with the oxidative phosphorylation enzyme system.

There are various theories regarding the mode of action of these hormones and at present it is considered likely that they influence enzymes, that they chelate with metal ions and that they have a direct effect on membrane permeability. Since the primary site of action of the hormones on the cells is unknown, investigation is difficult.

The hormones certainly affect a large number of enzymes; Tapley and Hatfield mention seventeen in their recent review (155). Some of the effects can be demonstrated both *in vivo* and *in vitro*. Thus the oxidation of succinate to fumaric acid is stimulated *in vivo* and by the addition of thyroxine to various mitochondrial preparations *in vitro*. The addition of thyroid hormones to normal mitochondria will uncouple oxidative phosphorylation while mitochondria isolated from thyrotoxic animals have a decreased ability to perform oxidative phosphorylation. The *in vivo* and *in vitro* results with some other enzymes, however, are at variance with one another, and it should be mentioned that all the *in vitro* effects on enzymes require concentrations of thyroxine many times greater than those found in tissue; it may be therefore that the effects noted are secondary to others.

Thyroxine forms complexes with bivalent metal ions such as Mn^{2+}, Ca^{2+}, Mg^{2+} and Zn^{2+}, the alanine side chain and the diphenyl ether groups being involved (35, 54, 58). Although there is no evidence for a direct interaction between thyroxine and a metal-containing enzyme, some of the *in vitro* effects can be explained by an interaction of the hormone with metal ions in the medium. Thus the copper-containing enzyme, ascorbic acid oxidase, is stimulated by thyroxine (58) but there is no evidence that this is due to a direct action on the metal in the enzyme; it seems more likely that it combines with excess copper or other metal impurities in the medium (53). Several other enzymes which have been shown to be dependent on Mg^{2+} or Zn^{2+} for activation are inhibited by thyroxine (54, 83, 173). Again the inhibition may result from the removal of soluble ions from the medium.

Not all inhibitory effects of thyroxine on enzymes can be attributed to chelation however; acetyl phosphatase is apparently not dependent on any of the ions likely to chelate with thyroxine and yet is markedly inhibited by the hormone (67).

The swelling induced by thyroid hormones to mitochondria isolated from rat liver has been extensively studied. The process is associated with the uptake of water and electrolytes and with the release of protein into the suspending medium. Thyroxine causes swelling *in vitro* at a concentration of 10^{-8} M which is within the physiological range (86). Mitochondria isolated from rats which have been treated with thyroxine are found to be more fragile than normal (153). It may be that the effects on enzymes therefore are a result of the action on the mitochondrial membrane where the passage of substances involving respiratory activity and energy transfer is affected. Tapley and Hatfield (155) consider that much of the evidence at present points to the mitochondrial membrane as the primary site of action of the hormones.

In recent work, however, the interesting observation has been made that small amounts of thyroid hormones cause an early and substantial increase in the rate of protein synthesis without altering the efficiency of oxidative phosphorylation (161). It may be that both the calorigenic and growth-promoting actions are secondary manifestations of a primary action, at the cellular level, which influences the rate of protein synthesis (160).

It is known that actinomycin D inhibits protein synthesis by suppressing the formation of messenger RNA and puromycin inhibits the assembly of new protein at the ribosome (76, 104, 131). Starvation also suppresses protein synthesis by the deprivation of essential amino acids and lowers the level of RNA in the cell. Each of these inhibitory agents interrupts the action of thyroid hormones, particularly actinomycin D; this suggests that the hormones may act by controlling the availability of messenger RNA rather than by direct stimulation of protein synthesis.

CHEMICAL STRUCTURE AND BIOLOGICAL ACTIVITY

Many analogues of thyroxine have been investigated for biological activity, and it is possible to draw certain conclusions regarding the relationship between chemical structure and biological activity. However, assessment of this relationship is complicated by the fact that relative biological potencies may vary according to the biological assay used.

The main structural requirements needed for biological activity appear to be:

1. The phenolic group must be free. The role of the hormones in oxidative processes has focused attention to the redox potentials of these compounds. The free phenolic group could participate in reversible quinonoid formation and in accordance with this theory it is found that 3-hydroxylated analogues which cannot undergo quinone-formation are inactive (110). Moreover, polarographic evidence shows that thyroxine has a reduction wave (17, 143); it is a good electron acceptor and this capacity in different hormones is related to their respective biological activities (94).
2. The asymmetry of the alanine side chain is important. D-thyroxine possesses only a fraction of the activity of L-thyroxine *in vivo*, but in many *in vitro* studies the isomers are equally effective. This is probably explained by the fact that after intravenous injection the D-isomer disappears more rapidly and is less concentrated in the peripheral tissues than the L-isomer (154). Analogues with propionic, formic or acetic acids instead of alanine have only a fraction of the activity of thyroxine. However, in amphibia the analogues may be even more potent, possibly because of their rapid diffusion into tadpole tissues (55).
3. At least one substituent in each benzene ring is required at the 3- or 5-position. Substitution with iodine generally yields compounds with higher activity than with other halogens or with methyl, butyl or isopropyl groups. There are exceptions, however. 3,5-diiodo-3',5'-dimethylthyropropionic acid has 30–40 per cent more calorigenic activity than the 3,3',5,5'-tetraiodo analogue (120). Moreover a number of alkyl substituents at position 3' give highly active compounds: L-3'-isopropyl-3,5-diiodothyronine is three times as active as triiodothyronine itself in tadpoles (167).
4. The diphenyl ether linkage appears to be essential for activity.

ANTAGONISTS TO THYROID HORMONES

The term 'antithyroid compound' is used for drugs of the thiouracil type (I, Fig. 7.3) which permit the accumulation of iodide in the thyroid gland but block the formation of organic iodine compounds. Included in this class of compound are many substituted derivatives of thiouracil and thiourea and other sulphur-containing compounds. They are thought to prevent the oxidation of iodide and the subsequent iodination of the thyroid proteins. Since monoiodotyrosine may form in the presence of thiouracil the inhibitory action may occur somewhere between mono- and diiodotyrosine (144).

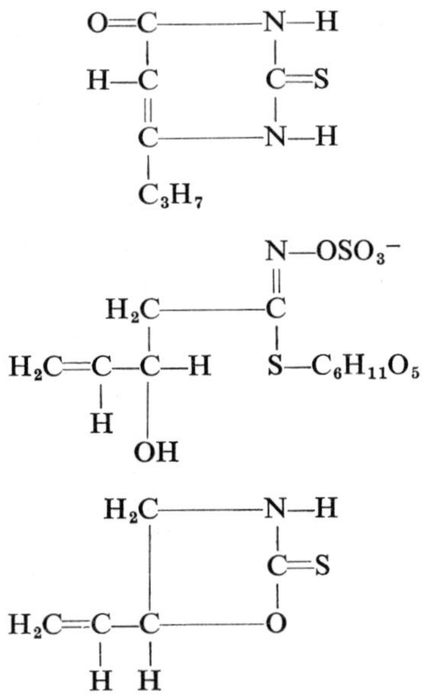

$$
\begin{array}{lll}
O{=}C\text{------}N{-}H & & \\
\quad| \qquad\quad | & & \\
H{-}C \qquad\quad C{=}S & & \mathrm{I} \\
\quad\|\qquad\qquad | & & \\
\quad C\text{------}N{-}H & & \\
\quad| & & \\
\quad C_3H_7 & &
\end{array}
$$

$$
\begin{array}{ll}
\qquad\qquad\quad N{-}OSO_3{}^- \\
\qquad\qquad\qquad \| \\
\quad H_2C\text{------}C \qquad\qquad\qquad \mathrm{II} \\
\qquad\quad | \qquad\quad | \\
H_2C{=}C{-}C{-}H \quad S{-}C_6H_{11}O_5 \\
\qquad | \qquad | \\
\qquad H \quad OH
\end{array}
$$

$$
\begin{array}{ll}
\quad H_2C\text{------}N{-}H \\
\qquad | \qquad\quad | \\
\qquad | \qquad\quad C{=}S \qquad\qquad \mathrm{III} \\
\qquad | \qquad\quad | \\
H_2C{=}C{-}C\text{------}O \\
\quad | \quad | \\
\quad H \ H
\end{array}
$$

FIG. 7.3. Antagonists to thyroid hormones

I propyl thiouracil
II progoitrin
III goitrin

There are a number of naturally-occurring substances possessing goitrogenic properties which appear to act similarly to thiouracil. An extensive review of such compounds has appeared recently (63). They are contained in foods, particularly in vegetables of the brassica family. Several thiooxazolidones and isothiocyanates have been isolated in addition to polysulphides and thiocyanates. Weak goitrogens have also been isolated from peanuts, soybeans and possibly milk.

A particularly interesting substance, 5-vinyl-2-thiooxazolidine (III Fig. 7.3), 'goitrin', has been extracted from a variety of swede, *rutabaga*, and from rape seed. The racemic and optically active forms are even more active than propyl thiouracil in man. Goitrin does not occur free in an active form but its precursor, progoitrin, (II, Fig. 7.3), has been isolated from rutabaga seeds. It is a mustard oil glycoside which gives 2-hydroxy-3-butenyl isothiocyanate on enzymic hydrolysis (62). The secondary hydroxyl group is unstable and rapidly cyclizes to give goitrin.

Certain structural analogues of thyroxine inhibit the action of the thyroid hormones. Examples are the *p*-nitrophenylethyl ether and the *p*-nitrobenzyl ether of *N*-acetyldiiodotyrosine which were synthesized by Woolley (174) and the benzyl ether of 3,5-diiodo-4-hydroxybenzoic acid (56).

The compound n-butyl-4-hydroxy-3,5-diiodobenzoate (BHDB) inhibits the calorigenic effect of thyroxine in mice and in amphibia although a much higher ratio of BHDB to thyroxine is required in the former (95, 141). The inhibition is attributed to interference in the deiodination of thyroxine; the deiodination from the 3' and 5' positions is inhibited and from the 3 and 5 positions is accelerated, thereby rendering it inactive (50).

BHDB is also found to stimulate the conjugation of thyroxine with glucuronic and sulphuric acids and greatly increases its secretion in the bile. It alters the binding of thyroxine to plasma proteins, probably improving thereby its transport to the sites in the cell where the enzyme systems for conjugation are located.

REFERENCES

1 ADAMS, D. D. *J. clin. Endocr.* **18**, 699 (1958).

2 ADAMS, D. D., KENNEDY, T. H., PURVES, H. D. and SIRETT, N. E. *Endocrinology* **70**, 801 (1962).

3 BAKKE, J. L., HEIDEMAN, M. L., LAWRENCE, N. and WIBERG, C. *Endocrinology* **61**, 352 (1957).

4 BAKKE, J. L. and LAWRENCE, N. *J. clin. Endocr.* **19**, 35 (1959).

5 BAKKE, J. L., LAWRENCE, N., ARNETT, F. and MACFADDEN, W. *J. clin. Endocr.* **21**, 1280 (1961).

6 BAKKE, J. L., LAWRENCE, N. and ROY, S. *J. clin. Endocr.* **22**, 352 (1962).

7 BARKER, S. B. *Ciba Fdn Colloq. Endocr.* **10**, 253 (1957).

8 BARKER, S. B. In *Methods in Hormone Research* (edited by R. I. Dorfman) vol. 1, p. 351, Academic Press, New York (1962).

9 BARKER, S. B. *Biochem. J.* **90**, 214 (1964).

10 BARNES, J. H., BORROWS, E. T., ELKS, J., HEMS, B. A. and LONG, A. G. *J. chem. Soc.* 2824 (1950).

11 BATES, R. W. and CONDLIFFE, P. G. *Recent Prog. Horm. Res.* **16**, 309 (1960).

12 BATES, R. W. and CORNFIELD, J. *J. Endocr.* **60**, 225 (1957).

13 BATES, R. W., GARRISON, M. M. and HOWARD, T. B. *Endocrinology* **65**, 7 (1959).

14 BEALE, D. and WHITEHEAD, J. K. *Clin. Chim. Acta* **5**, 150 (1960).

15 BECK, J. C., MCKENZIE, J. M., FISHMAN, J., GOSSELIN, L. and MCGARRY, E. E. *Ciba Fdn Colloq. Endocr.* **14**, 238 (1962).

16 BIRD, R. and JACKSON, D. F. *Clin. Chem.* **8,** 389 (1962).

17 BORROWS, E. T., HEMS, B. A. and PAGE, J. E. *J. chem. Soc.* S204 (1949).

18 BOTTARI, P. M. *Ciba Fdn Colloq. Endocr.* **13,** 275 (1960).

19 BOTTARI, P. M. and DONOVAN, B. T. *J. Physiol.* **140,** 36P (1957).

20 BOUCHILLOUX, S., ROLLAND, M., TORRESANI, J., ROQUES, M. and LISSITZKY, S. *Biochim. biophys. Acta* **93,** 15 (1964).

21 BOWDEN, C. H., MACLAGAN, N. F. and WILKINSON, J. H. *Biochem. J.* **59,** 93 (1955).

22 BRONK, J. R. *Biochem. J.* **89,** 16P (1963).

23 CARSTEN, M. E. and PIERCE, J. G. *J. biol. Chem.* **235,** 78 (1960).

24 CARSTEN, M. E. and PIERCE, J. G. *J. biol. Chem.* **238,** 1724 (1963).

25 CHALMERS, J. R., DICKSON, G. T., ELKS, J. and HEMS, B. A. *J. chem. Soc.* 3424 (1949).

26 CHRISTENSEN, L. K. and LITONJUA, A. D. *J. clin. Endocr.* **21,** 104 (1961).

27 CHURCHILL, W. H. and TAPLEY, D. F. *Nature, Lond.* **202,** 29 (1964).

28 CIERESZKO, L. S. *J. biol. Chem.* **160,** 585 (1945).

29 CLAYTON, J. C. and HEMS, B. A. *J. Chem. Soc.* 840 (1950).

30 CONDLIFFE, P. G. *Endocrinology* **72,** 893 (1963).

31 CRISPELL, K. R., COLEMAN, J. and HYER, H. *J. clin. Endocr.* **17,** 1305 (1957).

32 CRISPELL, K. R., PARSON, W. and HOLLIFIELD, G. *J. clin. Invest.* **35,** 164 (1956).

33 CROOKE, A. C. and MATTHEWS, J. D. *Ciba Fdn Colloq. Endocr.* **5,** 25 (1953).

34 D'ANGELO, S. A. and GORDON, A. S. *Endocrinology* **46,** 39 (1950).

35 DAVIS, S. *J. biol. Chem.* **224,** 759 (1957).

36 DEDMAN, M. L., FAWCETT, J. S. and MORRIS, C. J. O. R. *Biochem. J.* **78,** 34P (1961).

37 DE GROOT, L. J. and CARVALHO, E. *J. clin. Endocr.* **20,** 21 (1960).

38 DERRIEN, Y., MICHEL, R. and ROCHE, J. *Biochim. biophys. Acta* **2,** 454 (1948).

39 DIMITRIADOU, A., TURNER, P. C. R., SLATER, J. D. H. and FRASER, R. *Biochem. J.* **82,** 20P (1962).

40 DOPHEIDE, T. A. A. and TRIKOJUS, V. M. *Nature, Lond.* **201,** 1128 (1964).

41 DORRINGTON, K. J. and MUNRO, D. S. *Clin. Sci.* **28,** 165 (1965).

42 DUNN, J. T. and WERNER, S. C. *J. clin. Endocr.* **24,** 460 (1964).

43 EDELHOCH, H. *J. biol. Chem.* **235,** 1326 (1960).

44 EDELHOCH, H. *J. biol. Chem.* **237,** 2778 (1962).

45 EDELHOCH, H. and LIPPOLDT, R. E. *J. biol. Chem.* **235,** 1335 (1960).

46 ELKS, J. and WALLER, G. *J. chem. Soc.* 2366 (1952).

47 FARRELL, L. P. and RICHMOND, M. H. *Clin. Chim. Acta* **6,** 620 (1961).

48 FEUER, G. *Biochem. J.* **73,** 349 (1959).

49 FLOCK, E. V. and BOLLMAN, J. L. *Biochem. J.* **84,** 621 (1962).
50 FLOCK, E. V. and BOLLMAN, J. L. *Endocrinology* **75,** 721 (1964).
51 FONTAINE, Y. A. and CONDLIFFE, P. G. *Biochemistry* **2,** 290 (1963).
52 FOSS, O. P., HANKES, L. V. and VAN SLYKE, D. D. *Clin. Chim. Acta* **5,** 301 (1960).
53 FRIEDEN, E. *Biochim. biophys. Acta* **9,** 696 (1952).
54 FRIEDEN, E., FORSBLAD, K. and EZELL, A. L. *Archs. Biochem. Biophys.* **96,** 423 (1962).
55 FRIEDEN, E. and WESTMARK, G. W. *Science* **133,** 1487 (1961).
56 FRIEDEN, E. and WINZLER, R. J. *J. biol. Chem.* **179,** 423 (1949).
57 GELOTTE, B. *J. Chromat.* **3,** 330 (1960).
58 GEMMILL, C. L. *J. biol. Chem.* **192,** 749 (1951).
59 GESCHWIND, I. I. and LI, C. H. *Endocrinology* **63,** 449 (1958).
60 GILLILAND, I. C. and STRUDWICK, J. I. *Clin. Sci.* **12,** 265 (1953).
61 GOTTSCHALK, A. and ADA, G. L. *Biochem. J.* **62,** 681 (1956).
62 GREER, M. A. *J. Amer. chem. Soc.* **78,** 1260 (1956).
63 GREER, M. A. *Recent Prog. Horm. Res.* **18,** 187 (1962).
64 GROSS, J. and PITT-RIVERS, R. *Lancet* i, 593 (1952).
65 GROSS, J. and PITT-RIVERS, R. *Biochem. J.* **53,** 645 (1953).
66 GROSS, J. and LEBLOND, C. P. *J. biol. Chem.* **184,** 489 (1950).
67 HARARY, I. *Biochim. biophys. Acta* **25,** 193 (1957).
68 HARINGTON, S. R. and BARGER, G. *Biochem. J.* **21,** 169 (1927).
69 HARTREE, A. S., BUTT, W. R. and KIRKHAM, K. E. *J. Endocr.* **29,** 61 (1964).
70 HAYNIE, T. P., WINZLER, R. J., MATOVINOVIC, J., CARR, E. A. and BEIERWALTES, W. H. *Endocrinology* **71,** 782 (1962).
71 HAYS, M. T., SOLOMON, D. H. and WERNER, S. C. *J. clin. Endocr.* **21,** 1475 (1961).
72 HEIDEMAN, M. L. *Endocrinology* **53,** 640 (1953).
73 HEIDEMAN, M. L., BAKKE, J. L. and LAWRENCE, N. L. *J. clin. Endocr.* **19,** 831 (1959).
74 HEIDEMAN, M. L., LEVY, R. P., McGUIRE, W. L. and SHIPLEY, R. A. *Endocrinology* **76,** 828 (1965).
75 HOCH, F. L. *Physiol. Rev.* **42,** 605 (1962).
76 HURWITZ, J., FURTH, J. J., MALAMY, M. and ALEXANDER, M. *Proc. natn. Acad. Sci. U.S.A.* **48,** 1222 (1962).
77 JORGENSEN, E. C., LEHMAN, P. A., GREENBERG, C. and ZENKER, N. *J. biol. Chem.* **237,** 3832 (1962).
78 JORGENSEN, E. C., ZENKER, N. and GREENBERG, C. *J. biol. Chem.* **235,** 1732 (1960).
79 KEATING, F. R., RAWSON, R. W., PEACOCK, W. and EVANS, R. D. *Endocrinology* **36,** 137 (1945).
80 KENDALL, E. C. *J. Amer. med. Ass.* **64,** 2042 (1915).

81 KERKOF, P. R., RAGHUPATHY, E. and CHAIKOFF, I. L. *Endocrinology* **75,** 537 (1964).
82 KIRKHAM, K. E. *J. Endocr.* **25,** 259 (1962).
83 KUBY, S. A., NODA, L. and LARDY, H. A. *J. biol. Chem* **210,** 65 (1954).
84 LAMEYER, L. D. F., KASSENAAR, A. A. H. and QUERIDO, A. *Nature, Lond.* **175,** 685 (1955).
85 LEE, N. D., HENRY, R. J., and GOLUB, O. *J. J. clin. Endocr.* **24,** 486 (1964).
86 LEHNINGER, A. L. and RAY, B. L. *Biochim. biophys. Acta* **26,** 643 (1957).
87 LEPP, A. and STARR, P. *J. clin. Endocr.* **22,** 800 (1962).
88 LIMONOVA, E. E. *Problemy̆ Éndokr. Gormonoter.* **8,** 41 (1962).
89 LINDSAY, R. H. and BARKER, S. B. *Endocrinology* **62,** 513 (1958).
90 LISSITZKY, S., BÉNÉVENT, M.-T. and ROQUES, M. *C.R. Soc. Biol. Paris* **154,** 755 (1960).
91 LISSITZKY, S. and BISMUTH, J. *Clin. Chim. Acta* **8,** 269 (1963).
92 LISSITZKY, S., BISMUTH, J. and ROLLAND, M. *Clin. Chim. Acta* **7,** 183 (1962).
93 LOBO, L. C. G., DA SILVA, M. M., HARGREAVES, F. B. and COUCEIRO, A. M. *J. clin. Endocr.* **24,** 285 (1964).
94 LOVELOCK, J. E. *Nature, Lond.* **189,** 729 (1961).
95 MACLAGAN, N. F., SHEEHAN, M. M. and WILKINSON, J. H. *Nature, Lond.* **164,** 699 (1949).
96 MAJOR, P. W. and MUNRO, D. S. *Clin. Sci.* **23,** 463 (1962).
97 MALOOF, F. and SOODAK, M. *Pharmacol. Rev.* **15,** 43 (1962).
98 McGARRY, E. E., AMBE, L., NAYAK, R., BIRCH, E. and BECK, J. C. *Metabolism* **13,** 1154 (1964).
99 McKENZIE, J. M. *Endocrinology* **63,** 372 (1958).
100 McKENZIE, J. M. *Proc. R. Soc. Med.* **55,** 539 (1962).
101 McKENZIE, J. M. and FISHMAN, J. *Proc. Soc. exp. Biol. Med.* **105,** 126 (1960).
102 MICHEL, R., ROCHE, J. and TATA, J. R. *Bull. Soc. Chim. biol. Paris* **34,** 466 (1952).
103 MORREALE DE ESCOBAR, G., LLORENTE, P., JOLIN, T. and ESCOBAR DEL REY, F. *Biochem. J.* **88,** 526 (1963).
104 MORRIS, A., FAVELUKES, S., ARLINGHAUS, R. and SCHWEET, R. B. *Biochem. biophys. Res. Commun.* **7,** 326 (1962).
105 MORRIS, C. J. O. R. *Proc. R. Soc. Med.* **55,** 540 (1962).
106 MORTON, M. E. and CHAIKOFF, I. L. *J. biol. Chem.* **147,** 1 (1943).
107 MUNRO, D. S. *Proc. R. Soc. Med.* **55,** 542 (1962).
108 MUNRO, D. S. *J. Endocr.* **19,** 64 (1959).
109 MUSSETT, M. V. and PERRY, W. L. M. *Bull. Wld Hlth Org.* **13,** 917 (1955).
110 NIEMANN, C. and REDEMANN, C. E. *J. Amer. chem. Soc.* **63,** 1549 (1941).

110a ODELL, W. D., WILBER, J. F. and PAUL, W. E. *Endocrinology* **25,** 1179 (1965).

111 O'DONNELL, I. J., BALDWIN, R. C. and WILLIAMS, J. W. *Biochim. biophys. Acta* **28,** 294 (1958).

112 OPPENHEIMER, J. H., SQUEF, R., SURKS, M. I. and HAVER, H. *J. clin. Invest.* **42,** 1769 (1963).

113 OPPENHEIMER, J. H. and SURKS, M. I. *J. clin. Endocr.* **24,** 785 (1964).

114 OSORIO, C. and MYANT, N. B. *Nature, Lond.* **182,** 866 (1958).

115 PARLOW, A. F., CONDLIFFE, P. G., REICHERT, L. E. and WILHELMI, A. E. *Endocrinology* **76,** 27 (1965).

116 PEARSE, A. G. E. and NOORDEN, S. VAN. *Can. med. Ass. J.* **88,** 462 (1963).

117 PIERCE, J. G. and CARSTEN, M. E. *J. Amer. chem. Soc.* **80,** 3482 (1958).

118 PIERCE, J. G., CARSTEN, M. E. and WYNSTON, L. K. *Annls. N. Y. Acad. Sci.* **86,** 613 (1960).

119 PILEGGI, V. J., SEGAL, H. A. and GOLUB, O. J. *J. clin. Endocr.* **24,** 273 (1964).

120 PITTMAN, C. S., SHIDA, H. and BARKER, S. B. *Endocrinology* **68,** 248 (1961).

121 PITT-RIVERS, R. *Biochem. J.* **82,** 108 (1962).

122 PITT-RIVERS, R., NIVEN, J. S. F. and YOUNG, M. R. *Biochem. J.* **90,** 205 (1964).

123 PITT-RIVERS, R. and SACKS, B. I. *Biochem. J.* **82,** 111 (1962).

124 PLASKETT, L. G. *Biochem. J.* **78,** 652 (1961).

125 PLASKETT, L. G. *Biochem. J.* **78,** 657 (1961).

126 PLASKETT, L. G., BARNABY, C. F. and LLOYD, G. I. *Biochem. J.* **87,** 473 (1963).

127 PLASKETT, L. G. and BARNABY, C. F. *Nature, Lond.* **204,** 1271 (1964).

128 PLASKETT, L. G., BARNABY, C. F. and LLOYD, G. I. *Biochem. J.* **89,** 479 (1963).

129 QUERIDO, A., KASSENAAR, A. A. H. and LAMEYER, L. D. F. *Acta endocr. Copenh.* **12,** 335 (1953).

130 RALL, J. E., ROBBINS, J. and EDELHOCH, H. *Ann. N.Y. Acad. Sci.* **86,** 373 (1960).

131 REICH, E., GOLDBERG, I. H. and RABINOWITZ, M. *Nature, Lond.* **196,** 745 (1962).

132 ROBBINS, J. *J. biol. Chem.* **208,** 377 (1954).

133 ROBBINS, J. and RALL, J. E. *Physiol. Rev.* **40,** 415 (1960).

134 ROCHE, J., LISSITZKY, S. and MICHEL, R. *C. R. Acad. Sci. Paris* **234,** 1228 (1952).

135 ROCHE, J. and MICHEL, R. *Adv. Protein Chem.* **6,** 253 (1951).

136 ROCHE, J., MICHEL, R., WOLF, W. and NUNEZ, J. *Biochim. biophys. Acta* **19,** 308 (1956).

137 ROITT, I. M. and DONIACH, D. *Lancet* ii, 1027 (1958).

138 ROSENBERG, L. L. and LA ROCHE, G. *Endocrinology* **75,** 776 (1964).
139 SCHNEIDER, P. B. *Endocrinology* **74,** 973 (1964).
140 SELENKOW, H. A., PASCASIO, F. M. and CLIVE, H. J. *Ciba Fdn Colloq. Endocr.* **14,** 248 (1962).
141 SHEAHAN, M. M., WILKINSON, J. H. and MACLAGAN, N. F. *Biochem. J.* **48,** 188 (1951).
142 SHULMAN, S., ROSE, N. R. and WITEBSKY, E. *J. Immunol.* **75,** 291 (1955).
143 SIMPSON, G. K. and TRAILL, D. *Biochem. J.* **40,** 116 (1946).
144 SLINGERLAND, D. W., GRAHAM, D. E., JOSEPHS, R. K., MULVEY, P. F., TRAKAS, A. P. and YAMAZAKI, E. *Endocrinology* **65,** 178 (1959).
145 SOKOLOFF, L. and KAUFMAN, S. *J. biol. Chem.* **236,** 795 (1961).
146 SOKOLOFF, L., KAUFMAN, S., CAMPBELL, P. L., FRANCIS, C. M. and GELBOIN, H. *J. biol. Chem.* **238,** 1432 (1963).
147 SONENBERG, M. *Vitams. Horm.* **16,** 205 (1958).
148 SONENBERG, M. and MONEY, W. L. *Ann. N. Y. Acad. Sci.* **86,** 625 (1960).
149 STEINER, R. F. and EDELHOCH, H. *J. Amer. chem. Soc.* **83,** 1435 (1961).
150 STERLING, K. and HEGEDUS, A. *J. clin. Invest.* **41,** 1031 (1962).
151 SURKS, M. I. and OPPENHEIMER, J. H. *J. clin. Endocr.* **24,** 794 (1964).
152 TABACHNICK, M. and STERLING, K. *Fed. Proc.* **20,** 205 (1961).
153 TAPLEY, D. F. *J. biol. Chem.* **222,** 325 (1956).
154 TAPLEY, D. F., DAVIDOFF, F. F., HATFIELD, W. B. and ROSS, J. E. *Amer. J. Physiol.* **197,** 1021 (1959).
155 TAPLEY, D. F. and HATFIELD, W. B. *Vitams and Horm.* **20,** 251 (1962).
156 TATA, J. R. *Biochem. J.* **72,** 214 (1959).
157 TATA, J. R. *Clin. Chim. Acta* **6,** 819 (1961).
158 TATA, J. R. *Biochem. J.* **77,** 214 (1960).
159 TATA, J. R. *Recent Prog. Horm. Res.* **18,** 221 (1962).
160 TATA, J. R. *Nature, Lond.* **197,** 1167 (1963).
161 TATA, J. R., ERNSTER, L., LINDBERGH, O., ARRHENIUS, E., PEDERSEN, S. and HEDMAN, R. *Biochem. J.* **86,** 408 (1963).
162 TATA, J. R., WIDNELL, C. C. and GRATZER, W. B, *Clin. Chim. Acta* **6,** 597 (1961).
163 TEPPERMAN, J. and TEPPERMAN, H. M. *Pharmacol. Rev.* **12,** 301 (1960).
164 TONG, W. and CHAIKOFF, I. L. *J. biol. Chem.* **232,** 939 (1958).
165 UI, N., TARUTANI, O., KONDO, Y. and TAMURA, H. *Nature, Lond.* **191,** 1199 (1961).
166 UTIGER, R. D., ODELL, W. D. and CONDLIFFE, P. G. *Endocrinology* **73,** 359 (1963).
167 WAHLBORG, A., BRIGHT, C. and FRIEDEN, E. *Endocrinology* **75,** 561 (1964).
168 WERNER, S. C. *Ciba Fdn Colloq. Endocr.* **14,** 225 (1962).
169 WERNER, S. C. and BLOCK, R. J. *Nature, Lond.* **183,** 406 (1959).
170 WERNER, S. C. and RADICHEVICH, I. *Nature, Lond.* **197,** 877 (1963).

171 WERNER, S. C., TIERNEY, J. and TALLBERG, T. *J. clin. Endocr.* **24,** 339 (1964).
172 WITEBSKY, E., ROSE, N. R., TERPLAN, K., PAINE, J. R. and EGAN, R. W. E. *J. Amer. med. Ass.* **164,** 1439 (1957).
173 WOLFF, J. and WOLFF, E. C. *Biochim. biophys. Acta* **26,** 387 (1957).
174 WOOLLEY, D. W. *J. biol. Chem.* **164,** 11 (1946).
175 WYNSTON, L. K., FREE, C. A. and PIERCE, J. G. *J. biol. Chem.* **235,** 85 (1960).

8

PARATHYROID HORMONE AND CALCITONIN

THE PARATHYROID GLANDS

The parathyroids are the smallest of the endocrine glands and were over-looked for many years. There are usually four glands situated one at each of the upper and lower poles of the two lobes of the thyroid gland. When first recognized they were considered to have no functional significance but later it was shown that their removal from immature animals was often followed by the onset of tetany, convulsions and death.

Parathyroid hormone

BIOLOGICAL FUNCTION AND ACTIVITY

The parathyroid hormone is concerned with the regulation of calcium and phosphate metabolism. Removal of the parathyroid glands from experimental animals leads to a fall in the level of calcium and to an increase in the level of phosphorus in the plasma. Overactivity of the glands leads to a withdrawal of calcium from the bones, produces an excess in the blood, and causes increased excretion of phosphate by the kidney. The calcium-mobilizing and the phosphaturic activities have at times been ascribed to two different hormones but all the most recent work suggests that only one hormone, the parathyroid, is responsible.

The level of calcium in the blood is regulated within very narrow limits. Any change in the level affects the release of parathyroid hormone by a negative 'feed-back' mechanism (25); thus a fall in calcium stimulates further secretion of the hormone. However, it is difficult to explain the remarkably constant level of calcium in the blood by this simple mechanism since the hormone is relatively slow-acting. The position is now clarified by the discovery of another hormone, 'calcitonin', which is also involved in the regulation of calcium. This is a fast-acting hormone which lowers the level of calcium in the plasma; it will be discussed separately later in this chapter (p. 182).

The mechanism by which the hormone exerts its effects are still incompletely understood; there are several recent reviews where current theories are discussed at length (2a, 26, 28). Some authorities believe that the activities of the hormone can best be explained by action at the cellular level, and that the transport of inorganic phosphates into and across cells is enhanced (28); others, however, contend that action is at the organ level rather than the cellular level (33). The regulation of calcium is certainly the result of influence upon at least four different sites—the bones, kidneys, lactating mammary glands and the gastrointestinal tract where vitamin D also plays a part. The effect on the renal excretion of phosphate has been known for a long time and the experiments of Pullman et al. (30) demonstrate clearly that the hormone acts directly on mammalian renal tubules. However, it is now clear that the hormone influences the metabolism of other tissues and other ions, notably magnesium, potassium, hydrogen and sulphate, the uptake of sulphate being affected in cartilage, soft tissues and kidney homogenates.

Now that highly purified preparations of the hormone are available, it may not be long before the biochemical mechanisms become clearer. In this respect it is relevant to mention two recent experiments where in vitro techniques were employed. Rasmussen et al. (38) have shown that the hormone affects the uptake not only of phosphate but of sulphate ($^{35}SO_4^{2-}$) and of arsenate ($^{76}AsO_4^{3-}$) by rat liver mitochondria. Although the liver is not regarded as a major site of parathyroid hormone activity, and large doses of hormone were employed, a study of the effects on sulphate metabolism in vivo would be interesting. Secondly Gordon (18) has shown that the active peptide hormone plus a factor in serum albumin is able to release calcium from dead bone. This, taken in conjunction with the observations of MacIntyre et al. (24) on calcium and magnesium regulation, has led Gordon to suggest that the albumin-peptide complex binds or chelates certain divalent cations; it remains to be seen if this concept explains the mechanism of action of the hormone in vivo.

CELLULAR ORIGIN

Studies with the electron microscope reveal cytoplasmic occlusions in the parathyroid cells in which groups of Golgi membranes are surrounded by numerous secretory droplets. These consist of smooth envelopes which enclose a substance opaque to the electron microscope. The number of these droplets correlates with the experimental stimulation of the gland and the inclusions are considered to represent the intracellular precursor of the hormone.

Davis and Enders (14) have recently reviewed results obtained by means of electron microscopy and light microscopy. At present there is no satisfactory method of identifying the cellular origin of the hormone by the latter technique; studies by the fluorescent antibody method are therefore awaited with interest.

BIOLOGICAL ASSAY

Methods of assay usually depend on the measurement of calcium, phosphate or both ions in the plasma or urine of experimental animals.

In the method of Clark *et al.* (5) intact rats are injected with ^{45}Ca for at least forty days before the assay commences. By this time the isotope is distributed almost entirely into the stable fraction of bone. Injection of parathyroid hormone releases ^{45}Ca from the bone, and it may be measured in the urine. The assay is sensitive to about 40 USP units per 100 g body weight and the index of precision (λ) is about 0·3.

The official USP method also employs intact animals; the serum calcium is measured 18 hours after subcutaneous injection in dogs (29). Other assays employ parathyroidectomized animals. The method of Munson (27) is based on the maintenance of the serum calcium in the 6 hours after injection, while that of Davies *et al.* (12) depends on the change in serum calcium after 18 hours. The animals may be used again, so that cross-over designs are possible (40).

Assays in which phosphate is measured are rather similar. Davies *et al.* (13) use normal mice loaded with saline in a twin cross-over design and measure the increase in the rate of phosphate excretion during the $3\frac{1}{2}$ hours after injection.

In other methods parathyroidectomized rats are used. The excretion of inorganic phosphate (21) or of ^{32}P-labelled phosphate (17) over 6 hours gives an index of activity. The working range for the latter assay is between 5 and 40 USP units and λ for both is about 0·3.

Measurement of the increase in the ratio of phosphate to calcium in the urine of mice during 4 hours following injection affords a sensitive method of assay, 1–3 USP units being detectable (23).

METHODS OF EXTRACTION

Most commercial preparations of parathyroid hormone are of bovine origin; it is difficult to locate the glands in the pig. Recently a few attempts have been made to extract the hormone from human glands but at present little is known of its chemistry.

There are three important methods for the initial extraction from parathyroid tissue. The earliest depended on extraction with hot 0·2 N-hydrochloric acid and was widely used for some years (6). Because it was felt that the hydrochloric acid might damage the hormone and be disadvantageous in later purification, Davies and Gordon (11) adopted 80 per cent (v/v) acetic acid as the extracting agent. Thirdly, Aurbach (1) used concentrated phenol at room temperature instead of acid.

Purification

Extracts obtained by each of these methods have been purified by all the usual techniques including dialysis, ultrafiltration, electrophoresis and column chromatography. Countercurrent distributions and, recently, gel filtration on Sephadex, have proved most generally useful, however.

After extraction in 80 per cent (v/v) acetic acid at 70–75° Davies and Gordon (11) precipitated the active material by 86 per cent (v/v) acetone. It was then shown that some 60-65 per cent of the activity appeared in the ultrafiltrate through a cellophane membrane from solution at pH 2·4. Later it was shown that a rather higher yield was obtained by using formic, instead of acetic, acid (40). The product contained about 40 USP units per mg and although it gave a single boundary in the ultracentrifuge, it contained three electrophoretic peaks. The molecular weight of the ultrafiltered material was considered to be not greater than 5,000.

Some improvement in specific activity was obtained by ion-exchange chromatography on Dowex 50 resin (40). The extract was applied in 0·2 N-hydrochloric acid and was displaced from the resin by sodium chloride. Preparations possessing between 75 and 100 USP units per mg were obtained.

Rasmussen and Craig (32, 34, 35, 36) have purified extracts obtained by each of the three methods of extraction by precipitation with salt and tri-chloroacetic acid, by countercurrent distribution and by gel filtration. Typical solvent systems for countercurrent distribution are pyridine–n-butanol–0·1 M-acetic acid (3·5:5:12 by volume) and 4 volumes of 1:1 (v/v) n-butanol–n–propanol and 6 volumes of 6 per cent (v/v) acetic acid containing 1 per cent (w/v) sodium chloride.

Final purification on Sephadex gels G-25, G-50 and G-100 has been reported (2, 37, 39). The retention volume of the smaller polypeptides is altered by change of pH and of ionic strength on G-25, probably due to a change in the shape of the polypeptides (37) but change of pH was without effect on the larger peptides (2).

As a result of these fractionations a family of polypeptides with hormonal activity has been isolated. They vary in molecular weights from 3,800 to 8,500, with specific activities from 800 to 3,000 USP units per mg. There is a close correlation between the molecular size and the biological activity, the smallest polypeptides having the least and the largest polypeptides having the greatest calcium-mobilizing and phosphaturic activities.

Similar methods have been applied to the extraction of parathyroid hormone from human glands, but the hormone has not been purified (21, 42).

The yield varies widely from 0–500 USP units per g of fresh tissue, compared with 300–400 USP units per g of fresh bovine tissue.

Extraction of the hormone from blood has been attempted by the phenol method (17a). Plasma is mixed with an equal volume of phenol heated to 55°. After shaking for one hour ten volumes of a mixture of acetic acid and acetone (1:4 v/v) containing sodium chloride are added and the precipitate which forms at 5° is removed after 12 hours. An equal volume of ether is then added to the extract to precipitate the active material. In another method active material has been separated from rat and human plasma by ammonium sulphate precipitation and cold ethanol fractionation (41). The normal circulating level estimated by this method is 40 USP units per ml human plasma.

When parathyroid hormone is injected into rats, it becomes associated with the α-globulin fraction of the plasma. *In vitro* experiments have shown that excess also becomes associated with albumin. When incubated with human plasma, it is attached to *β* and *γ* globulins.

Extraction of the hormone from urine is possible by adsorption to benzoic acid at pH 3·5 (10). The normal excretion is in the range 10 to 30 USP units per 24 hours, although occasionally no activity can be detected by the method depending on the excretion of ^{32}P by parathyroidectomized mice (17).

CHEMICAL AND PHYSICAL PROPERTIES

Six different polypeptides have been isolated by Rasmussen and Craig (37). The largest of these have molecular weights of about 8,500 and were obtained both by the phenol and the acetic acid methods of extraction. They contain no sugars or lipids; the *N*-terminal amino acid is alanine. The amino acid compositions vary slightly according to the method of extraction as shown in Table 8.1.

A smaller peptide with molecular weight of 5,200 has valine at the *N*-terminus, which suggests that the *N*-terminal residue is not essential for biological activity.

The smallest peptide with biological activity contains 33 amino acids and has a molecular weight of 3,800. Its activity is only about one sixth of that of the largest peptides calculated on a molecular basis.

Chemical modifications and biological activity

One of the most interesting features of the chemistry of the active peptides is the presence of an oxidation-reduction centre, methionine, as in corticotrophin. When oxidized with peroxide or performic acid the activity drops. The loss of activity is initially more rapid than the rate of oxidation of methionine in those peptides containing two methionine residues. It is probable that only one of these residues is at the active centre, or 'core'. If this is oxidized more readily than the second, the initially high rate of loss of activity is readily explained. Some of the activity is regenerated by reduction of the

TABLE 8.1

Amino acid analysis of preparations of parathyroid hormone

| | Number of residues | | |
	(*a*)	(*b*)	(*c*)
Lysine	7	7	8
Histidine	3	3	4
Ammonia	—	7	7
Arginine	4	4	5
Aspartic acid	8	8	7
Threonine	1	1	1
Serine	7	7	5
Glutamic acid	10	10	9
Proline	3	2	3
Glycine	4	4	4
Alanine	6	6	7
Valine	6	6	6
Methionine	2	2	2
Isoleucine	3	3	3
Leucine	7	7	7
Tyrosine	1	1	1
Phenylalanine	2	2	2
Tryptophan	1	1	1
Total amino acids	75	74	75

(*a*) Preparation (a), reference 37.
(*b*) Preparation (c), reference 37.
(*c*) AURBACH, G. D. and POTTS, J. T. *Proc. Second International Congress Endocrinology*, p. 1260 (1964).
N-terminal amino acids: Ala-Val-
C-terminal amino acids: . . . -Ser-Leu.

oxidized product (37). Reaction with cyanogen bromide causes cleavage of the peptide chains at the methionine residues, the methionine being converted to homoserine. Thus each end of the hormone is removed leaving the central 'core' which has been found to retain *in vitro* activity (2a).

Another chemical modification leading to loss of biological activity is acetylation. Complete inactivation occurs within 30 minutes at room temperature when the hormone is treated with acetic anhydride in trimethylamine (37).

The hormone appears to be stable in bovine glands maintained at 30° for 24 hours (22). The presence of cysteine has been stated to enhance its activity but this is not a universal finding (22, 31).

Antisera to bovine parathyroid hormone have been produced in rabbits (4, 41a, 43). When non-specific antibodies are removed by suitable absorption, a single precipitin line is obtained in double diffusion and immuno-electrophoretic experiments. The antisera specifically inhibit the biological activity of the hormone.

Preliminary experiments indicate apparent antigenic differences between the bovine and the human hormones; difficulties may therefore arise in the application of the immunological technique to clinical studies unless sufficient quantities of the human hormone can be obtained in a purified state. The results of Berson and Yalow (4) are encouraging, however; using the sensitive ^{131}I method, they have shown a weak reaction between the human hormone and the antiserum to bovine hormone. In this way 0·15–0·6 mUSP unit is detectable and preliminary results for normal serum are in the range 0·3–3·0 mUSP units per ml which is a hundredfold less than by the bioassay described on page 178.

Calcitonin

A second hormone affecting calcium metabolism, calcitonin, acts more rapidly than parathyroid hormone and has the reverse effect, since it causes a decrease in the calcium content of the plasma.

ORIGIN

An ingenious series of experiments was devised by Copp et al. (7, 8, 9) to study the origin of calcitonin. They perfused blood of high and of low calcium content through the thyroid and parathyroid glands of dogs. The hormone was liberated when the glands were perfused with blood of high calcium content. From the results of further experiments in which the parathyroid glands were removed they concluded that these, rather than the thyroid glands, were the source of calcitonin and presented further confirmation of this by similar experiments in sheep. In this animal, the superior parathyroid is located at some distance from the upper pole of the thyroid and has a separate blood supply so that it can be perfused separately. Copp et al. have also reported that some commercial preparations of parathyroid hormone contain a hypocalcaemic factor which is recognized by the prompt drop in the calcium level of plasma after intravenous injection. This drop is followed later by the usual rise attributable to parathyroid hormone.

As a result of perfusion experiments in dogs, Foster et al. (15) confirmed the existence of calcitonin but neither they nor other workers found any evidence to support the views of Copp et al. on the origin of the hormone. Rather they found that thyroid extracts contained a potent plasma calcium-lowering agent. It is possible to perfuse the parathyroid glands separately from the thyroid in the goat as well as in the sheep; a perfusion with plasma containing a high concentration of calcium of a single parathyroid gland, after removal of the thyroid and the other parathyroids, produced no change in systemic calcium (15). When the thyroid was included in the perfusion, a significant fall in the plasma level of calcium occurred. The name 'thyro-calcitonin' has been suggested for this hormone (19).

The cellular origin of the hormone has been investigated in the canine thyroid (16). As in the human gland, there are two types of cell in the acini of the canine thyroid, the *principal* cells and the *mitochondrian-rich* cells. These latter cells are present not only in the acini but in groups between adjacent acini, a position described as 'parafollicular'. They may be recognized histochemically since they contain a much higher level of α-glycerophosphate dehydrogenase than the acinar principal cells. In glands perfused with blood containing a high concentration of calcium, a definite increase in acid phosphatase was noted in the mitochondrian-rich cells and to a lesser extent in the principal cells also. The α-glycerophosphate levels were lower in the mitochondrian-rich cells which secrete calcitonin. Evidence from electron microscopy or from fluorescent-antibody methods is not yet available.

BIOASSAY

Calcitonin can be recognized by its effect on the circulating level of calcium in the rat. After an infusion of one hour into the tail vein the calcium level is measured by flame fluorimetry in the method of Baghdiantz et al. (3). Until a standard preparation becomes available the unit has been defined as one tenth of the amount required to produce a fall of 0·5 m-equiv. calcium per litre.

METHODS OF EXTRACTION AND PURIFICATION

Porcine thyroid glands are a richer source of calcitonin than bovine glands, and they do not contain parathyroid glands (3). Extracts of these glands may be purified considerably by centrifugation at 100,000 g followed by gel filtration on Sephadex G-50 (20).

A precipitation method has also been described (3). The glands are extracted by 0·2 N-HCl at 60–70° for five minutes, and after one hour at room temperature the extract is filtered. At this stage the filtrate contains about 180 units per mg protein nitrogen.

The extract is now dialysed at 4° for 48 hours against 0·1 M-acetate buffer, pH 4·6. All the active material remains in the non-dialysable fraction. On adding an equal volume of 2 M-sodium chloride an inactive precipitate forms overnight at 4°. It is removed by centrifugation and an equal volume of 3 M-sodium chloride is added and stored at 4° for 12 hours. Active material is now precipitated and at this stage contains about 1,200 units per mg protein nitrogen.

This material is further purified by gel filtration on Sephadex G-100 in acetate buffer at pH 4·6 containing 0·2 M-sodium chloride. The main active band is separated from the main protein fraction and then contains about 23,000 units per mg protein nitrogen.

It is interesting to note that the purified preparation now passes membranes which retained the activity of crude extracts. This suggests that calcitonin is associated with larger molecules in the crude extract.

CHEMICAL PROPERTIES

Relatively crude extracts of calcitonin from thyroid glands are stable for up to two weeks at 4° in buffers of below pH 4·9. At pH 7·2 a precipitate forms at 4° and some activity is lost.

Partially purified preparations (1,200 units per mg protein nitrogen) are relatively stable to boiling in acetate buffer at pH 4·6. There is a 12 per cent loss of activity after 15 minutes, 46 per cent in 40 minutes and 77 per cent loss after 2 hours. Boiling in N-hydrochloric acid or sodium hydroxide for one hour completely inactivates the hormone.

The biological activity is completely destroyed within 6 hours by the action of pepsin at pH 3 and of trypsin at pH 7.

Chemically, therefore, calcitonin is a polypeptide or a low molecular weight protein. Since it is extracted from the thyroids, the question arises as to whether it may be one of the thyroid hormones. Thyroxine, however, is inert in assays for calcitonin (19). In addition, calcitonin is soluble in acid and is destroyed by trypsin and pepsin in contrast to thyroxine. Thyroglobulin is also excluded from consideration since calcitonin is of much smaller molecular weight, and is retained on Sephadex G-100.

REFERENCES

1 AURBACH, G. D. *Arch. Biochem. Biophys.* **80,** 466 (1959).
2 AURBACH, G. D. and POTTS, J. T. *Endocrinology* **75,** 290 (1964).
2a AURBACH, G. D. and POTTS, J. T. *Proc. Second International Congress Endocrinology*, 1260 (1964).
3 BAGHDIANTZ, A., FOSTER, G. V., EDWARDS, A., KUMAR, M. A., SLACK, E., SOLIMAN, H. A. and MACINTYRE, I. *Nature, Lond.* **203,** 1027 (1964).
4 BERSON, S. A., YALOW, R. S., AURBACH, G. D. and POTTS, J. T. *Proc. natn. Acad. Sci. U.S.A.* **49,** 613 (1963).
5 CLARK, I., BOWERS, W. and GEOFFROY, R. *Endocrinology* **66,** 527 (1960).
6 COLLIP, J. B. *J. biol. Chem.* **63,** 395 (1925).
7 COPP, D. H., CAMERON, E. C., CHENEY, B. A., DAVIDSON, A. G. F. and HENZE, K. G. *Endocrinology* **70,** 638 (1962).
8 COPP, D. H. *Recent Prog. Horm. Res.* **20,** 59 (1964).
9 COPP, D. H. and HENZE, K. G. *Endocrinology* **75,** 49 (1964).

10 DAVIES, B. M. A. *J. Endocr.* **16**, 369 (1957).
11 DAVIES, B. M. A. and GORDON, A. H. *Biochem. J.* **61**, 646 (1955).
12 DAVIES, B. M. A., GORDON, A. H. and MUSSETT, M. V. *J. Physiol.* **125**, 383 (1954).
13 DAVIES, B. M. A., GORDON, A. H. and MUSSETT, M. V. *J. Physiol.* **130**, 79 (1955).
14 DAVIS, R. and ENDERS, A. C. In *The Parathyroids* (edited by R. O. Greep and R. V. Talmage), p. 76, C. C. Thomas, Springfield, Ill. (1961).
15 FOSTER, G. V., BAGHDIANTZ, A., KUMAR, M. A., SLACK, E., SOLIMAN, H. A. and MACINTYRE, I. *Nature, Lond.* **202**, 1303 (1964).
16 FOSTER, G. V., MACINTYRE, I. and PEARSE, A. G. E. *Nature, Lond.* **203**, 1029 (1964).
17 FUJITA, T., MORII, H., IBAYASHI, H., TAKAHASHI, Y. and OKINAKA, S. *Acta endocr. Copenh.* **38**, 321 (1961).
17a FUJITA, T., MORII, H. and OKINAKA, S. *Endocrinology* **70**, 711 (1962).
18 GORDON, G. S. *Acta endocr. Copenh.* **44**, 481 (1963).
19 HIRSCH, P. F., GAUTHIER, G. F. and MUNSON, P. L. *Endocrinology* **73**, 244 (1963).
20 HIRSCH, P. F., VOELKEL, E. F., SAVERY, A. and MUNSON, P. L. *Fedn. Proc.* **23**, 204 (1964).
21 KENNY, A. D. and MUNSON, P. L. *Endocrinology* **64**, 513 (1959).
22 KENNY, A. D., ROTH, S. I. and CASTLEMAN, B. *J. clin. Endocr.* **24**, 375 (1964).
23 LEMON, H. M. *Boston med.* **13**, 107 (1962).
24 MACINTYRE, I., BOSS, S. and TROUGHTON, V. A. *Nature, Lond.* **198**, 1058 (1963).
25 MCLEAN, F. C. *Clin. Orthopaed.* **9**, 46, 1957.
26 MCLEAN, F. C. and BUDY, A. M. *Vitams. Horm.* **19**, 165 (1961).
27 MUNSON, P. L. *Annls N.Y. Acad. Sci.* **60**, 776 (1955).
28 NEUMAN, W. F. and DOWSE, C. M. In *The Parathyroids* (edited by R. O. Greep and R. V. Talmage), p. 310, C. C. Thomas, Springfield, Ill. (1961).
29 *Pharmacopoeia of the U.S.A.* (16th Revision), 491 (1960).
30 PULLMAN, T. N., LAVENDER, A. R., AHO, I. and RASMUSSEN, H. *Endocrinology* **67**, 570 (1960).
31 RASMUSSEN, H. *Endocrinology* **64**, 367 (1959).
32 RASMUSSEN, H. *J. biol. Chem.* **235**, 3442 (1960).
33 RASMUSSEN, H. *Amer. J. Med.* **30**, 112 (1961).
34 RASMUSSEN, H. and CRAIG, L. C. *J. Amer. chem. Soc.* **81**, 5003 (1959).
35 RASMUSSEN, H. and CRAIG, L. C. *J. biol. Chem.* **236**, 759 (1961).
36 RASMUSSEN, H. and CRAIG, L. C. *J. biol. Chem.* **236**, 1083, 1961.
37 RASMUSSEN, H. and CRAIG, L. C. *Recent Prog. Horm. Res.* **18**, 269 (1962).
38 RASMUSSEN, H., SALLIS, J., FANG, M., DE LUCA, H. F. and YOUNG, H. *Endocrinology* **74**, 388 (1964).

39 RASMUSSEN, H., SZE, Y.-L. and YOUNG, R. *J. biol. Chem.* **239,** 2852 (1964).

40 RASMUSSEN, H. and WESTALL, R. G. *Biochem. J.* **67,** 658 (1957).

41 REICHERT, L. E. and L'HEUREUX, M. V. *Endocrinology* **68,** 1036 (1961).

41a TASHJIAN, A. H., LEVINE, L. and MUNSON, P. L. *Biochem. biophys. Res. Commun.* **8,** 259 (1962).

42 TISELIUS, P., ENGFELDT, B., PORATH, J., WALLENIUS, G. and WERNER, I. *Metabolism* **13,** 929 (1964).

43 WILLIAMS, G. A., HARGIS, G. K., SIDWELL, C. G. and YAKULIS, V. J. *Proc. Soc. exp. Biol. Med.* **115,** 61 (1964).

9

INSULIN AND GLUCAGON

Diabetes has been recognized from the time of the ancient Egyptians and a description of the disease which laid emphasis on the large amounts of urine passed appeared in the first century A.D. That the disease is associated with the pancreas was recognized towards the end of the eighteenth century and two types of the disease were described, one in which the urine tasted sweet—*diabetes mellitus*—and the other in which the sweet taste was lacking—*diabetes insipidus*. Eventually in 1916 Shafer noted that the cells of the pancreas known as the 'islets of Langerhans' secreted the active substance controlling the metabolism of carbohydrates which he called *insulin*, meaning 'in an islet'.

When the supply of insulin is deficient, the amount of sugar in the blood increases (hyperglycaemia) and it appears in the urine—originally described as 'urine with honey'. Eventually ketone bodies appear in the blood which result chiefly from the incomplete oxidation of fatty acids. Formerly the disease was progressive and rapidly fatal due to the failure to use glucose and to the toxic effects of the ketone bodies. The picture is now completely changed, due to the isolation of insulin in 1922 by Banting and Best and to the successful use of the hormone by replacement therapy.

Soon after the first successful use of insulin in the treatment of diabetes, it was observed that when given intravenously there was a marked but transitory period of hyperglycaemia. Kimball and Murlin (65) rightly suggested that this effect was not due to insulin but to an impurity which they named *glucagon*. At the time, this view was not generally accepted but later when insulin was isolated in crystalline form it no longer caused any initial rise in blood sugar. For some time interest in insulin overshadowed interest in glucagon and it was much later that glucagon was isolated in pure form and recognized as a hormone of the pancreas. It has also been known as the *hyperglycaemic glycogenolytic factor*, the hyperglycaemic action being due to the liberation of glucose from the liver.

Origin

Although many reagents precipitate insulin, most of the complexes are redissolved by the solvents used in histology. Romeis's fluid which is a mixture of saturated mercuric chloride, picric acid, formaldehyde and acetic acid precipitates it in an insoluble form, however, and has proved useful in studies of the cellular origin of insulin (7).

Insulin is rich in disulphide, but deficient in sulphydryl groups; when the disulphide groups are reduced to sulphydryls with thioglycollic acid, the insulin in a histological section not only becomes even more insoluble but may also be stained with the reagent, 2,2'-dihydroxy-6,6'-dinaphthyldisulphate (8). In this way it has been shown that the β-cells of the islets stain with this reagent whereas the α-cells do not. Further evidence that the hormone is located in the β-cells is obtained from experiments in which the histological reagents are modified so that insulin does not form an insoluble complex; the resultant staining of the β-cells is much weaker.

Numerous studies in support of this conclusion by the fluorescent-antibody method have been reported since the technique was first applied to insulin by Lacy and Davies (70). It appears that the formalin, the various alcohols and the xylol used for the preparation of the sections cause no loss in the ability of the antibody to bind insulin (10). In a study of the foetal pancreas of rodents, fluorescent staining was detected from the fourteenth day of gestation onwards in the rat, at a stage when staining with the thiol reagent was still negative (42). In the mouse, no differentiation between the α- and β-cells could be made at this stage although electron microscopy revealed occasional cells containing a few dense granules which might represent the earliest stages of differentiation of the β-cells (88). By the sixteenth day, insulin activity has actually been demonstrated (42) and by the eighteenth day the characteristic β-cells are noted by light microscopy.

There is much evidence to suggest that the α-cells produce glucagon. There are several means whereby selective damage to the β-cells may be effected. Treatment with the simple chemical alloxan is one of the best known methods (34); the action of this and related substances is probably due to oxidation of essential thiol groups in the β-cells. There follows a marked reduction in the amount of insulin, but no corresponding decrease in the amount of glucagon that can be extracted from the pancreas.

Selective destruction of the α-cells gives conflicting results, mainly because none of the substances used causes uniform or complete destruction of these cells. However, the experiments of Bencosme et al. (for summary see (9)) with cobalt chloride have shown convincingly that in guinea-pigs in which only a few normal α-cells remain, no glucagon was detected. In animals with less damage to the α-cells, glucagon was still extractable. Furthermore, the uncinate process of the pancreas, whether in normal animals or in those treated with alloxan, contains no α-cells and no glucagon.

BIOLOGICAL ACTIVITY

The action of insulin in the regulation of carbohydrate metabolism has been recognized for many years, but the importance of its actions on fat and protein metabolism has been more slowly realized and the actions were, in fact, first thought to be secondary effects.

Carbohydrate metabolism

Insulin adjusts the rate at which glucose is utilized by body tissues, particularly muscle; when it is lacking there is a slower rate of utilization and an accumulation of sugar in the blood. It affects the first step in the conversion of glucose to glycogen:

$$\text{Glucose} + \text{ATP} \xrightarrow[\text{insulin}]{\text{hexokinase}} \text{glucose-6-phosphate} + \text{ADP}$$

Probably the chief determinant in this reaction is hexokinase, and insulin may modify its activity. Once this step has occurred, the synthesis of glycogen and fatty acids proceeds in the absence of insulin.

The action of glucagon on the other hand is to release glucose from the glycogen in the liver (112). It affects the rate-limiting phosphorylase step whereby units of glucose are split off from the glycogen molecule giving glucose-1-phosphate (Fig. 9.1). The phosphorylase is present in the liver in an

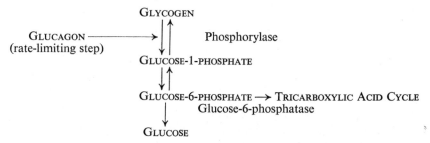

FIG. 9.1. The influence of glucagon on the release of glucose from glycogen

active and an inactive form (dephosphophosphorylase). The inactive form is produced from the active under the influence of phosphatase; it is re-phosphorylated by a phosphokinase and so converted back to the active form. Glucagon causes an increase in the active form either by inhibiting the phosphatase or by enhancing the action of phosphokinase.

Fat metabolism

The conversion in the liver and adipose tissue of carbohydrate to neutral fat is dependent on the presence of insulin and the mobilization of fat from that stored in adipose tissue is prevented by insulin. Glucagon has a lipolytic action on adipose tissue, similar to that of other hormones such as corticotrophin, adrenaline and growth hormone, but it is not a potent lipolytic agent in intact animals, probably because its effect is efficiently counteracted by insulin.

The direct effect of insulin *in vitro* on the uptake of glucose by adipose tissue has been widely studied (55, 69, 95). It increases the incorporation of glucose carbon into long chain fatty acids (120, 126, 127) but its capacity to incorporate labelled acetate, pyruvate, malonate, acetaldehyde, citrate, α-ketoglutarate, succinate and fumarate is dependent on the presence of glucose in the medium (125).

Protein metabolism

Insulin has a protein-anabolic action, while glucagon is associated with protein catabolism, the breakdown of amino acids and the synthesis of urea. Thus the two hormones have powerful antagonistic effects not only concerned with carbohydrate but with nitrogen metabolism as well. These effects can be shown to be independent since the catabolic action of glucagon may be abolished by insulin while its glycogenolytic activity remains unimpaired (82).

Insulin stimulates the incorporation of labelled amino acids into protein in experiments with the isolated rat diaphragm (77). The point of action is closely related to the process of incorporation of activated amino acids into peptide chains. In common with other protein anabolic hormones, it can influence the activity of intracellular structures such as ribosomes and may stimulate the synthesis of RNA (68).

The effects of these hormones on the urea cycle have been carefully studied (79). Rats were made diabetic by treatment with alloxan, to destroy the β-cells, the source of insulin, and leave only glucagon; other rats were treated with glucagon. Similar effects were noted in each group of animals; the activity of three of the enzymes concerned in this cycle, the mitochondrial-linked carbamoyl phosphate synthetase and the two supernatant enzymes, arginino succinase and argino-succinate synthetase (the rate-limiting factor), were increased, whereas the activities of the remaining mitochondrial enzyme, ornithine transcarbamoylase, and of the remaining supernatant enzyme, arginase, were unchanged. Glucagon has also an *in vitro* effect, promoting the synthesis of urea in the isolated, perfused, liver (82).

Other effects

In addition to the above metabolic effects, glucagon has an independent action on the renal tubules, which leads to an increased renal excretion of sodium, potassium, chloride, inorganic phosphorus, iodine and bicarbonate in dog (110) and in man (35). There is also a rapid increase in the renal excretion of uric acid (36). An increase in hepatic blood flow is also reported following intravenous administration of glucagon (102).

MODES OF ACTION

Many attempts have been made to explain the various activities associated with insulin in terms of a single effect on some particular metabolic process. Hechter and Lester (53) have discussed at length the effect on cellular permeability. It has been established that insulin regulates this in muscle and certain other tissues. This holds for carbohydrates such as D-galactose, L-arabinose, D-xylose (66, 72) and glucose (90), for amino acids such as α-aminobutyric acid (25, 67) and for cations such as sodium and potassium. Since the transport of substrate into the cell is an obligatory prelude to subsequent metabolism, it was originally suggested that this single action on permeability might account for all the known physiological effects of the hormone. This now seems rather unlikely; certainly some *in vitro* effects on the metabolism of muscle and liver are difficult to explain on this basis. Instead, it is interesting to consider the effect on certain enzymic activities (77, 114).

The transport of glucose across the cell membrane is normally inhibited when high-energy phosphate-containing substances are readily available which can phosphorylate and thus inactivate the carrier in the cell membrane. Insulin may prevent the phosphorylation or de-phosphorylate the inactivated carrier. Now the biosynthesis of protein is also dependent on the availability of high-energy phosphate-containing substances and insulin may direct these away from the carrier involved in sugar transport to the site of protein biosynthesis. If the action on carbohydrates is sufficient to promote lipogenesis also, a single point of action on the three metabolic actions may exist. This is an attractive hypothesis and it should stimulate further work in this field.

A number of interesting interactions between insulin and other hormones are discussed in the review of Manchester and Young (77). Here there is only space to mention that the growth-promoting action of growth hormone itself depends on the availability of insulin; furthermore, growth hormone is necessary for the growth-promoting action of insulin.

CLINICAL APPLICATIONS

Insulin itself (soluble insulin) is rapidly absorbed and is effective for only a few hours; hence many modified insulins have been investigated. There are the slow-acting preparations, protamine zinc insulin (47) and crystalline or amorphous insulin zinc suspensions (48). The latter are not prepared in the usual phosphate buffers but in acetate, since this medium keeps the insulin in suspension without the use of protamine. Intermediate in effect are globin insulin and isophane insulin, a mixture of insulin and protamine with no excess of either.

Insulin is destroyed by the digestive juices and is therefore ineffective by mouth; glucagon is even more rapidly destroyed. There are two known processes, the reduction of disulphide bonds and proteolysis. Only the latter process occurs with glucagon, which lacks cystine residues. Experimental work on the metabolism of these hormones has been reviewed by Kenny (64).

There has been some interest in other hypoglycaemic agents which may be active by mouth (75). These include salicylates, guanidine derivatives, biguanides and sulphanilyl derivatives. The biguanides are somewhat toxic but some derivatives are useful antidiabetic agents. Certain sulphonamides are safe to use, including tolbutamide (Fig. 9.2, I) and chlorpropamide (Fig. 9.2, II) which has a longer life in the body. These two compounds have been widely used but are effective in lowering the blood sugar only in patients able to secrete some insulin.

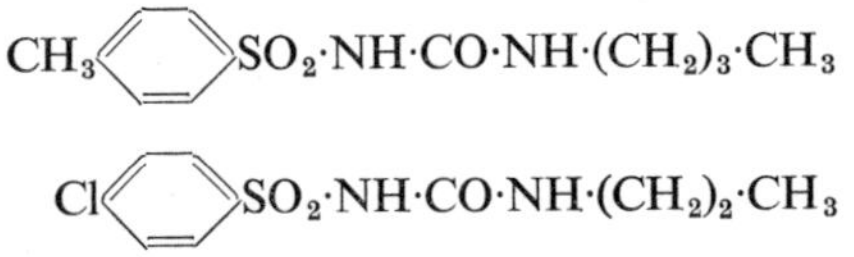

$$CH_3 \langle\!\!\bigcirc\!\!\rangle SO_2 \cdot NH \cdot CO \cdot NH \cdot (CH_2)_3 \cdot CH_3 \qquad\qquad I$$

$$Cl \langle\!\!\bigcirc\!\!\rangle SO_2 \cdot NH \cdot CO \cdot NH \cdot (CH_2)_2 \cdot CH_3 \qquad\qquad II$$

FIG. 9.2

The mode of action of these compounds is still uncertain. They do not appear to have any common structural features and are not as effective or safe as insulin.

BIOLOGICAL ASSAY

(a) *Insulin*

The accurate standardization of insulin is particularly important since it is a potent drug, self-administered daily by many patients of variable intelligence; moreover its action is rapid, and it produces unpleasant and dangerous effects if dosages exceed very narrow limits.

The original method was based on the effect of insulin on the blood sugar of the rabbit. Early preparations were standardized by finding the amount required to lower the blood sugar of a normal 2 kg rabbit to 45 mg per 100 ml within 5 hours. There is much variation between animals and usually cross-over designs are employed (111).

A similar test may be performed in mice, the fall in blood sugar being recognized by the onset of convulsions (105). When the preparation is injected subcutaneously, glucagon does not interfere. A carefully standardized version of this method has been described (133).

These two methods were used in the collaborative assays of the fourth international standard of insulin when it was found that twin cross-over tests on 24 rabbits, each used twice, gave about three times the precision obtained from the convulsion test on 96 mice (5). Even so the simplicity of the latter method makes it more convenient both practically and economically in spite of the need for more replication.

Greater sensitivity is obtained by using hypophysectomized or adrenalec-tomized mice or rats, or by removing endogenous insulin by treatment with alloxan. By this means it is possible to detect between 0·05 and 0·5 mU insulin (19, 20).

There are several *in vitro* methods of assay including those employing rabbit liver slices (112), rat adipose tissue (78, 96, 103) and rat diaphragm (27, 45, 94, 117, 128). 10 mU of insulin produces a significant increase in the utilization of glucose by adipose tissue, ^{14}C-labelled glucose being converted to $^{14}CO_2$ (78). With high doses the metabolism of glucose is increased about tenfold.

The isolated rat diaphragm method is also convenient for measuring small quantities of insulin. Cunningham (27) incubates rat hemi-diaphragms in a buffer containing glucose and gelatin, and insulin is estimated by its effect on the uptake of glucose. Gelatin is included to prevent the adsorption of the small amounts of insulin on to the glassware. Concentrations of 10 to 1,000 μU per ml give fairly reproducible results and over the most sensitive part of the concentration-response curve, 10 to 150 μU per ml, there is a straight-line relationship between concentration and effect.

STANDARDS   The fourth international standard preparation is now avail-able (5). The starting material consisted of 52 per cent bovine and 48 per cent porcine insulins. Protamine-splitting enzymes were removed and the material was recrystallized several times as zinc insulin. It contains only 0·069 per cent glucagon.

The assays were performed in twenty different laboratories, the agreed potency is 24 i.u. per mg and the unit is defined as the activity in 0·04167 mg.

(b) *Glucagon*

The lack of a simple and reliable method of assay explains why it took so long to isolate and purify glucagon. Both *in vivo* and *in vitro* methods have been described, the former depending on the measurement of the increased blood sugar and the latter on the stimulation of glycogenolysis or of phos-phorylase in liver slices or homogenates.

An *in vivo* assay of reasonable precision has been developed by Staub and Behrens (107) in which the blood sugar is determined in fasted, anaesthetized cats at 5-minute intervals during the 25 minutes following injection of the test material. This is compared with the effect of standard glucagon and the ratio of the response is linearly related to the potencies. The effect of insulin in the unknown preparation may be destroyed by incubation with cysteine.

The *in vitro* method of Vuylsteke and de Duve (122) is rather more sensi-tive and is shorter than the *in vivo* but is more complex. The amount of glu-cose is determined after incubation of rabbit liver slices with standard glucagon and the test substances. Even greater sensitivity (0·035 μg per ml is

o

the median effective dose) is obtained by measuring the liver phosphorylase before and after a 10-minute incubation with glucagon (16, 93). It is doubtful if these methods are completely specific, and they may be subject to inference from some constituents of plasma (15).

Immunological methods

INSULIN

Antibodies have been detected in the sera of patients treated with preparations of insulin, but it does not follow that the antibodies are to insulin itself (129). However, guinea-pigs readily produce antibodies to bovine insulin (59) and there is good evidence that the antisera neutralize the biological activity of insulin and therefore contain antibodies to the hormone. This has been demonstrated in a variety of assay methods including *in vivo* effects on blood sugar in rats (2), the induction of signs of diabetes in the mouse (86) and *in vitro* effects on isolated rat diaphragm (28).

The chemical structures of the insulins from different species are discussed on p. 199. Only the dog, pig (24) and whale possess identical amino acid structures, but immunological differences concerned with the free energy changes in the formation of the antigen-antibody complex can be detected between insulins, not only with different amino acids (11, 12, 131), but even between porcine and cetacean (13). Since the latter have the same primary structure, presumably they have distinct conformations.

The energy with which a particular antiserum reacts with an antigen has an important bearing on the choice of antiserum for immunoassay. This subject has been discussed at length by Yalow and Berson (130). Antisera from guinea-pigs immunized with bovine insulin react more weakly with human insulin than with bovine or porcine insulins. Guinea-pig antiserum to porcine insulin, however, reacts often identically with human or porcine. In an assay based on the ^{131}I-radioimmunoassay, the method of choice with regard to insulin, it is undesirable for the labelled hormone to react more energetically than the unlabelled hormone since the principle of the assay is the displacement of the labelled by the unlabelled antigen. When anti-porcine serum is used it does not matter whether porcine or human ^{131}I]insulin is used since they react identically; anti-bovine serum, however, with labelled bovine insulin would not be suitable for the assay of human insulin since the small quantities of human insulin it is desired to measure would not displace the labelled bovine insulin.

Several satisfactory radioimmunoassay methods have been developed (18, 46, 87, 130). The labelling of the antigen presented some difficulties initially. There were reports that insulin suffered damage and failed to bind to antibody satisfactorily, and methods were investigated for removing the damaged components. However, the difficulties have now been overcome either by the preparation of insulin which has high specific activity and which has suffered little or no loss of hormonal or antigenic activity (56, 57), or by the development of assay methods which, while being of the required sensitivity, do not require insulin of very high specific activity (46).

The iodination depends upon the use of iodine monochloride prepared by the reaction:

$$2KI + KIO_3 + 6HCl \longrightarrow 3ICl + 3KCl + 3H_2O.$$

free iodine being removed by extraction in carbon tetrachloride. Labelled iodine is added to borate buffer at pH 8, any hydrogen peroxide produced by β-radiation being destroyed by sodium sulphite. The insulin and freshly prepared iodine monochloride is now added, the ^{131}I present as iodide exchanging with the iodine in the reagent to form ^{131}ICl. This in turn reacts with the tyrosine residues of insulin to attach ^{131}I by stable, covalent bonds, the reaction taking less than a minute. Serum albumin is added as a protective diluent and the product is dialysed against a solution of serum albumin. In this way specific activities of 100–125 mc of ^{131}I per mg insulin are obtained (56). Such preparations are suitable for immunoassay and contain approximately 0·65 atom of iodine per molecule. Much higher specific activities can be obtained in the range 237–409 mc of ^{131}I per mg with up to 11 atoms of iodine per molecule. However, as more than 1 atom per molecule is introduced, there is a progressive loss of hormonal activity, although up to 6 atoms have no effect on the capacity of the labelled insulin to bind antibody.

The iodination method of Hales and Randle (46) is similar but these workers are content with specific activities within the range of 5–20 mc per mg.

The insulin-antibody complex is separated from free insulin in the immunoassay by fractional precipitation with salt, by electrophoresis with solvent flow (chromatoelectrophoresis) (130) or by means of a second antibody to γ-globulin which precipitates specifically the insulin–anti-insulin complex (46). The second and third methods have been used most widely.

In the chromatoelectrophoretic method free insulin adsorbs firmly to the paper at the site of application while insulin bound to antibody migrates as a single peak away from the origin. The separation is complete within about 90 minutes at 4°.

There are several versions of the third method. The labelled insulin, the test material and the antibody may be incubated together and then the antibody complex is precipitated by the anti-γ-globulin (Fig. 9.3,a). In assays in plasma the plasma γ-globulin may interfere by cross-reacting with the precipitating antiserum. The antibody to insulin is still reactive towards antigen, however, even after reaction with anti-γ-globulin so in a second method the labelled and unlabelled antigens are added last (Fig. 9.3,b). The sensitivity of the reaction is increased by allowing the unlabelled antigen to react before

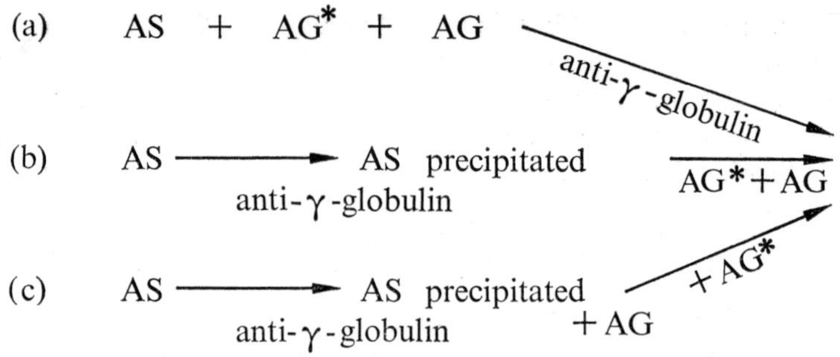

(a)   AS + AG* + AG

anti-γ-globulin

(b)   AS ⟶ AS precipitated
anti-γ-globulin $\overline{AG*+AG}$

(c)   AS ⟶ AS precipitated   + AG*
anti-γ-globulin   + AG

AS–AG complex with a proportion of the AG*. The measurement of this proportion
bound to antibody permits the determination of unlabelled AG by reference to a standard
curve.

FIG. 9.3. Three methods for the immunoassay of insulin

AS = antiserum to insulin; AG* = insulin labelled with ^{131}I; AG = unknown or
standard insulin. For explanation see text.

adding the labelled (Fig. 9.3,c). The latter method is capable of measurements down to 6 mU insulin per ml which is of comparable sensitivity with
other methods.

Specificity

The specificity of the immunoassay is high. Serum proteins do not interfere
and there are several examples of chemical modifications of the antigen
which have the same effect on biological and immunological activities. Thus
the separate A- and B-chains of insulin are completely without biological or
immunological activity (11) while if alanine is removed from the C-terminus
of porcine insulin both activities are retained (14, 43). In this respect it is
interesting to note that porcine or human insulins differ only in the C-terminal amino acid, which is alanine in the former and threonine in the latter.
Porcine is antigenic in man, however, in spite of the fact that the antibodies
are not directed against this part of the molecule since, as we have seen
above, removal of the alanine does not alter the immunological activity.
The immunological potency is retained even when eight amino acids (B
23–30) are removed (132) although the desoctapeptide insulin lacks biological
activity (52).

GLUCAGON

Bovine and porcine glucagons are antigenic in rabbits but not in guinea-
pigs (116). The antibodies are reasonably specific for glucagon, and show no
cross-reaction with insulin or other protein hormones. By use of the radioimmunoassay, it is possible to measure as little as 50 μg per ml of glucagon;
no doubt the clinical application of such a method will help to clarify the
present rather uncertain hormonal status of glucagon.

Chemical properties of insulin

(a) METHODS OF EXTRACTION

(1) *From the pancreas*

Most commercial preparations of insulin are obtained from bovine or porcine pancreatic tissue. The first methods of extraction were by neutral or acidic solvents followed by aqueous ethanol (17). There have since been many modifications and in one of the most recent (76), for rat insulin, the frozen pancreas is extracted in 80 per cent ethanol containing sufficient phosphoric acid to bring the pH finally to 3. After allowing an adequate time for extraction, the crude extract is brought to pH 8 with ammonia. Inactive material which comes out of solution is removed and then insulin is precipitated by the addition of ethanol and ether. Next, salt and fatty impurities are removed by separating insulin as the picrate (39). Finally the picrate is dissolved in acidified acetone, and crude insulin hydrochloride is precipitated by adding excess acetone, after which it is washed with ether and dried.

(2) *From blood*

Methods have been devised for the extraction of insulin from blood both for clinical and for veterinary purposes (4, 28). Plasma, to which a little N-HCl has been added, is extracted with a mixture of ethanol, toluene and n-butanol (10:1:1 by vol.). The residue, separated by centrifugation, is extracted exhaustively with the same mixture of solvents and the combined extracts are then treated with acetone to precipitate the insulin. Recoveries of between 34 and 41 per cent of insulin added to plasma have been reported.

(b) METHODS OF PURIFICATION

Practically all methods are based on fractional precipitation with alcohol, isoelectric precipitation or salting-out procedures. Thus insulin was crystallized for the first time in 1926 by isoelectric precipitation from buffered acetic acid brought to pH 5·6 by the addition of weak base.

The addition of certain metals such as zinc, cobalt, nickel or cadmium facilitates precipitation. The crystals normally contain some zinc, between 0·15 and 0·60 per cent, according to the method of purification.

Paper chromatographic methods, particularly with the system s-butanol–1 per cent v/v acetic acid (1:1, v/v), have been used widely for experimental work on the purification of insulin (39, 40, 44, 113). In this system it has an R_F of 0·3; it may be stained with bromocresol green and may be estimated quantitatively following elution in relatively pure extracts. This method is not specific since other substances of pancreatic origin have the same R_F.

There are several column chromatographic methods available (30, 38,

81, 91, 106) including some interesting partition methods (92). Here the solvents are mixtures of salts and ethylene glycol monoethyl and monobutyl ethers (ethyl and butyl cellosolves) with Celite as the inert supporting material. In 2·5 M-potassium phosphate, pH 7·6,–water–ethyl cellosolve–butyl cellosolve (15:13:5·33:2·67 by vol.) the distribution is 25:1 in favour of the upper phase (which is therefore used as the stationary phase on silane-treated Celite) and the rate of flow with respect to the solvent front is 0·15. A column containing 6 g Celite was calculated to contain 400 theoretical plates. Other systems include 5 M-sodium dihydrogen phosphate adjusted to pH 3 with phosphoric acid–ethyl cellosolve–butyl cellosolve–water (9:6·67:3·33:15 by vol, $R_F = 0·38$) and water–butyl cellosolve–2·5 M-potassium phosphate, pH 7·6 (83:45·5:10, $R_F = 0·8$). Crude insulin fractionated by such systems has been purified to give a potency of 24 i.u. per mg equal to the international standard.

The solvents, n-butanol and dichloroacetic acid, are suitable for the countercurrent distribution of insulin. A highly purified insulin containing 27 i.u. per mg which was homogeneous by several criteria was resolved into two components differing in the number of amide groups by this system, without, however, increasing the specific activity (50, 51).

Gel filtration is now proving useful for the purification of insulins of various species. Sephadex G-50, equilibrated in ammonium bicarbonate buffer at pH 7·8, has been used for bovine insulin (38). Following crystallization from zinc acetate at pH 5·9 a yield of 5·5 mg per 100 g pancreas was obtained.

Sephadex G-50 has also been employed for the purification of feline (30) and human insulins (84). Here the columns were run in 1 N-acetic acid. Human insulin was subsequently crystallized from citrate buffer and was relatively free from glucagon; when crystallized from ammonium acetate buffers, it may not be. Alternatively gel filtration combined with electrophoresis on cellulose acetate furnishes a simple method for obtaining experimental amounts of the two hormones free of one another (74).

CHEMICAL STRUCTURE

The elucidation of the structure of insulin by Sanger and his colleagues is one of the great chemical achievements of this century. It was during this work that the fluoro-dinitrobenzene (FDNB) method was developed for the determination of the N-terminal amino acids.

The scheme adopted was to determine the amino acid composition of the molecule as a whole, then the N-terminal and C-terminal amino acids and then to break up the molecule into small peptides, determine the structure of each and so eventually arrive at the complete structure.

The N-terminal amino acids determined by the FDNB method were found to be glycine and phenylalanine; the reagent also reacted with the ε-amino group of lysine in the polypeptide chain. On the basis of an assumed molecular weight of 12,000 there were calculated to be 2 residues each of glycine and phenylalanine suggesting that there were 4 polypeptide chains (97).

The separation of these chains, which were assumed to be joined together by the disulphide bridges of the cystine known to be present in the molecule, presented some difficulties initially. Eventually the problem was solved by the use of performic acid which produces two cysteic acid residues from each cystine:

$$
\begin{array}{ccc}
CH_2{-}S{-}S{-}CH_2 & & CH_2{-}SO_3H \\
| \qquad\qquad | & \xrightarrow{\text{H.CO}_3\text{H}} & | \\
CH{\cdot}NH_2 \quad CH{\cdot}NH_2 & & 2\ CH{\cdot}NH_2 \\
| \qquad\qquad | & & | \\
CO_2H \qquad CO_2H & & CO_2H
\end{array}
$$

The reagent also reacts with methionine and tryptophan but these amino acids are not present in insulin.

Two fractions were obtained after this treatment, fraction A containing the N-terminal glycine and fraction B the N-terminal phenylalanine. The former is acidic, containing no basic amino acids, while the latter is basic.

Each was now submitted to mild acid hydrolysis to give peptides, the structures of which were each determined separately. It was soon noted that if the molecular weight was indeed 12,000 there must be two identical halves since the molecule appeared to be built from two types of chain, not four. The molecular weight of the monomer is in fact now known to be 6,000.

The complete structure of fraction B, known as the B-chain, was worked out first, proving rather easier than the A-chain. The first four N-terminal amino acids were identified using the FDNB method; then the chain was submitted to partial hydrolysis with acid and the 50 or so fragments produced were each analysed, together with 10 more produced by enzymic hydrolysis. The peptides were separated by ion-exchange chromatography, ionophoresis on paper or silica gel or by adsorption on charcoal (100, 101). The effect of enzymic hydrolysis on the B-chain is shown in Fig. 9.4 (101).

The structure of the A-chain was rather more difficult to elucidate since it is much less susceptible to enzymic hydrolysis (98, 99). It is not attacked by trypsin and there is a sequence of 13 amino acids not split by either chymotrypsin or pepsin. A further difficulty was the separation of the cysteic acid peptides from this chain. Paper ionophoresis at pH 2·75 was found to be the solution since carboxylic acid groups are uncharged, $-SO_3H$ groups carry negative charges and the $-NH_2$ groups carry positive charges.

The structure of bovine insulin was finally determined and is shown in Fig. 9.5. There are slight differences in structure in insulins of other species (49). In the A-chain these variations mainly concern the disulphide ring. Position 8 is occupied by threonine except in the ox, sheep or whale when it is alanine instead. Serine is usually at position 9 but there is glycine in sheep and

		Pepsin	Chymotrypsin	Trypsin
1	H.Phe			
		←--		
2	Val			
3	Asp(NH$_2$)			
4	Glu(NH$_2$)			
		←--		
5	His			
6	Leu			
7	CySO$_3$H			
8	Gly			
9	Ser			
10	His			
11	Leu			
		←		
12	Val			
13	Glu			
		←--		
14	Ala			
		←--		
15	Leu			
		←--	←--	
16	Tyr			
		←	←	
17	Leu			
18	Val			
19	CySO$_3$H			
20	Gly			
21	Glu			
22	Arg			
				←
23	Gly			
		←--		
24	Phe			
		←		
25	Phe			
		←	←	
26	Tyr			
			←	
27	Thr			
28	Pro			
29	Lys			
				←
30	Ala.OH			

Fig. 9.4. Enzymic hydrolysis of the B chain of insulin (101)

← major sites of action
←-- other bonds split

the horse. Position 10 is occupied by valine in the ox and sheep, threonine in the whale and isoleucine in other species (49). Finally glutamic acid is at position 4 except in the rat when it is aspartic acid.

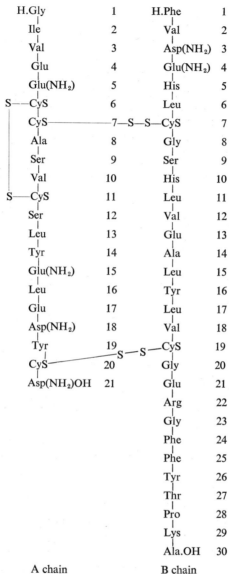

A chain		B chain	
H.Gly	1	H.Phe	1
Ile	2	Val	2
Val	3	Asp(NH₂)	3
Glu	4	Glu(NH₂)	4
Glu(NH₂)	5	His	5
CyS	6	Leu	6
CyS	7	CyS	7
Ala	8	Gly	8
Ser	9	Ser	9
Val	10	His	10
CyS	11	Leu	11
Ser	12	Val	12
Leu	13	Glu	13
Tyr	14	Ala	14
Glu(NH₂)	15	Leu	15
Leu	16	Tyr	16
Glu	17	Leu	17
Asp(NH₂)	18	Val	18
Tyr	19	CyS	19
CyS	20	Gly	20
Asp(NH₂)OH	21	Glu	21
		Arg	22
		Gly	23
		Phe	24
		Phe	25
		Tyr	26
		Thr	27
		Pro	28
		Lys	29
		Ala.OH	30

FIG. 9.5. Amino acid sequence of bovine insulin

In the B-chain asparagine is at position 3, but rat insulin contains lysine instead. Lysine is at position 29 except in one form of rat insulin which contains methionine—a most unusual amino acid to occur in insulin. Three different amino acids are found at position 30; there is usually alanine, but serine occurs in the rabbit and rat and threonine in the human. Furthermore, there are other differences in insulins from fish.

Structure and biological activity

Some of the amino acids in insulin may be modified without loss of bio-logical activity while others must remain intact if full activity is to be re-tained. When the N-terminal amino acids and the ε-amino groups of lysine are acetylated the product is still active. Since there is a possibility, however, that these groups are de-acetylated *in vivo*, Mills (83) prepared polynitro derivatives by treating insulin with 2:4:5-trinitrotoluene and found that extensive substitution destroyed activity. The reaction with the free amino groups and also with the phenolic groups of tyrosine was found to be markedly influenced by pH. By stopping the reaction at appropriate times it was found that some substitution was possible without loss of biological activity. When less than two amino groups were masked by dinitrotolyl groups no loss of activity occurred, but the activity fell to zero when rather less than three residues were introduced.

The phenolic groups of tyrosine appear to be important since iodination causes loss of activity while the disulphide bridges are essential and when broken by reduction or oxidation there is complete inactivation. The effect of iodination has been studied by using labelled iodine monochloride in alkaline glycine buffer (41). No loss of activity in the isolated rat diaphragm method was noted when up to 3·2 atoms of iodine were introduced per molecule. As more iodine is introduced there is a rapid decline in activity until at 6·8 atoms per molecule no activity remains. During the reaction the A-chain is iodinated preferentially to the B-chain. Comparatively little di-iodotyrosine is formed until most of the tyrosine has been mono-iodinated. In the initial stages of iodination 50 per cent of the iodine is at position 19 in the A-chain and only 12·4 per cent in the whole of the B-chain. Then an increasing proportion enters the tyrosine at position 14 in the A-chain and when 3 atoms of iodine per molecule are introduced there is still only 21 per cent in the B-chain. Lee (71) considers that inactivation occurs when iodine enters position 26 of the B-chain.

Some interesting observations regarding structure and activity have been made as a result of the use of enzymic hydrolysis. Carboxypeptidase (and trypsin) removes the alanine from the C-terminus of the phenylalanine chain with no loss of activity (52, 89). The other C-terminal residue, asparagine, is more resistant to the enzyme but it is released more rapidly from zinc-free insulin rather than from zinc-insulin and at pH 9·4 rather than pH 7·4. The desalanine-desasparagine insulin produced contains less than 5 per cent of the original activity, which indicates that the C-terminal asparagine is much more important for biological activity than is C-terminal alanine.

Continued treatment with trypsin slowly splits the arginine-glycine bond in the B-chain (positions 22–23) so that the products are free alanine (from the C-terminus), a heptapeptide (positions 23–29) and the remainder of the molecule (which has been called DHA-insulin (89). The heptapeptide is inactive but DHA-insulin contains about 15 per cent of the activity of insulin itself. This could not be accounted for by the presence of unchanged insulin as a contaminant so that it appears that the amino acids 23–30 are not essential for biological activity but they clearly have some influence on it.

Finally in considering enzymic reactions, it is possible to remove the first six N-terminal residues of the B-chain by the action of leucine aminopeptidase (52). Since the product is still active it appears that this part of the molecule is not essential for biological activity.

From the results of these experiments it appears that a very important part of the molecule is the sequence Tyr-Cys-Asp-NH$_2$ (positions 19–21 of the A-chain). Each of these amino acids appears to be essential for biological activity and the same sequence occurs in insulins of all species examined. Since there are differences between the various insulins in the amino acids elsewhere in the molecule, and each insulin is active, it could be concluded that these particular amino acids are not essential for activity. The differences are concerned particularly with the interesting intra-chain disulphide bridge in the A-chain which, although always containing the same number of residues (which incidentally is the same number as in oxytocin and vasopressin), occurs with five different combinations of amino acids.

FACTORS AFFECTING THE ACTION OF INSULIN

Several factors have been described which inhibit the action of insulin. Thus the insulin-like activity found in blood, and measured by its effect in the isolated rat diaphragm method, is apparently increased if the blood is diluted (28, 123) or is extracted (29). This could be explained by the presence of a factor which opposes the action of insulin in this assay or by the binding of part of the insulin to a factor which renders it biologically inactive.

Such a factor has been termed the *synalbumin* insulin antagonist. It is elevated in diabetic subjects (119) and it may be a polypeptide (118). Some interesting experiments have been carried out by Ensinck *et al.* (37) who have pointed out that the B-chain of insulin becomes bound to albumin under certain conditions and that this chain may conceivably act as an inhibitor to the parent insulin.

Now there are several ways of separating the B-chain from insulin. Oxidation with performic acid has already been mentioned. There is also the method of treatment with sodium sulphite–copper sulphate–urea at pH 10·2 for 8–10 hours (32), the chain being separated by subsequent chromatography on Dowex 50W–X2 with 2·7 M-formic acid–8 M-urea and 10 N-ammonia–8 M-urea (3, 32). The sulpho B-chain so obtained may then be reduced by thioglycollic acid or by sodium in liquid ammonia. An enzymic method involves incubation with glutathione and glutathione-insulin trans-hydrogenase (115), an enzyme isolated from mammalian liver.

In order to study the effect of serum albumin in conjunction with the B-chain, it was necessary to prepare albumin free of inhibiting factors. When isolated from serum, albumin may oppose the action of insulin, but when passed through columns of partially acetylated cellulose or Dowex 50 resin or when treated with thioglycollic acid it no longer shows this property. It seems therefore that the anti-insulin activity is not an intrinsic property of albumin but is rather a factor retained by the columns or a factor depending on the presence of disulphide bonds.

A small but significant anti-insulin effect was noted with both sulpho B- and reduced B-chains but not with oxidized B-chain. The same effects were noted in the presence of albumin which had previously been passed through an acetylated cellulose column to remove its anti-insulin effect. If maximum binding to albumin had occurred it was calculated that 6 μg of the B-chain associated with albumin caused an inhibition comparable with that obtained with 100 μg of the B-chain in buffer alone. The increase in activity in the presence of albumin may be partly due to the increased solubility of the B-chain in the presence of protein.

Since anti-insulin activity is thus shown to be a property of the sulpho and reduced B-chains and not of the B-chain obtained by irreversible oxidation with performic acid it may be suggested that the thiol groups are responsible. Other evidence that this is so is provided by experiments which show that loss of activity occurs after reaction with alkylating agents. Thus treatment with iodoacetamide or N-ethyl maleimide destroys all anti-insulin activity.

The mode of action of the anti-insulin factor is unknown but it is interesting to note that the disulphide bonds of insulin are essential for activity; the B-chain may therefore inhibit the action of insulin by competing for available thiol receptor sites.

Labelled preparations of insulin have been used to study the binding of insulin to serum proteins (1, 6, 26, 85) in normal and abnormal states. Immunoelectrophoretic experiments have shown that insulin is normally bound to α- and β-macroglobulins while in insulin-resistant diabetics it is bound to γ- or β-globulins.

Insulin complexes may be adsorbed from serum by cationic exchange resins in the sodium form from which insulin is eluted in acid or alkali (1). When it is bound in this way it does not exert its full biological effect so the binding protein may act as a regulatory mechanism for insulin activity.

Synthesis of insulin

BIOSYNTHESIS

The incorporation of ³H- and ¹⁴C-labelled amino acids into insulin has been demonstrated on several occasions in experiments with isolated pancreatic tissue (54, 73, 76, 121). It is interesting to note that when segments of rat pancreas are incubated with [³H]leucine the B-chain becomes labelled, but when isoleucine, an amino acid which does not occur naturally in this chain, is used instead, no label appears in the B-chain.

CHEMICAL SYNTHESIS

The total synthesis of insulin has now been reported (61, 62, 63, 80). Although the original yields reported are extremely small, this is a remarkable achievement, since it is the first and only time a naturally occurring protein hormone has been synthesized. This development has been made possible by the improved methods (see Chapter 1) for the protection of specific groups in peptide chains and for the condensation of the fragments.

The synthesis of the A-chain was given as an example of a synthesis on p. 16 and the B-chain has been synthesized in a similar fashion (60, 62). There remains the problem of joining the two chains correctly—a formidable task when one considers all the possible ways of joining together the different disulphide linkages.

The feasibility of such a combination has been demonstrated in experiments with the A- and B-chains from natural insulin (33, 58). Treatment of insulin with sodium sulphite and sodium tetrathionate (sulphitolysis) breaks the disulphide bridges converting them to thiol groups. They are next converted to S-sulphonates ($-SH \rightarrow -S-SO_3H$) in which form the chains are separated and purified. The thiol form of each chain is then regenerated by treatment with mercaptoethanol or thioglycollic acid. Oxidation in air of a mixture of the two chains gives insulin in yields of about 10 per cent of the theoretical.

In the synthesis of the A- and B-chains the thiol groups are protected by benzylation. The protecting groups are removed by sodium in liquid ammonia and then the chains are treated as above, i.e. by sulphitolysis followed by purification, reduction and then oxidation in air (61). The efficiency of the synthesis is reported to be about 10 per cent of that using the natural chains.

Some interesting combinations of natural A- and B-chains from different species to produce active products have been reported, e.g. cod-bovine hybrid insulins (31, 124).

Chemical properties of glucagon

METHODS OF PREPARATION

Glucagon was first prepared in crystalline form from crude porcine insulin (109). The method depended on precipitation from acetone and salts at low pH values and finally on crystallization from 0·033 M-glycine buffer at pH 8·6 containing 0·67 M-urea.

Repeated recrystallizations of this material did not alter the biological activity significantly. Additional evidence of purity was the finding of a single *N*- and a single *C*-terminal amino acid residue. Starch zone electrophoresis, however, revealed two components in the proportion of 9:1. When the major component was submitted to a second electrophoresis the minor component again appeared in the same proportion. The two components appear to be identical in amino acid composition.

CHEMICAL PROPERTIES

Glucagon crystallizes in the form of rhombic dodecahedra. The crystals often contain traces of copper, cobalt and other metals. The water content is about 13 per cent and may be removed by drying at 100° without loss of biological activity.

When warmed at 40° in dilute HCl glucagon readily forms fibrils which retain full biological activity. The hormone is in fact remarkably stable in acid solution (e.g. at pH 2) and is much more stable in alkali than is insulin; it is almost insoluble between pH 6 and pH 8. Since it contains no cystine, it is very resistant to treatments which destroy disulphide bridges; in this way it again differs from insulin.

There are 15 different amino acids in the total of 29 residues from which the estimated molecular weight of glucagon is about 3,500. It is completely hydrolysed by leucine amino-peptidase into its component amino acids, all being of the L-configuration (104).

End group analysis by the FDNB procedure indicates that the *N*-terminal amino acid is histidine (23, 108) while the hydrazinolysis and carboxy-peptidase methods show that the *C*-terminal amino acid is threonine (22).

The partial structure of glucagon was determined by identifying the peptides produced following enzymic hydrolysis of the protein (21). The amino acid composition is given in Figure 9.6.

	Calculated number of residues to the nearest integer assuming a molecular weight of 3550
Aspartic acid	4
Glutamic acid	3
Threonine	3
Serine	4
Glycine	1
Alanine	1
Valine	1
Leucine	2
Lysine	1
Arginine	2
Histidine	1
Tyrosine	2
Tryptophan	1
Phenylalanine	2
Methionine	1
Ammonia	4

FIG. 9.6. The amino acid composition of bovine glucagon (22)

It will be noted that three common amino acids, cystine, isoleucine and proline which are present in insulin are lacking in glucagon but it contains tryptophan and methionine which are not present in insulin.

REFERENCES

1 ANTONIADES, H. *Endocrinology* **68**, 7 (1961).

2 ARQUILLA, E. R. *Ciba Fdn Colloq. Endocr.* **14**, 146 (1962).

3 BAILEY, J. L. and COLE, R. D. *J. biol. Chem.* **234**, 1733 (1959).

4 BAIRD, C. W. and BORNSTEIN, J. *Lancet* i, 1111 (1957).

5 BANGHAM, D. R. and MUSSET, M. V. *Bull. Wld Hlth Org.* **20**, 1209 (1959).

6 BARRETT, J. L. and BOSHELL, B. R. *Diabetes* **11**, S35 (1962).

7 BARRNETT, R. J., MARSHALL, R. B. and SELIGMAN, A. M. *Endocrinology* **57**, 419 (1955).

8 BARRNETT, R. J. and SELIGMAN, A. M. *Science* **116**, 323 (1952).

9 BEHRENS, O. K. and BROMER, W. W. *Vitam Horm.* **16**, 263 (1958).

10 BERNS, A. W., HIRATA, Y. and BLUMENTHAL, H. T. *J. Lab. clin. Med.* **60**, 535 (1962).

11 BERSON, S. A. and YALOW, R. S. *J. clin. Invest.* **38**, 2017 (1959).

12 BERSON, S. A. and YALOW, R. S. *J. clin. Invest.* **40**, 1803 (1961).

13 BERSON, S. A. and YALOW, R. S. *Nature, Lond.* **191**, 1392 (1961).

14 BERSON, S. A. and YALOW, R. S. *Science* **139**, 844 (1963).

15 BERTHET, J. *Amer. J. Med.* **26**, 703 (1959).

16 BERTHET, J., SUTHERLAND, E. W. and RALL, T. W. *J. biol. Chem.* **229**, 351 (1957).

17 BEST, C. H. *Br. med. Bull.* **16**, 179 (1960).

18 BODA, J. M. *Amer. J. Physiol.* **206**, 419 (1964).

19 BORNSTEIN, J. and LAWRENCE, R. D. *Br. med. J.* i, 732 (1951).

20 BORNSTEIN, J. and LAWRENCE, R. D. *Br. med. J.* ii, 1541 (1951).

21 BROMER, W. W., SINN, L. G. and BEHRENS, O. K. *J. Amer. chem. Soc.* **79**, 2807 (1957).

22 BROMER, W. W., STAUB, A., DILLER, E. R., BIRD, H. L., SINN, L. G. and BEHRENS, O. K. *J. Amer. chem. Soc.* **79**, 2794 (1957).

23 BROMER, W. W., STAUB, A., SINN, L. G. and BEHRENS, O. K. *J. Amer. chem. Soc.* **79**, 2801 (1957).

24 BROWN, H., SANGER, F. and KITAI, R. *Biochem. J.* **60**, 556 (1955).

25 CHRISTENSEN, H. N. *Perspect. Biol. Med.* **2**, 228 (1958).

26 CLAUSEN, J., GJEDDE, F. and JØRGENSEN, K. *Proc. Soc. exp. Biol. Med.* **112**, 778 (1963).

27 CUNNINGHAM, N. F. *J. Endocr.* **25**, 35 (1962).

28 CUNNINGHAM, N. F. *J. Endocr.* **25**, 43 (1962).

29 CUNNINGHAM, N. F. *J. Endocr.* **31**, 1 (1964).

30 DAVOREN, P. R. *Biochim. biophys. Acta* **63**, 150 (1962).

31 Dixon, G. H. *Proc. 2nd Int. Congr. Endocr.* 1207 (1965).

32 Dixon, G. H. and Wardlaw, A. C. *Nature, Lond.* **188,** 721 (1960).

33 Du, Y.-C., Zhang, Y.-S., Lu, Z.-X. and Tsou, C.-L. *Scientia sin.* **10,** 84 (1961).

34 Dunn, J. S. and McLetchie, N. G. B. *Lancet* ii, 384 (1943).

35 Elrick, H., Huffman, E. R., Hlad, C. J., Whipple, N. and Staub, A. *J. clin. Endocr.* **18,** 813 (1958).

36 Elrick, H., Whipple, N., Arai, Y. and Hlad, C. J. *J. clin. Endocr.* **19,** 1274 (1959).

37 Ensinck, J. W., Mahler, R. J. and Vallance-Owen, J. *Biochem. J.* **94,** 150 (1965).

38 Epstein, C. J. and Anfinsen, C. B. *Biochemistry* **2,** 461 (1963).

39 Fenton, E. L. *Biochem. J.* **71,** 507 (1959).

40 Fenton, E. L. *Biochem. J.* **81,** 570 (1961).

41 Garratt, C. J. *Nature, Lond.* **201,** 1324 (1964).

42 Grillo, T. A. I. *J. Endocr.* **31,** 67 (1964).

43 Grodsky, G. M., Peng, C. T. and Forsham, P. H. *Archs. Biochem. Biophys.* **81,** 264 (1959).

44 Grodsky, G. M., Tarver, H., Light, A. and Simpson, M. V. *Nature, Lond.* **177,** 223 (1956).

45 Groen, J., Kamminga, C. E., Willebrands, A. F. and Blickman, J. R. *J. clin. Invest.* **31,** 97 (1952).

46 Hales, C. N. and Randle, P. J. *Biochem. J.* **88,** 137 (1963).

47 Hallas-Møller, K., Jersild, M., Petersen, K. and Schlichtkrull, J. *J. Amer. med. Ass.* **150,** 1667 (1952).

48 Hallas-Møller, K., Petersen, K. and Schlichtkrull, J. *Science* **116,** 394 (1952).

49 Harfenist, E. J. *J. Amer. chem. Soc.* **75,** 5528 (1953).

50 Harfenist, E. J. and Craig, L. C. *J. Amer. chem. Soc.* **73,** 878 (1952).

51 Harfenist, E. J. and Craig, L. C. *J. Amer. chem. Soc.* **74,** 3083 (1952).

52 Harris, J. I. and Li, C. H. *J. Amer. chem. Soc.* **74,** 2945 (1952).

53 Hechter, O. and Lester, G. *Recent Prog. Horm. Res.* **16,** 139 (1960).

54 Humbell, R. E., Renold, A. E., Herrera, M. G. and Taylor, K. W. *Endocrinology* **69,** 874 (1961).

55 Itzhaki, S. and Wertheimer, E. *Endocrinology* **61,** 72 (1957).

56 Izzo, J. L., Bale, W. F., Izzo, M. J. and Roncone, A. *J. biol. Chem.* **239,** 3743 (1964).

57 Izzo, J. L., Roncone, A., Izzo, M. J. and Bale, W. F. *J. biol. Chem.* **239,** 3749 (1964).

58 Jiang, R.-Q., Du, Y.-C. and Tsou, C.-L. *Scientia sin.* **12,** 542 (1963).

59 Jones, V. E. and Cunliffe, A. C. *Nature, Lond.* **192,** 136 (1961).

60 Katsoyannis, P. G. *Metabolism* **13,** 1059 (1964).

61 Katsoyannis, P. G. *Proc. 2nd Int. Congr. Endocr.* 1216 (1965).

62 KATSOYANNIS, P. G., FUKUDA, K., TOMETSKO, A., SUZUKI, K. and TILAK, M. *J. Amer. chem. Soc.* **86**, 930 (1964).

63 KATSOYANNIS, P. G., TOMETSKO, A. and FUKUDA, K. *J. Amer. chem. Soc.* **85**, 2863 (1963).

64 KENNY, A. J. *Br. Med. Bull*, **16**, 202 (1960).

65 KIMBALL, C. P. and MURLIN, J. R. *J. biol. Chem.* **58**, 337 (1923).

66 KIPNIS, D. M. and CORI, C. F. *J. biol. Chem.* **224**, 681 (1957).

67 KIPNIS, D. M. and NOALL, M. W. *Biochim. biophys. Acta* **28**, 226 (1958).

68 KORNER, A. *Biochem. J.* **92**, 449 (1964).

69 KRAHL, M. E. *Ann. N. Y. Acad. Sci.* **54**, 649 (1951).

70 LACY, P. E. and DAVIES, J. *Stain Technol.* **34**, 85 (1959).

71 LEE, N. D. *Fedn Proc.* **18**, 271 (1959).

72 LEVINE, R. and GOLDSTEIN, M. S. *Recent Prog. Horm. Res.* **11**, 343 (1955).

73 LIGHT, A. and SIMPSON, M. N. *Biochim. biophys. Acta* **20**, 251 (1956).

74 LOCHNER, J. DE V., ESTERHUIZEN, A. C. and UNGER, R. H. *Diabetes* **13**, 387 (1964).

75 MAHLER, R. F. *Brit. med. Bull.* **16**, 250 (1960).

76 MALLORY, A., SMITH, G. H. and TAYLOR, K. W. *Biochem. J.* **91**, 484 (1964).

77 MANCHESTER, K. L. and YOUNG, F. G. *Vitams Horm.* **19**, 95 (1961).

78 MARTIN, D. B., RENOLD, A. E. and DAGENAIS, Y. M. *Lancet* ii, 76 (1958).

79 MCLEAN, P. and NOVELLO, F. *Biochem. J.* **94**, 410 (1965).

80 MEINHOFER, J., SCHNABEL, E., BREMER, H., BRINKOFF, O., SROKA, R., KLOSTERMEYER, H., BRANDENBURG, D., OKUDA, T. and ZAHN, H. *Z. Naturforsch.* **186**, 1120 (1963).

81 MENDIOLA, L. and COLE, R. D. *J. biol. Chem.* **235**, 3484 (1960).

82 MILLER, L. L. *Recent Prog. Horm. Res.* **17**, 539 (1961).

83 MILLS, G. L. *Biochem. J.* **53**, 37 (1953).

84 MIRSKY, I. A., JINKS, R. and PERISSUTTI, G. *J. clin. Invest.* **42**, 1869 (1963).

85 MITCHELL, M. L. *J. clin. Endocr.* **23**, 1001 (1963).

86 MOLONEY, P. J. *Ciba Fdn Colloq. Endocr.* **14**, 169 (1962).

87 MORGAN, C. R. and LAZAROW, A. *Proc. Soc. exp. Biol. Med.* **110**, 39 (1962).

88 MUNGER, B. L. *Amer. J. Anat.* **103**, 275 (1958).

89 NICOL, D. S. H. W. *Biochem. J.* **75**, 395 (1960).

90 PARK, C. R., JOHNSON, L. H., WRIGHT, J. H. and BATSEL, H. *Amer. J. Physiol.* **191**, 13 (1957).

91 PORATH, J. and LI, C. H. *Biochim. biophys. Acta* **13**, 268 (1954).

92 PORTER, R. R. *Biochem. J.* **53**, 320 (1953).

93 RALL, T. W., SUTHERLAND, E. W. and BERTHET, J. *J. biol. Chem.* **224**, 463 (1957).

94 RANDLE, P. J. *Br. med. J.* i, 1237 (1954).

P

95 RENOLD, A. E., MARTIN, D. B., DAGENAIS, Y. M., STEINKE, J., NICKER-SON, R. J. and SHEPS, M. C. *J. clin. Invest.* **39,** 1487 (1960).

96 SAMAAN, N. A., DEMPSTER, W. J., FRASER, R., PLEASE, N. W. and STILLMAN, D. *J. Endocr.* **24,** 263 (1962).

97 SANGER, F. *Br. med. Bull.* **16,** 183 (1960).

98 SANGER, F. and THOMPSON, E. O. P. *Biochem. J.* **53,** 353 (1953).

99 SANGER, F. and THOMPSON, E. O. P. *Biochem. J.* **53,** 366 (1953).

100 SANGER, F. and TUPPY, H. *Biochem. J.* **49,** 463 (1951).

101 SANGER, F. and TUPPY, H. *Biochem. J.* **49,** 481 (1951).

102 SHOEMAKER, W. C., VAN ITALLIE, T. B. and WALKER, W. F. *Amer. J. Physiol.* **196,** 315 (1959).

103 SLATER, J. D. H., SAMAAN, N., FRASER, R. and STILLMAN, D. *Br. med. J.* i, 1712, (1961).

104 SMITH, E. L., HILL, R. L. and BORMAN, A. *Biochim. biophys. Acta* **29,** 207 (1958).

105 SMITH, K. L. In *Hormone Assay* (edited by C. W. Emmens), p. 35, Academic Press, New York (1950).

106 SMITH, L. F. *Biochim. biophys. Acta* **82,** 231 (1964).

107 STAUB, A. and BEHRENS, O. K. *J. clin. Invest.* **33,** 1629 (1954).

108 STAUB, A., SINN, L. C. and BEHRENS, O. K. *Fedn. Proc.* **13,** 303 (1954).

109 STAUB, A., SINN, L. C. and BEHRENS, O. K. *J. biol. Chem.* **214,** 619 (1955).

110 STAUB, A., SPRINGS, V., STOLL, F. and ELRICK, H. *Proc. Soc. exp. Biol. Med.* **94,** 57 (1957).

111 STEWART, G. A., *Br. med. Bull.* **16,** 196 (1960).

112 SUTHERLAND, E. W. and CORI, C. F. *J. biol. Chem.* **172,** 737 (1948).

113 TAYLOR, K. W., HUMBELL, R. E., STEINKE, J. and RENOLD, A. E. *Biochim. biophys. Acta* **54,** 391 (1961).

114 TEPPERMAN, J. and TEPPERMAN, H. M. *Pharmac. Rev.* **12,** 301 (1960).

115 TOMIZAWA, H. H. *J. biol. Chem.* **237,** 428 (1962).

116 UNGER, R. H., EISENTRAUT, A. M., McCALL, M. S. and MADISON, L. L. *Ciba Fdn Colloq. Endocr.* **14,** 212 (1962).

117 VALLANCE-OWEN, J. and HURLOCK, B. *Lancet* i, 68 (1954).

118 VALLANCE-OWEN, J. and LILLEY, M. D. *Lancet* i, 804 (1961).

119 VALLANCE-OWEN, J. and LILLEY, M. D. *Lancet* i, 806 (1961).

120 VAUGHAN, M. *J. biol. Chem.* **236,** 2196 (1961).

121 VAUGHAN, M. and ANFINSEN, C. B. *J. biol. Chem.* **211,** 367 (1954).

122 VUYLSTEKE, C. A. and DE DUVE, C. *Archs int. Pharmacodyn. Thér.* **109,** 437 (1957).

123 WILLEBRANDS, A. F., GELD, H. V. D. and GROEN, J. *Diabetes* **7,** 119 (1958).

124 WILSON, S., DIXON, G. H. and WARDLAW, A. C. *Biochim. biophys. Acta* **62,** 483 (1962).

125 WINEGRAD, A. I. *Vitams Horm.* **20,** 141 (1962).

126 WINEGRAD, A. I. and RENOLD, A. E. *J. biol. Chem.* **233,** 267 (1958).
127 WINEGRAD, A. I. and RENOLD, A. E. *J. biol. Chem.* **233,** 273 (1958).
128 WRIGHT, P. H. *Lancet* ii, 621 (1957).
129 WRIGHT, P. H. *Brit. med. Bull.* **16,** 219 (1960).
130 YALOW, R. S. and BERSON, S. A. *J. clin. Invest.* **39,** 1157 (1960).
131 YALOW, R. S. and BERSON, S. A. *J. clin. Invest.* **40,** 2190 (1961).
132 YALOW, R. S. and BERSON, S. A. *Amer. J. Med.* **31,** 882 (1961).
133 YOUNG, D. M. and LEWIS, A. H. *Science* **105,** 368 (1947).

10

CATECHOLAMINES

A number of cells in the adrenal medulla and in the peripheral sympathetic ganglia contain catecholamines and are recognized by staining with dichromate; they have been called 'chromaffin cells'. In mammals the medulla contains the bulk of the chromaffin cells which were originally thought to secrete only adrenaline (epinephrine). Later noradrenaline was recognized as the transmitter substance liberated by post-ganglionic sympathetic nerves and it was found to occur with adrenaline in the chromaffin cells in many parts of the body.

Substances acting like adrenaline (and there are many) have been called 'sympathomimetic amines' while the terms 'adrenergic' and 'cholinergic' were introduced originally to distinguish nerves liberating a substance like adrenaline from those liberating acetyl choline. Gaddum and Holzbauer (25) have drawn attention to the fact that the term 'adrenergic' is sometimes applied to drugs as if it meant the same thing as sympathomimetic.

Biosynthesis

The metabolic pathways leading to adrenaline have been carefully studied, lately, by the use of labelled preparations (e.g. 29). Much of the evidence for the pathway shown in Figure 10.1 has been reviewed by Gaddum and Holzbauer (25).

The decarboxylase necessary for the conversion of L-3,4-dihydroxy-phenylalanine (dopa) to 3-hydroxytyramine (dopamine) is inhibited by phenylpyruvate; L-phenylalanine has no effect. Metabolites of phenylalanine, however, do interfere in the synthesis of adrenaline and there is a decrease in the concentration of adrenaline in the plasma in the condition of phenylketonuria. Experimentally the production of labelled dopamine and adrenaline from L-[2-^{14}C]tyrosine is observed by *in vitro* experiments with adrenal

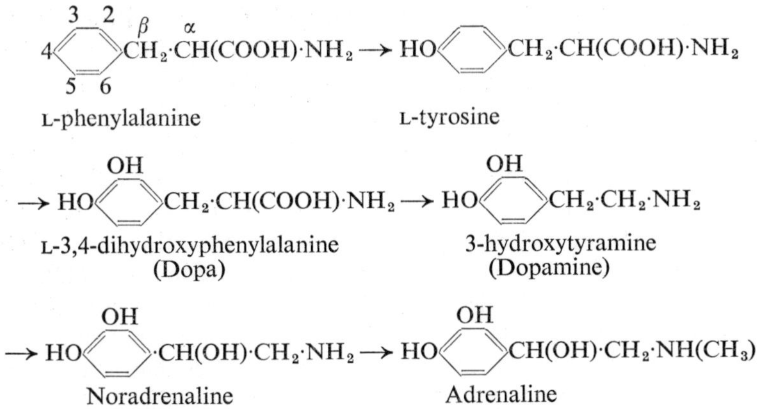

$$\underset{5\quad6}{\overset{3\quad2}{\bigcirc}}\beta\ \alpha\ CH_2\cdot CH(COOH)\cdot NH_2 \rightarrow HO\bigcirc CH_2\cdot CH(COOH)\cdot NH_2$$

l-phenylalanine   l-tyrosine

$$\rightarrow HO\overset{OH}{\bigcirc}CH_2\cdot CH(COOH)\cdot NH_2 \rightarrow HO\overset{OH}{\bigcirc}CH_2\cdot CH_2\cdot NH_2$$

l-3,4-dihydroxyphenylalanine   3-hydroxytyramine
(Dopa)   (Dopamine)

$$\rightarrow HO\overset{OH}{\bigcirc}\cdot CH(OH)\cdot CH_2\cdot NH_2 \rightarrow HO\overset{OH}{\bigcirc}CH(OH)\cdot CH_2\cdot NH(CH_3)$$

Noradrenaline   Adrenaline

Fig. 10.1

medullary tissue from guinea-pigs. The addition of sodium phenyl pyruvate, however, inhibits the synthesis considerably and results in the accumulation of labelled dopa instead (10). There are a number of competitive enzymes to this decarboxylase, one of the most potent being 5-(3,4-dihydroxy-cinnamoyl)-salicylic acid (33).

The final stage of the biosynthesis, the N-methylation of noradrenaline, requires the presence of adenosyl-S-methionine and ATP. Since N-methyl compounds are not decarboxylated it seems clear that methylation occurs after decarboxylation.

Biological activity

Adrenaline and noradrenaline have a wide variety of biological actions. Only the natural l-isomers are fully active, the d-forms being only 1/15th or so as active and the dl-forms having intermediate activities. A number of effects of adrenaline and noradrenaline were originally thought to be different but later several were shown to be quantitative rather than qualitative differences. These biological actions include effects on metabolism and circulation, on smooth and skeletal muscle, on peripheral nerves and the central nervous system as well as an influence on the release of hormones from the anterior pituitary and the adrenal gland (25).

Among the metabolic effects there is much evidence both from *in vivo* and *in vitro* experiments that adrenaline causes liver glycogen to be liberated as glucose; noradrenaline is less active in this respect. Thus muscular activity increases glucose metabolism and, as the blood sugar falls, adrenaline is secreted and not only releases sugar from the liver but also prevents the uptake of sugar by the muscles.

Both hormones increase the mobilization of lipids from adipose tissue *in vivo* and *in vitro* (60). This effect may be recognized by the release of non-esterified fatty acids (NEFA) from the epididymal fat pads of rats, an action similar to that of corticotrophin or cortisone (see p. 57). The effect of each is antagonized if the pad is pretreated with adrenergic blocking agents; this suggests that the catecholamines play an intermediary role in the release of NEFA by corticotrophin. Now the alkaloid, reserpine, depletes adipose and other tissue of noradrenaline (9, 43); after such treatment the effect of corticotrophin is abolished, and this again suggests that the release of NEFA by corticotrophin is by a mechanism which involves noradrenaline (48).

The action on the circulation is well known. Adrenaline causes constriction of the arteries and a very considerable rise in blood pressure; nanogram quantities can be recognized by this effect in the cat. Noradrenaline is a general vasoconstrictor and controls the blood pressure by regulating the tone of the arterioles. Both hormones stimulate the formation of the cyclic adenylate, adenosine-3′,5′-monophosphate (50); this produces an increased concentration of phosphorylase in several organs including the heart, whose force of contraction is thereby increased.

The action of the catecholamines on the release of hormones from the anterior pituitary has been much studied, and there is a good deal of evidence that they play some part in the release of corticotrophin, thyrotrophin (49) and luteinizing hormone. There is some suggestion also that they may directly stimulate the production of corticosteroids from the adrenal cortex.

METHODS OF BIOLOGICAL ASSAY

Several of the above biological properties have been used to develop sensitive assay procedures. The pressor effect in the cat or rat is suitable for the assay of noradrenaline, as little as 5 ng being detectable in the rat (52). Adrenaline is rather less active in this test.

A second action concerns the inhibition of the movements of the isolated uterus of the rat. This is a particularly sensitive assay for adrenaline and is much less sensitive for noradrenaline (26).

An assay was described by Armin and Grant (1) which is capable of detecting 0·002 ng of adrenaline. This depends on the constrictor action on the artery of a denervated ear of the rabbit, the end point being the measurement of the diameter of the artery.

DISTRIBUTION AND FUNCTION

The proportion of noradrenaline to adrenaline differs in the adrenal and other organs between the species (for summary see (18)) and even in different animals of the same species. In man there is about 0·6 g of catecholamines per g adrenal tissue, 16–17 per cent of this being noradrenaline. The adrenal cortex contains some of both, roughly in the same ratio as in the medulla.

The proportion is markedly different in the foetus, however, where there is practically only noradrenaline.

It is well known that the production of adrenaline from the adrenal increases in stress—it has been termed the 'emergency hormone'. There has been much discussion whether it influences the production of corticotrophin from the pituitary or directly stimulates the adrenal to produce corticosteroids.

The secretion of adrenaline may be induced by insulin hypoglycaemia. It is interesting to note that this occurs to an equal extent in normal and adrenalectomized subjects so that extra-adrenal cells may produce the hormone in response to insulin (22). Similar effects are noted in response to muscular work (7).

Catecholamines are widely distributed elsewhere in the body. In studies with tritiated preparations it has been shown that the anterior pituitary has a higher affinity for noradrenaline than for adrenaline and more tritiated material accumulates here than in the posterior pituitary, the brain or the hypothalamus (59). Here also there is a higher activity of catechol O-methyl transferase (3), an enzyme which seems to account for the inactivation of a large proportion of circulating catecholamines.

The concentrations of these hormones in the pituitary and gonads have been studied in the early stages of pregnancy in the rat (4). The hypothalamic stimulation of gonadotrophic secretion which occurs on the second and third days of pregnancy correlates with an increased concentration of catecholamines in the anterior pituitary as well as in the ovarian adrenergic nervous system; the surge of oestrogens which follows is accompanied by a reduction in the pituitary content and the release of adrenaline from the uterus.

Chromaffin cells are identified also in the liver capsule and the gut of the ox, cow and sheep (16). Sites where these cells are most numerous are shown to be rich in dopamine which is apparently stored in tissue mast cells (6).

The brain also contains adrenaline and noradrenaline, but the chief catecholamine appears to be dopamine which constitutes between 50 and 80 per cent of the total catecholamines (41). The human brain contains also dopa and an acidic catechol compound.

The catecholamines are stored in special granular structures in the chromaffin cells which are observed by staining with osmium. These granules contain a large amount of ATP which decreases when catecholamines are released. Isolated granules take up dopamine as well as adrenaline and noradrenaline, the uptake being activated by ATP and Mg^{2+} and being inhibited by reserpine (see 18).

Certain drugs cause the release of catecholamines from chromaffin cells by direct action on the cell membrane (nicotine, histamine and acetylcholine are examples) while others (tyrosine, phenylalanine) act on the granules (11).

Adrenaline and noradrenaline are metabolized firstly to 3,4-dihydroxy mandelic acid (Fig. 10.2a) under the influence of monoamine oxidase and aldehyde dehydrogenase and then to 3-methoxy-4-hydroxy mandelic acid (Fig. 10.2b) by catechol O-methyl transferase. This is a normal constituent of

(a)

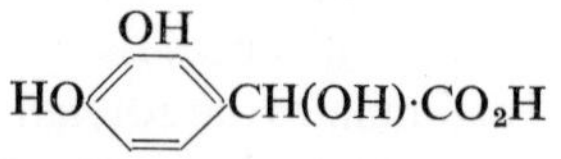

OH

HO⟨　⟩CH(OH)·CO₂H

3,4-dihydroxymandelic acid

(b)

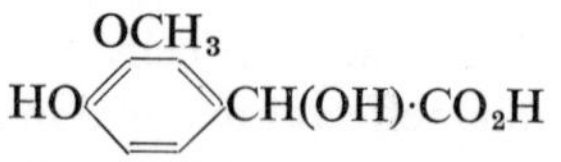

OCH₃

HO⟨　⟩CH(OH)·CO₂H

3-methoxy-4-hydroxymandelic acid

Fig. 10.2

urine, between 2 and 4 mg being excreted per 24 hours and is much increased in patients with tumours such as pheochromocytoma (35) or neuroblastoma (53, 54). It is usually extracted from urine by organic solvents after acid hydrolysis and is purified by paper chromatography (35). For identification on chromatograms and for colorimetric determination at 590 mμ the reagent, 2,6-dichloroquinonechloromide in alcohol, is suitable.

HISTOLOGICAL METHODS

Some of the reactions used for identifying chromaffin cells are given in Table 10.1. By a careful choice of reactions it may be possible to differentiate

TABLE 10.1

Staining reactions of chromaffin cells

Stain	Sections fixed in:	
	Formol-dichromate	Formalin
Giemsa (Gurr's R.66)	green or blue-green	red or red-purple
Toluidine blue	green or blue-green	negative or blue
Methylene blue in lithium carbonate	green or blue-green	negative or blue
Indophenol	negative	negative
Alkaline diazonium compounds	negative	negative
Hexamine silver (28)	positive	positive
Turnbull's blue	negative	negative
Ziehl-Nelson (44)	negative	negative
Schmorl's ferricyanide (44)	positive	weak
PAS	weak	negative

In addition to the references above, the stains are discussed in (15) and some modifications described in (37).

these cells from others such as mast cells and melanophores of the skin with which they may be confused. A critical survey of such methods has appeared (15). Melanophores chelate with ferrous ions and so give a positive Turnbull's blue reaction and a very strong positive reaction with Schmorl's reagent after fixing in formalin; chromaffin granules, however, react with Schmorl's reagent only after fixing in formalin and dichromate. Enterochromaffin cells contain 5-hydroxytryptamine and may be differentiated since they couple with alkaline diazonium compounds, give a positive indophenol reaction and a strongly positive Schmorl's reaction after fixing with formalin.

These techniques are reasonably sensitive, but some tissues may contain only a few chromaffin cells which are not sufficient to detect by these stains. Sometimes it is possible to detect such traces by extraction of the tissue followed by biological or chemical assay.

The terms chromaffin cells and catecholamine-containing cells are not too precise since they include those cells containing dopamine as well as adrenaline and noradrenaline; the differentiation between these catecholamines may be of great functional significance (18). Structurally, cells producing adrenaline and noradrenaline seem to be different from those producing dopamine. Originally dopamine was considered to serve as a store of precursor for noradrenaline (8). However, large amounts of dopamine are found in tissues such as lung and bronchi where it is unlikely to be required as a precursor for noradrenaline, which is present in only small amounts.

Chemical properties

The catecholamines are catechol-β-ethanolamines and therefore have the properties of phenols, alcohols and amines. Adrenaline is a crystalline, laevorotatory, secondary base (m.p. 215°), sparingly soluble in water, readily soluble in alkali. Loss of biological activity results from treatment at high pH and heat; heating even in acid solution causes racemization.

METHODS OF EXTRACTION

Methods are available for the extraction of the catecholamines from tissues, urine and blood. They may be extracted directly from tissues by acidic ethanol (10) or perchloric acid (5), but hydrolysis is first required with urine where conjugates occur (34). Some free compounds, probably from ethereal sulphates, are released by boiling at pH 2 for 20 minutes (21). Glucuronides certainly occur and adrenaline monoglucuronide has been isolated from urine after adrenaline is administered to rabbits (14). After hydrolysis n-butanol is a suitable solvent.

Dopamine has not been recognized in blood but several methods have been described for the extraction of adrenaline and noradrenaline. They are partly bound to protein when they are biologically inactive. Extraction by methods of precipitation leads to losses, but an alternative method giving reasonable recoveries has been described by Weil-Malherbe and Bone (58). Blood is collected in a solution containing fluoride and thiosulphate which act as anti-oxidant and anti-coagulant. The red cells are lysed by cetyltrimethyl-ammonium bromide or by freezing at $-40°$ and the plasma and lysate are extracted by n-butanol. The catecholamines are then extracted with 0·05 N-HCl and the extract is concentrated and brought to pH 6·5 with phosphate buffer.

Extracts from urine or blood are often next adsorbed on to alumina (56) from which they are eluted by 0·2 N-HCl. Starch has also been used as adsorbent with n-butanol–N-HCl as solvent (31).

Purification

Paper chromatography has been widely used with systems based on phenol or n-butanol–acetic acid (20, 41, 52, 58). In phenol–water (3:1 w/v) in an atmosphere saturated with 5N-HCl noradrenaline migrates with an R_F of 0·31, adrenaline 0·55 and dopamine 0·47. In n-butanol–acetic acid–water (4:1:5 by volume) the respective R_Fs are 0·24, 0·29 and 0·32. These systems are suitable for two-dimensional chromatography (10).

The catecholamines may be recognized on paper chromatograms by reaction with potassium ferricyanide at pH 7·8 (36). Alternatively the paper may be dried and sprayed with 10 per cent v/v ethylenediamine–ammonia (1:4 v/v) when they fluoresce under u.v. light. They also fluoresce after exposure to iodine vapour followed by ammonia (41).

Determination

The optical density at 279 mμ is occasionally useful for the determination of catecholamines and they also have a natural fluorescence which is activated at 285 mμ and measured at 325 mμ. More specific reactions are usually employed, however. Some of them make use of the coloured indole compounds produced by a variety of oxidizing agents whilst others rely on the fluorescence which is produced in alkali or after conjugation with ethylenediamine.

Oxidation of adrenaline and noradrenaline with iodine gives the corresponding iodochromes (19, 38 46, Fig. 10.3). The rates of oxidation are different for the two compounds, adrenaline being completely oxidized within $1\frac{1}{2}$ minutes at pH 4, while in this time only 10 per cent of noradrenaline is

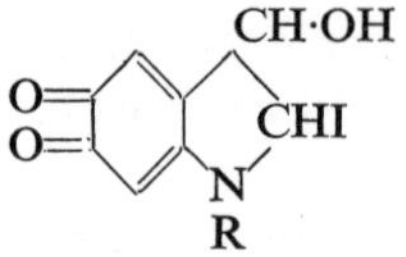

FIG. 10.3. Iodochromes (R = CH$_3$ for adrenaline, H for noradrenaline)

oxidized. The reaction may be stopped by thiosulphate and the colours read at 529 mμ. About 25 μg of the catecholamine is required for this reaction. Permanganate may be substituted for iodine when again adrenaline is oxidized at pH 3·6 in 2 minutes, while noradrenaline is only oxidized to the extent of 5–10 per cent. At pH 5·6 both are oxidized completely within 3 minutes (51).

Adrenaline reduces arsenomobybdic acid to a blue compound. This is not a specific reaction but it is very sensitive, especially if the adrenaline is first treated with alkali (45, 47).

The primary amine group of noradrenaline replaces the sulphonic acid group of 1,2-naphthoquinone-4-sulphonate in borate buffer at pH 8·6 giving a purplish-red derivative, soluble in organic solvents with maximum absorption at 540 mμ (2). Since secondary amines do not react, adrenaline does not interfere in this reaction.

Fluorescence methods

Fluorimetric determinations of the catecholamines are probably used more commonly than any others (see 17). Adrenaline gives a transient yellow-green fluorescence in the presence of strong alkali and oxygen, and this may be stabilized by the addition of ascorbic acid; under the same conditions noradrenaline fluoresces only slightly (23, 24, 27). The fluorescence is attributed to adrenolutine, a trihydroxyindole formed by the series of reactions shown in Fig. 10.4. The indole, adrenochrome, is not fluorescent and the leuco-adrenochrome is unstable and has not been isolated. Acetylation of the fluorescent compound by acetic anhydride in pyridine gives 3,5,6-triacetoxy-N-methyl indole (32) which may be extracted from the neutralized reaction mixture by ether and crystallized.

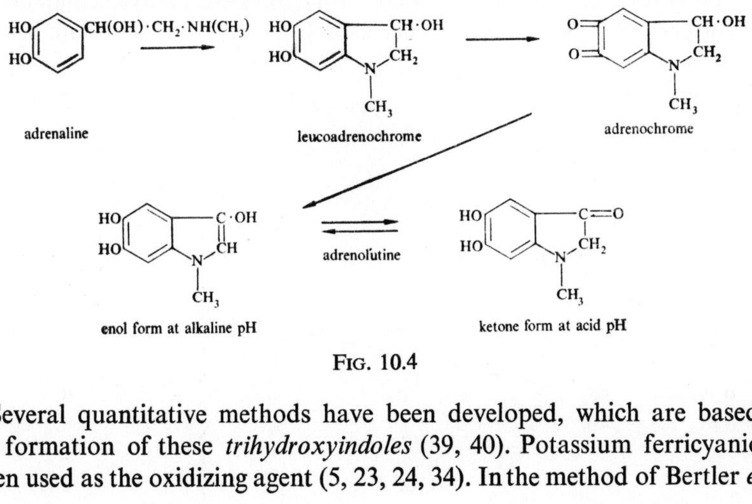

FIG. 10.4

Several quantitative methods have been developed, which are based on the formation of these *trihydroxyindoles* (39, 40). Potassium ferricyanide is often used as the oxidizing agent (5, 23, 24, 34). In the method of Bertler *et al.*

(5) the catecholamines are extracted in perchloric acid and then most of the perchlorate ions are removed as potassium perchlorate after the addition of potassium carbonate. Adrenaline and noradrenaline are then separated from dopa by ion-exchange chromatography on Dowex 50: they are eluted in 0·4–1·0 N-HCl and dopa in 2 N-HCl. Oxidation with potassium ferricyanide is then carried out in phosphate buffer at pH 6·5 in the presence of zinc sulphate. After 2 minutes 5 N-NaOH and ascorbic acid are added. The fluorescence is read after 5–30 minutes; adrenolutine gives maximum fluorescence at 545 mμ with an activating wavelength of 425 mμ, while noradrenolutine is activated at 410 mμ and read at 535 mμ. When these substances are present together, differential estimation is best obtained by using activating wavelengths of 410 and 455 mμ and taking readings at 540 mμ.

The blank values are kept to a minimum and the product is more stable if ethylenediamine is added to the mixture (23, 24): again mixtures can be · estimated by using two activating wavelengths.

Iodine is another oxidizing agent which has been used successfully (12). After transformation to the lutines the intensity of fluorescence is increased by adjusting the pH to 5·3. Readings are taken at 510 mμ with an activating wavelength of 510 mμ.

The trihydroxyindole methods are capable of measuring down to about 0·02 μg catecholamine per ml. Still higher sensitivity but rather less specificity is obtained in the *ethylenediamine method*. The catecholamines condense with this reagent to give strongly fluorescent compounds (42). Reactions between oxidized catechols and various amines and diamines have been widely studied and many give fluorescent products (30, 55). Substitution normally occurs in the para positions to the quinoid oxygens but when no such position is available condensation takes place with the quinoid oxygen. Thus adrenaline rapidly forms adrenochrome which condenses with ethylenediamine as shown in Fig. 10.5(a). Noradrenaline, however, cyclizes much more slowly

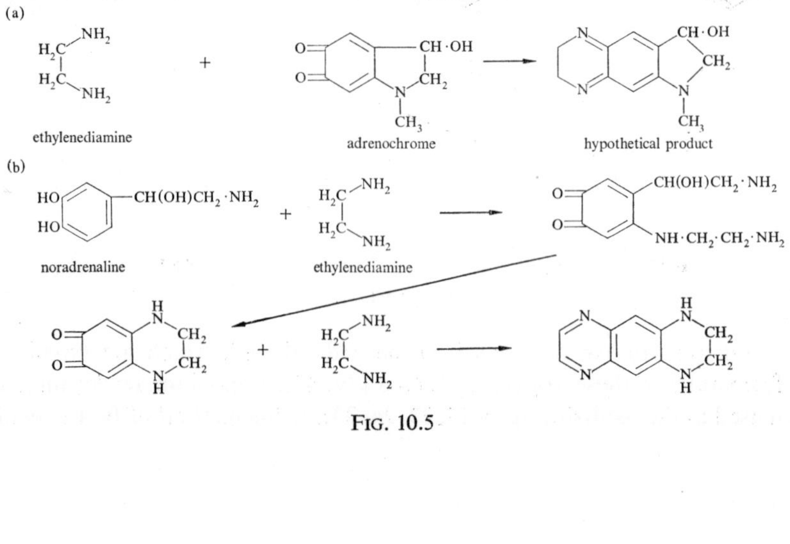

FIG. 10.5

than adrenaline, and ethylenediamine conjugates at the available *para* position to the quinoid oxygen (position 6). Then cyclization of the ethylenediamine side chain takes place and the β-ethanolamine portion of the molecule is eliminated (Fig. 10.5(b)). Another molecule of ethylenediamine then condenses with the quinoid oxygens and gives a product identical to that obtained by reaction of catechol and ethylenediamine.

After condensation with ethylenediamine the fluorescent compounds are extracted in organic solvents for quantitative determination (56, 57, 58). Adrenaline and noradrenaline can be differentiated by reading the fluorescence at 480 and 550 mμ. The intensity of fluorescence of noradrenaline is similar at both wavelengths but the fluorescence of adrenaline is four times stronger at 550 mμ.

A specific method has been described for dopamine (13). In this procedure there are three steps: (a) oxidation by iodine at pH 6·5, (b) molecular rearrangement by the addition of alkaline sulphite which at the same time prevents further oxidation and (c) adjustment of the pH to 5·3 producing a 5,6-dihydroxyindole (Fig. 10.6) which fluoresces at an activation (345 mμ) and

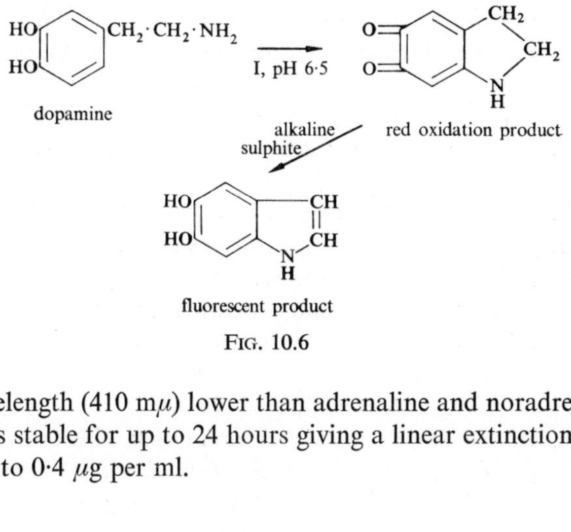

FIG. 10.6

emission wavelength (410 mμ) lower than adrenaline and noradrenaline. The fluorescence is stable for up to 24 hours giving a linear extinction curve with quantities up to 0·4 μg per ml.

REFERENCES

1 ARMIN, J. and GRANT, R. T. *J. Physiol.* **121**, 593 (1953).

2 AUERBACH, M. E. and ANGELL, E. *Science* **109**, 537 (1949).

3 AXELROD, J., ALBERS, R. W. and CLEMENTE, C. D. *J. Neurochem.* **5**, 68 (1959).

4 BARNEA, A. and SHELESNYAK, M. C. *J. Endocr.* **31**, 271 (1965).

5 BERTLER, Å., CARLSSON, A. and ROSENGREN, E. *Acta physiol. scand.* **44**, 273 (1958).

6 BERTLER, Å., FALCK, B., HILLARP, N.-Å., ROSENGREN, E. and TORP, A. *Acta physiol. scand.* **47,** 251 (1959).

7 BIRKE, G., EULER, U. S. VON and STROM, G. *Acta med. scand.* **164,** 219 (1959).

8 BLASCHKO, H. *Pharmac. Rev.* **11,** 307 (1959).

9 BLOOM, G., ÖSTLUND, E., EULER, U. S. VON, LISHAJKO, F., RITZEN. M. and ADAMS-RAY, J. *Acta physiol. scand.* **53,** Suppl. 185 (1961).

10 BOYLEN, J. B. and QUASTEL, J. H. *Biochem. J.* **80,** 644 (1961).

11 BURN, J. H. and RAND, M. J. *J. Physiol.* **144,** 314 (1958).

12 CARLSSON, A. *Pharmac. Rev.* **11,** 300 (1959).

13 CARLSSON, A. and WALDECK, B. *Acta physiol. scand.* **44,** 293 (1958).

14 CLARK, W. G. and DRELL, W. *Fedn Proc.* **13,** 343 (1954).

15 COUPLAND, R. E. and HEATH, I. D. *J. Endocr.* **22,** 59 (1961).

16 COUPLAND, R. E. and HEATH, I. D. *J. Endocr.* **22,** 71 (1961).

17 ELMADJIAN, F. In *Methods in Hormone Research* (edited by R. I. Dorfman) Vol. 1, Academic Press, New York (1962).

18 EULER, U. S. VON. In *Comparative Endocrinology* (edited by U. S. von Euler and H. Heller) p. 258, Academic Press, New York (1963).

19 EULER, U. S. VON and HAMBERG, U. *Acta physiol. scand.* **19,** 74 (1949).

20 EULER, U. S. VON, HAMBERG, U. and HELLNER, S. *Biochem. J.* **49,** 655 (1951).

21 EULER, U. S. VON and HELLNER, S. *Acta physiol. scand.* **22,** 161 (1951).

22 EULER, U. S. VON, IKKOS, D. and LUFTE, R. *Acta endocr. Copenh.* **38,** 441 (1961).

23 EULER, U. S. VON and LISHAJKO, F. *Acta physiol. scand* **45,** 122 (1959).

24 EULER, U. S. VON and LISHAJKO, F. *Acta physiol. scand.* **51,** 348 (1961).

25 GADDUM, J. H. and HOLZBAUER, M. *Vitams Horm.* **15,** 151 (1957).

26 GADDUM, J. H., PEART, W. S. and VOGT, M. *J. Physiol.* **108,** 467 (1949).

27 GADDUM, J. H. and SCHILD, H. *J. Physiol.* **80,** 9P (1934).

28 GOMORI, G. In *Microscopic Histochemistry, Principles and Practice,* University of Chicago Press, Chicago (1952).

29 GOODALL, M. and KIRSCHNER, N. *J. biol. Chem.* **226,** 213 (1957).

30 HACKMAN, R. H. and TODD, A. R. *Biochem. J.* **55,** 631 (1953).

31 HAMBERG, U. and EULER, U. S. VON *Acta chem. scand.* **4,** 1185 (1950).

32 HARLEY-MASON, J. *J. Chem. Soc.* 1276 (1950).

33 HARTMAN, W. J., AKAWIE, R. I. and CLARK, W. G. *J. biol. Chem.* **216,** 507 (1955).

34 JACOBS, S. L., SOBEL, C. and HENRY, R. J. *J. clin. Endocr.* **21,** 305 (1961).

35 JACOBS, S. L., SOBEL, C. and HENRY, R. J. *J. clin. Endocr.* **21,** 315 (1961).

36 JAMES, W. O. *Nature, Lond.* **161,** 851 (1948).

37 JOHNELS, A. G. and PALMGREN, A. *Acta zool., Stockh.* **41,** 313 (1960).

38 KUNTZMAN, R., SHORE, P. A., BOGDANSKI, D. and BRODIE, B. B. *J. Neurochem.* **6,** 226 (1961).

39 LUND, A. *Acta pharmac. tox.* **5,** 75 (1949).
40 LUND, A. *Acta pharmac. tox.* **6,** 137 (1950).
41 MONTAGU, K. *Biochem. J.* **86,** 9 (1963).
42 NATELSON, S., LUGOVOY, J. K. and PINCUS, J. B. *Archs Biochem.* **23,** 157 (1949).
43 PAOLETTI, R., SMITH, R. L., MAICKEL, R. P. and BRODIE, B. B. *Bioch. biophys. Res. Commun.* **5,** 424 (1961).
44 PEARSE, A. G. E. In *Histochemistry, Theoretical and Applied,* Churchill, London (1960).
45 RAAB, W. *Biochem. J.* 37, 470 (1942).
46 RICHTER, D. and BLASCHKO, H. *J. Chem. Soc.* 601 (1937).
47 SHAW, F. H. *Biochem. J.* **32,** 19 (1938).
48 SMITH, R. L., PAOLETTI, R. and BRODIE, B. B. *Biochem. J.* **84,** 51P (1962).
49 SONENBERG, M. *Vitams Horm.* **16,** 205 (1958).
50 SUTHERLAND, E. W. and RALL, T. W. *Pharmac. Rev.* **12,** 265 (1960).
51 SUZUKI, T. and OZAKI, T. *Tohuku J. exp. Med.* **54,** 332 (1951).
52 VOGT, M. *Br. J. Pharmac. Chemother.* **7,** 325 (1952).
53 VOORHESS, M. L. and GARDNER, L. I. *J. clin. Endocr.* **21,** 321 (1961).
54 VOORHESS, M. L. and GARDNER, L. I. *J. clin. Endocr.* **22,** 126 (1962).
55 WALLERSTEIN, J. S., ALBA, R. T. and HALE, M. G. *Biochim. biophys. Acta* **1,** 175 (1947).
56 WEIL-MALHERBE, H. and BONE, A. D. *Biochem. J.* **51,** 311 (1952).
57 WEIL-MALHERBE, H. and BONE, A. D. *Lancet* i, 974 (1953).
58 WEIL-MALHERBE, H. and BONE, A. D. *Biochem. J.* **58,** 132 (1954).
59 WEIL-MALHERBE, H., WHITBY, L. G. and AXELROD, J. *J. Neurochem.* **8,** 55 (1961).
60 WINEGRAD, A. I. *Vitams Horm.* **20,** 175 (1962).

11

THE STEROID HORMONES

All the steroid hormones have the perhydrocyclopentanephenanthrene ring system (Fig. 11.1) as the basic structure, the rings being identified by the letters A, B, C and D. The steroids considered here contain up to 21 carbon

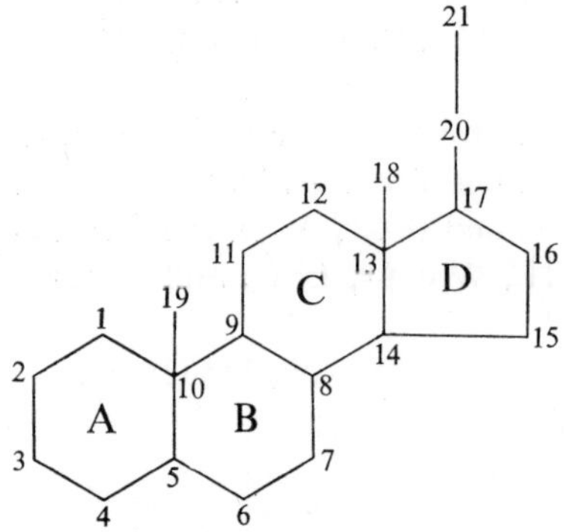

FIG. 11.1

atoms (C_{21} steroids) numbered as shown. Each carbon atom bears two hydrogen atoms except when it is common to two rings (i.e. at $C_{(5)}$, $C_{(10)}$, $C_{(8)}$, $C_{(9)}$, $C_{(13)}$, $C_{(14)}$). These hydrogen atoms are not usually written in the structure unless it is required to draw special attention to configuration. Positions 18 and 19 are usually occupied by angular methyl groups unless otherwise indicated.

Stereoisomerism

Each six-membered ring exists in one of two forms, usually as a chair, and rarely (48) as a boat which is thermodynamically less stable (7) (Fig. 11.2).

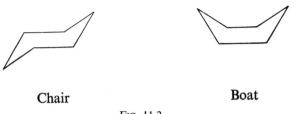

Chair   Boat

FIG. 11.2

Stereoisomerism can occur depending on the orientation in space of one ring to another. The two commonest structures in the natural steroids are shown in Fig. 11.3 where it is seen that they differ only in the manner by which rings A and B are joined at $C_{(5)}$. In the first, rings A and B have the *trans* or α configuration and in the second the *cis* or β configuration. In both structures rings B/C and C/D are *trans*. The conformations of ring D and of the

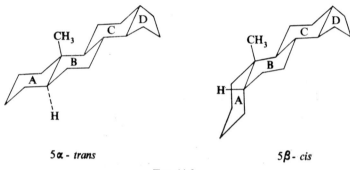

5α - *trans*   5β - *cis*

FIG. 11.3

2-carbon side chain at positions 20 and 21 are less certainly known than those of the C_{19} skeleton. Certain evidence from X-ray crystallography and optical rotation dispersion spectra (58) suggests that ring D is a strained half-chair with $C_{(15)}$ close to the line projected through $C_{(8)}$ and $C_{(10)}$, and $C_{(17)}$ close to the line parallel to this through $C_{(12)}$ and $C_{(16)}$.

Stereoisomerism also occurs due to groups attached to the ring carbon atoms, since they may be orientated below or above the plane of the ring (α and β respectively). Conventionally the α bonds are indicated by dashed, and the β bonds by solid lines, and the methyl group at position 19 is arbitrarily given the β configuration. Thus in the structures shown in Fig. 11.3 it is seen that in the first, where rings A and B are *trans* the H substituent at $C_{(5)}$ is *trans* and the isomer is accordingly the 5α isomer; in the second the H substituent is *cis* and is, therefore, the 5β isomer.

Distinction may also be made between equatorial bonds which lie close to the plane of the ring to which they are attached, and axial bonds which lie more or less perpendicular to the main plane of the ring (7) (Fig. 11.4).

Q

Absolute configuration

In Fig. 11.3 the methyl group at position 19 has been assigned the custo-mary β configuration. In a total synthesis of a steroid, the mirror image, dif-fering in absolute configuration from the β form, is also produced. The abso-lute configuration of nearly all steroids has now been established; only those with the β configuration are biologically active (88).

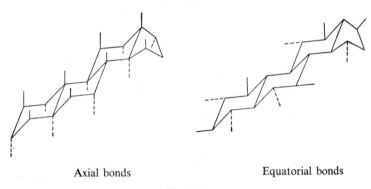

Axial bonds   Equatorial bonds

FIG. 11.4

Nomenclature

The names and formulae of the parent hydrocarbons are given in Fig. 11.5. It should be noted that whereas *androst*ane and *oestr*ane refer to the 5α isomers, pregnane refers to the 5β isomer.

Allo compounds refer to those which differ from the natural or typical steroids with reference to configuration at $C_{(5)}$ e.g. pregnanediol (5β) and allopregnanediol (5α). When the configuration differs at any other carbon atom, the prefix *epi* is used, e.g. testosterone (17β hydroxyl group) and epitestosterone (17α hydroxyl group).

The suffix, *-ane*, indicates a fully saturated nucleus, *-ene* the presence of one double bond, and *-diene*, two double bonds etc.; (the terminal 'e' is dropped before a vowel). The position of the double bond is indicated by the number of the carbon atom from which it originates and it is understood to terminate at the next higher carbon atom unless an alternative is possible, in which case it is indicated. Thus a bond originating at $C_{(5)}$ can terminate at $C_{(6)}$ or $C_{(10)}$ and is designated 5-ene or 5(10)-ene respectively. For convenience a double bond is often indicated by Δ, thus Δ^4- indicates a double bond originating from $C_{(4)}$.

Alcohols are indicated by the suffixes *-ol, -diol, -triol*, etc. or by the pre-fixes *hydroxy, dihydroxy, trihydroxy*, etc., and ketones by the suffixes *-one, -dione*, or prefix *oxo*. The prefix *dehydro* is used to indicate the elimination of two hydrogen atoms, e.g. in dehydroepiandrosterone (Fig. 11.6) and

5α-series   5β-series

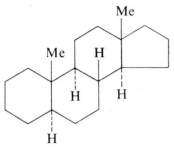

5α- androstane   5β- androstane (aetiocholane)

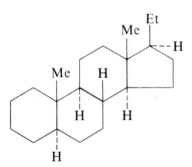

5α- pregnane (allopregnane)

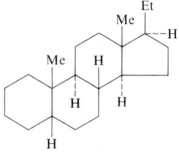

5β- pregnane

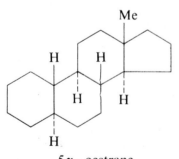

5α- oestrane

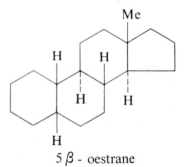

5 β - oestrane

Fig. 11.5. The names and formulae of the parent hydrocarbons of the steroid hormones. Trivial names used in this and following Chapters will be found in Appendix Table 2

di(tetra)hydro for the addition of two (four) hydrogen atoms, e.g. in tetra-hydrocortisol (Fig. 11.6).

Deoxy indicates the elimination of an oxygen atom; thus corticosterone is 11β, 21-dihydroxypregn-4-ene-3, 20-dione and deoxycorticosterone is 21-hydroxypregn-4-ene-3,20-dione, the 11β-ol being replaced by H.

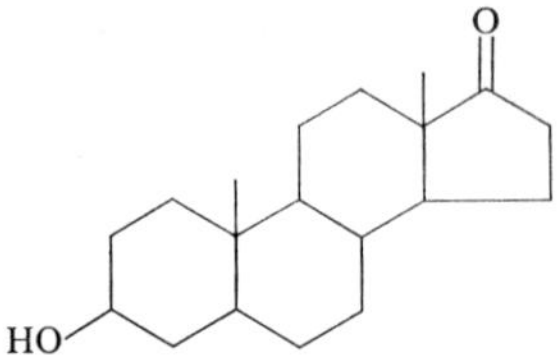

epiandrosterone
(3β-hydroxy-5α-androstan-17-one)

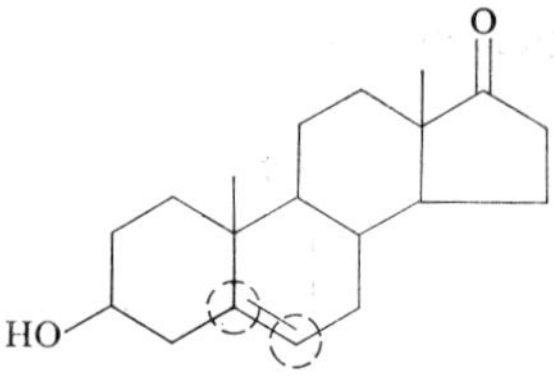

dehydroepiandrosterone
(3β-hydroxyandrost-5-en-17-one)

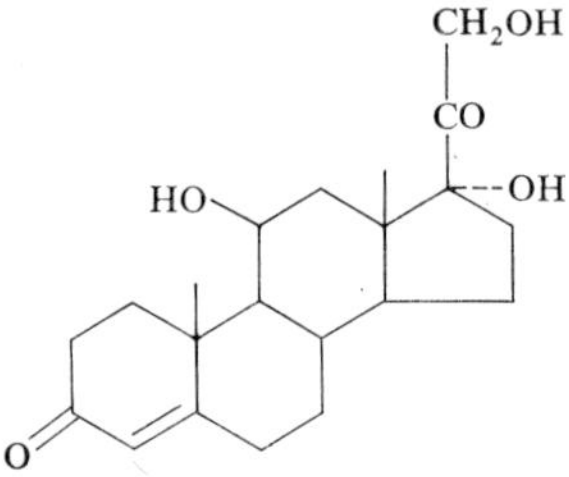

cortisol
(11β,17α,21-trihydroxypregn -4-
ene-3,20-dione)

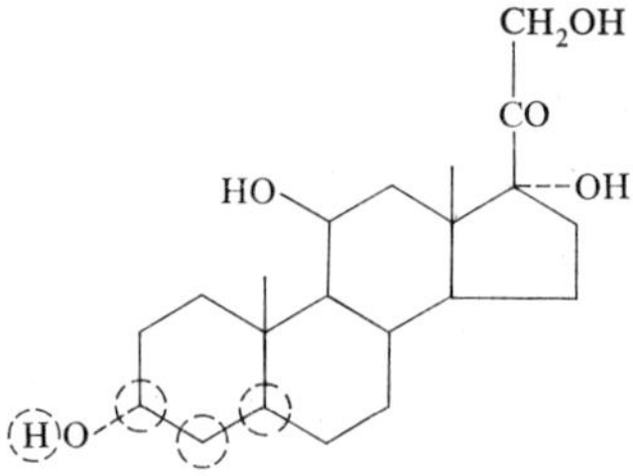

tetrahydrocortisol
(3α,11β,17α,21-tetrahydroxy-5β-
pregnan-20- one)

FIG. 11.6

The prefix *nor* indicates the elimination of a methyl group. Progesterone is pregn-4-ene-3,20-dione and nor-progesterone lacks the methyl group at $C_{(19)}$ and becomes an oestrane derivative, oestra-4-ene-3,20-dione.

The term *homo* indicates an enlargement of a ring. Many synthetic steroids are known with 6 carbons in ring D, e.g. D-homotestosterone.

Physical and chemical methods for the determination of structure

In order to establish with certainty the structure of a steroid, it is necessary to use several independent methods. The purpose of this section is to review briefly some of the more useful of these techniques.

In the technique of *rotatory dispersion*, the optical rotation is plotted against the wavelength of the incident light. Spectropolarimeters are now available which permit measurements to be taken from 700 mμ to about 270 mμ in about one hour.

Compounds which do not absorb light within the observed range give smooth absorption curves called 'plain' curves: the molecular rotation (symbol M, or preferably ϕ) increases in magnitude towards the lower wavelengths and the curves have no maxima or minima. Compounds which do absorb light give more complex curves, usually with one or more pronounced maxima or minima ('Cotton'-effect curves). These are called 'peaks' or 'troughs' and the curves are positive or negative, depending on whether the major feature of longer wavelengths is a peak or a trough. Examples of each of these curves are given in Figure 11.7.

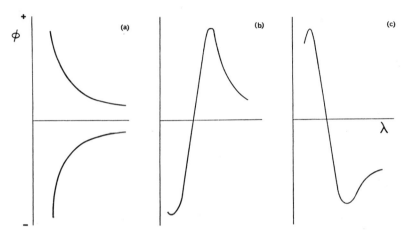

FIG. 11.7. Rotatory dispersion curves

(*a*) Plain curve
(*b*) Positive curve
(*c*) Negative curve

Ketones and aldehydes are convenient absorbing groups (λ max. 280–300 mμ) and may be recognized even if chemically they are rather inert. Djerassi has examined a complete range of steroids with ketone groups in all possible positions (49). Each position has its characteristic type of wave.

The technique is most valuable in problems concerned with *relative* stereochemistry of two or more centres in the same molecule. Thus reduction of Δ^4-3-ones can give 5α (A/B *trans*) or 5β (A/B *cis*) compounds and the two compounds have Cotton-effect curves with different signs; α is positive and β is negative.

For further information on this technique and on the results obtained the reader is referred to several recent reviews (46, 47, 77, 78).

A recent development is *circular dichroism*, which makes it possible to measure the difference in absorption coefficient between right-handed and left-handed circularly polarized light. The stereochemical information obtained is similar to that from rotatory dispersion measurements (22, 130).

Another physical method useful for structural investigations is *mass spectrometry*, which has the advantage that only a small quantity of steroid is required. A large number of deuterium-labelled steroids have been synthesized and used in this method for the investigation of hydrogen-transfer reactions, e.g. the enolization of 11-oxosteroids (139). Mass spectra of mono-ketones in all possible positions of the nucleus have been published (20).

From these it is possible to narrow down the possible points of attachment of the carbonyl groups and in combination with optical rotatory dispersion measurements the position can be established in virtually all instances.

The processes involved in mass spectrometry have been discussed in detail by Reed (98) and the application of the technique to the elucidation of structure has formed the subject of a recently published monograph (21).

Nuclear magnetic resonance is likely to be used a great deal in the future. Information is obtained about the local magnetic fields surrounding a given magnetic nucleus which arise from the movements of nearby electrons and from the magnetic dipoles of neighbouring nuclei. From this information deductions can be made about the distribution of these electrons and the arrangement and nature of the nuclei. The proton has a large magnetic moment and is easily recognized. Molecules with molecular weight of not less than 300 usually give sharp, well-resolved spectra with peaks associated with the various proton-containing linkages. The area under a peak gives a measure of the number of protons associated with the peak. The spectrum of a molecule is a characteristic 'fingerprint' of the molecule as is the infra-red spectrum; the hydrogen-containing functional groups giving rise to lines at characteristic values of the applied magnetic field for a given radiofrequency. Thus each group has its own characteristic chemical shift and the presence or absence of a group can often be indicated. Tables of these characteristics have been published (19, 33, 148, 149). Recent applications of the technique have been the determination of the configuration of 6-substituents in Δ^4-3-oxosteroids (39, 142), and investigations of the 18- and 19- methyl groups (148, 149).

A disadvantage of the technique at the present time is that up to 25–50 mg of material is required.

Infra-red spectrometry has been widely used in this field. The near infra-red absorption spectrum is one of the most highly characteristic physical properties of a molecule; quite minor changes in chemical structure or in stereochemical configuration alter the spectrum significantly. In the 'fingerprint' region (wave number about 1200–700cm^{-1}) the spectrum, with few exceptions, is absolutely specific for any one compound.

With modern instruments the quantity of sample required is small and, furthermore, it is unchanged during the analysis and can be recovered for further work. Compounds are normally examined in solvents such as carbon disulphide, bromoform or chloroform or in the solid state, e.g. in potassium bromide (101, 116). Measurements in solution are preferred because the spectra of solids may be complicated by intramolecular hydrogen bonding and by polymorphic effects (31, 44).

Tables listing the characteristic frequencies of the absorption bands for most steroids and derivatives are published (72, 102). The technique is particularly useful for detecting oxygen-containing groups in various positions on the steroid nucleus or for distinguishing equatorial and axial hydroxyl and other groups (96). Similar information about CH, CH_2 and CH_3 groups can more readily be obtained from nuclear magnetic resonance spectra.

The Δ^4-3-oxo group, common to so many biologically active steroids, absorbs strongly in the ultraviolet (λ max. about 240 mμ). The method of *ultraviolet spectroscopy* is commonly used for the quantitative estimation of certain steroids containing this group, notably progesterone. There has been a large number of publications dealing with u.v. absorption bands and correlation with structure: earlier literature was reviewed by Dorfman (51) and later by Dusza *et al.* (52). The absorption is usually measured in ethanol, but methanol, ether and chloroform have also been used. The presence of substituents in other positions of the steroid molecule may result in batho-chromic or hypsochromic effects on the absorption maximum of the Δ^4-3-one. Substitution of a halogen atom for the 9α-hydrogen atom in cortisol results in a hypsochromic effect (-3 mμ) with fluorine and this effect becomes bathochromic in proceeding from fluorine through chlorine to bromine. The introduction of an 11β-hydroxyl group has no influence on the absorption maximum of the Δ^4-3-ones. The presence of such a grouping may be recog-nized, however, since oxidation to the 11-oxo group has a hypsochromic effect (-3 to -5 mμ).

The ultraviolet absorption characteristics of double bonds in many other positions of the steroid nucleus have been reported (52). Notable advances have been made, in spite of practical difficulties, in the measurement of absorption in the region 190–210 mμ. Ellington and Meakins (54) have examined 47 steroids in this region. Double bonds of the type —HC = CH—, CH_2 = C<, —HC = C<, >C = C< and Δ^7 steroids all show maximum absorption between 195 and 197 mμ.

Polarography has been used both for qualitative and for quantitative work. Direct cathodic waves are given by Δ^4-3-oxosteroids but a far more satis-factory method is to use the water-soluble Girard hydrazones (4, 143). Cathodic waves are given in solutions of pH 5·6 by Δ^4-3-ones, 17-ones and 20-ones. The half-wave potentials are slightly different for each so that both the 3- and 20- waves are recognized in progesterone or deoxycorticosterone (Fig. 11.8). The 20-one wave, however, is absent in 17-hydroxysteroids; thus cortisol shows only a 3-one wave. Ketones at $C_{(11)}$ or at $C_{(3)}$ in a saturated ring A do not react.

A number of other steroid hydrazones give polarographic waves similar to the Girard T hydrazones (5). The only two substances tested which appear as possible practical alternatives to Girard T reagent, however, are maleic acid monohydrazide and aminoguanidine, but they appear to offer no advantages over the former reagent.

The absorption spectrum of a steroid in *concentrated sulphuric acid* is often useful to establish its identity, its purity or its concentration. An extensive

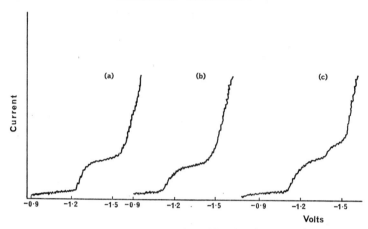

FIG. 11.8. Polarograms of the Girard hydrazones of:

(*a*) androsterone (17-ketone wave)
(*b*) cortisone (3-ketone wave)
(*c*) Progesterone (3- and 20-ketone waves)

review of these spectra appeared in 1950 (144) and lately the spectra of over 400 steroids have been published (112).

Usually a final concentration of 5–50 μg/ml is required, the acid being added to the dried steroid and allowed to stand for two hours at room temperature in the dark. The spectra are then recorded between 220 and 600 mμ. The spectra of some steroids alter remarkably with time and this property may be useful in distinguishing epimeric pairs of hydroxysteroids. Thus 11α- and 11β-hydroxyandrost-4-ene-3,17-dione show dissimilar spectra for the first two hours, but become virtually identical by four hours (11). In other cases the extinction coefficient at a particular wavelength may be useful: by this means testosterone may be distinguished from its $C_{(17)}$ epimer.

An extensive investigation of the correlation of structure with sulphuric acid spectra has been made by Bernstein and Lenhard (10). Some of their findings relevant to the steroids discussed in this book are shown in Table 11.1. There is considerable overlapping of absorption bands for various structural groups, and in addition to the details given it is found that hydroxyl groups give fairly general absorption between 300 and 600 mμ. Thus interpretation of an unknown curve may be very difficult by this technique.

Many steroids *fluoresce*, particularly in concentrated sulphuric acid or phosphoric acid. Now that sensitive and accurate spectrofluorimeters are available, methods have been developed for the quantitative estimation of several steroids in blood and urine. For basic reading on the subject of fluorescence the reader is referred to the article of Bowen (15).

A major advantage of the technique is its great sensitivity which is usually several times greater than the corresponding colorimetric procedure. How-

TABLE 11.1

*The absorption maxima of the sulphuric acid chromogens of structures
commonly occurring in steroid hormones*

Structure	Sulphuric acid chromogen. Absorption maximum (mμ)
$\Delta^{1,4}$-3-one	247–267 and 295–318
Δ^4-3-one	279–302
3-ol	300–350
Δ^4-6β-hydroxy-3-one $\Delta^{4,6}$-3-one	343–346
17α-hydroxy-17-acetyl side chain 17-ketol side chain	400–499
17-dihydroxyacetone side chain	450–549

ever, the fluorescence spectra usually vary less from one steroid to another than do the absorption spectra. The problem of *quenching* has received a great deal of attention and methods for its correction have included the use of internal standards (17, 68), the use of correction formulae (16) and the differential quenching of the fluorescence of the steroid and of the non-specific material (86). In the latter method, for example, the fluorescence of pure steroids in strong acid is quenched by nitrate or hydrogen peroxide at a different rate to the quenching of the non-specific fluorescence, and such a method has been applied to the estimation of oestrogens.

Biosynthesis and metabolism of steroids

In vitro STUDIES

In order to study the biosynthesis and metabolism of steroids, it is convenient to use *in vitro* techniques with homogenates, minces or slices of isolated organs. Such studies are carried out in artificial media which must inevitably contain very different relative concentrations of proteins, hormones, co-factors etc. to those which are present *in vivo*. It may be quite wrong, therefore, to believe that the reactions observed even remotely resemble those in intact animals. It is not surprising that the apparent activity of certain steroids is different *in vitro* from the activity *in vivo* (12, 61). In spite of this, considerable knowledge of steroid metabolism in endocrine tissue has been gained by such studies.

Labelled steroids

Labelled steroids are almost indispensable for metabolic studies both *in vivo* and *in vitro*. They also play an important part in isotopic dilution methods of estimation and as internal standards.

TABLE 11.2

Determination of plasma progesterone by a double isotope derivative method (100)

Steps in method	Unknown 10 ml plasma containing P_p μg progesterone	Standard P_s μg progesterone
Addition of internal indicator (0·075 μC, 0·9 mμg of [1,2-³H]progesterone)	X_p counts per minute (cpm)	X_s cpm
Extraction in ether and washing		
Formation of derivative ([3,20-bis-³⁵S]-thiosemicarbazone) by reaction at 48° for 16 hours with 1 mg [³⁵S]thiosemi-carbazide		
Thin layer chromatography (benzene–acetone–methanol, 89 : 1 : 10 by vol. in two dimensions)		
Paper chromatography (propylene glycol : toluene)		
Hydrolysis to [3-³⁵S]thiosemicarbazone by reaction with pyruvic acid at 45° for 1 hour		
Thin layer chromatography (benzene–acetone–methanol, 96 : 1 : 3 by vol. and dichloromethane–acetone–methanol, 98 : 1 : 1 by vol.)		
Acetylation to [3-³⁵S]thiosemicarbazone-2,4-diacetate by reaction with acetic anhydride in pyridine		
Thin layer chromatography (benzene–methanol, 90 : 10 v/v and methylene dichloride–methanol, 95 : 5 v/v)		
Paper chromatography (propylene glycol–toluene)		
Final counting of ³⁵S and ³H	S_p cpm H_p cpm	S_s cpm H_s cpm

At each chromatography the appropriate inert derivative is added as a carrier. **Calculation of result:** the percentage recovery is obtained from the ³H counts, i.e. $\dfrac{H_p \times 100}{X_p}$ for the unknown and $\dfrac{H_s \times 100}{X_s}$ for standard.

(The mean recovery reported for the method is 3%)

The final ³⁵S counts reflect the amount of progesterone originally present in the

In metabolic studies they avoid the use of massive, unphysiological doses. Ring-labelled ^{14}C compounds are useful since the label is not lost during metabolism but such compounds may be difficult to prepare and have low specific activity. Tritium-labelled compounds are easier to prepare and can be made with very high specific activity, but they are less satisfactory in some metabolic experiments unless the isotope is in an inactive part of the molecule so that it is not lost. There are also certain difficulties in counting tritium in biological fluids such as urine. Numerous examples of the use of both isotopes will be given in the later chapters.

The *secretion rate* of a steroid is often of more value clinically than the concentration in plasma or urine (18). The determination of secretion rate becomes a relatively simple problem by the use of a labelled steroid. It is given by injection or by infusion and the specific activities of the metabolites are measured in the urine. Reviews describing the use of labelled steroids in the measurement of secretion rates have appeared (120, 129).

The use of radioactive steroids as internal standards is necessary in order to correct for the large and variable losses that may be encountered in complicated methods. Thus in the determination of testosterone in plasma recoveries as low as 13 per cent have been recorded.

Labelled derivatives are frequently prepared in order to increase the specificity of methods. Tritium-labelled acetic anhydride and [^{35}S]thiosemicarbazide are examples of reagents that have been used. They may be usefully employed in combination with an internal standard labelled with a different isotope. An example of the use of these techniques is shown in Fig. 11.9 which describes the steps involved in a recent method for plasma progesterone (100).

BIOSYNTHESIS OF CHOLESTEROL

The synthesis of cholesterol is an integral part of the processes leading up to the formation of the physiologically active steroids. It has been established that acetate is the primary carbon source of cholesterol, there being probably about thirty separate reactions involved in the pathway through squalene and lumisterol to cholesterol. Much of the experimental work has been done

---

plasma and in the standard. The amount originally present in the standard is known (P_s) and therefore the amount in the plasma (P_p) can be calculated:

$$P_p = \frac{X_p}{H_p} \times \frac{H_s}{X_s} \times \frac{S_p}{S_s} \times P_s$$

The non-specific blank values are between 0·02 and 0·029 μg per 100 ml. The levels of progesterone found in human plasma by this method are:

Females, luteal phase   1·04 μg per 100 ml.
          follicular phase   0·113 μg per 100 ml.
Males   0·028 μg per 100 ml.

by *in vitro* studies using rat liver slices incubated with acetate labelled with ^{14}C both at the methyl and the carboxyl groups, or doubly-labelled acetate as in $^{13}CH_3$ $^{14}COOH$ (41, 84). By this means, and by degradation of the product, it is possible to find out which carbon atoms in cholesterol originate from the methyl groups and which from the carboxyl groups of acetate. The origin of all 27 carbon atoms is now known (Fig. 11.9).

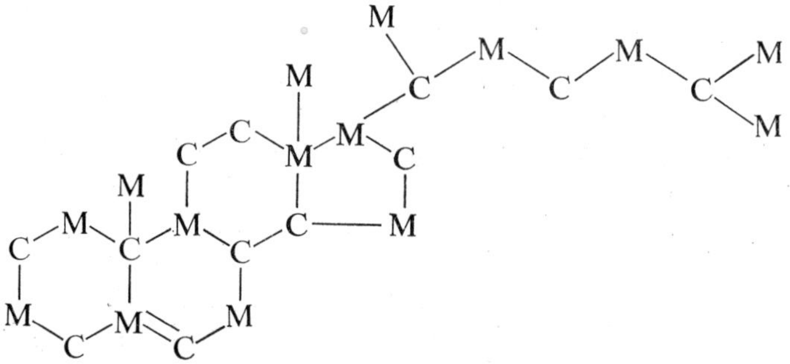

Fig. 11.9. Biosynthesis of cholesterol: carbon atoms C originate from carboxyl groups and M originate from methyl groups

Total synthesis has also been shown to occur in a variety of other tissues such as the adrenal cortex and the gonads.

Extensive reviews on the synthetic pathways have appeared (13, 37) but our chief interest in this book is concerned with the role of cholesterol as a hormone precursor rather than on the mechanism of cholesterol synthesis itself.

Steroids and enzymes

The principal metabolic changes undergone by steroids are oxidation and reduction, conjugation and hydrolysis. Oxidation and reduction may be classified into (1) interconversions of alcohols and ketones, (2) introduction or hydrogenation of C=C bonds, (3) hydroxylations and (4) oxidative scission of the side chain. These reactions may occur in the liver and many peripheral tissues as well as in the adrenals and gonads.

It has been found that catalytic amounts of some steroids mediate the transfer of hydrogen between NAD and NADP in the presence of some mammalian hydroxysteroid dehydrogenases. The term *hydroxysteroid dehydrogenase* was proposed for those pyridine-nucleotide linked enzymes which catalyse reversible oxidations of hydroxyl groups on the steroid nucleus or side chain (121). These catalysts exhibit high specificity with respect to the position and steric configuration of the hydroxyl group undergoing oxidation. The reaction may be represented as:

steroid alcohol + NAD(NADP)⇌

steroid ketone + $NADH_2(NADPH_2)$ + H^+

Several of these enzymes have been purified. A 3α-hydroxysteroid dehydrogenase *Pseudomonas testosteroni* (85) reacts with NAD but not with NADP. It oxidizes 3α-hydroxyl groups of C_{19} and C_{21} steroids in which the A/B ring junction is either *cis* or *trans*, although *cis* steroids react more slowly. Another 3α-hydroxysteroid dehydrogenase purified from rat liver (125) reacts equally well with NAD and NADP and A/B *cis* steroids react more rapidly than *trans*. A 3β-hydroxysteroid dehydrogenase also occurs in rat liver and this converts testosterone to androstenedione. Human placentae contain a 17β-hydroxysteroid dehydrogenase capable of converting oestradiol-17β to oestrone with either NAD or NADP as co-enzyme (80). By coupling the two co-enzymes with the dehydrogenase and oestradiol-17β the system can act as a transhydrogenase:

$$\text{-diol} + \text{NAD} \longrightarrow \text{-one} + \text{NADH}_2$$
$$\text{-one} + \text{NADPH}_2 \longrightarrow \text{-diol} + \text{NADP}$$

$$\overline{\text{NAD} + \text{NADPH}_2 \longrightarrow \text{NADP} + \text{NADH}_2}$$

An 11β-hydroxysteroid dehydrogenase obtained from rat liver is effective with both NAD and NADP (69) and converts cortisol to cortisone. In this case, however, there is no evidence that the system acts as a transhydrogenase.

Certain transformations in steroids have long been known to occur by the action of yeasts and bacteria. Such *microbiological methods* are often used for reactions which are otherwise difficult to carry out (56, 119, 133). Thus the hydrolysis of the 11β-acetoxy group is achieved under the influence of *Flavobacterium dehydrogenans* but is difficult by chemical means (35). There are many examples of hydroxylations including the 16α-hydroxylation of oestrone or oestradiol (75) and testosterone (67). The introduction of oxygen

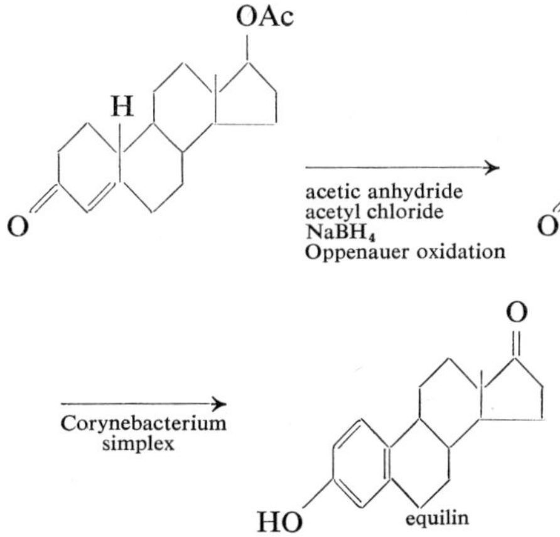

Fig. 11.10

at $C_{(11)}$ is also particularly useful for the production of steroids such as cortisone from natural products.

A microbiological reaction was used in the first synthesis of equilin (146): (Fig. 11.10).

The stereo-specificity of these reactions is well illustrated by the synthesis of two 5β-pregnanediones containing one atom of deuterium in place of the 11α- or the 11β-hydrogen (40). The product from 11α-hydroxylation of [11β-D]5β-pregnanedione with the enzyme from *Rhizopus nigricans* is 11α-hydroxy-5β-pregnanedione with no change in the deuterium content:

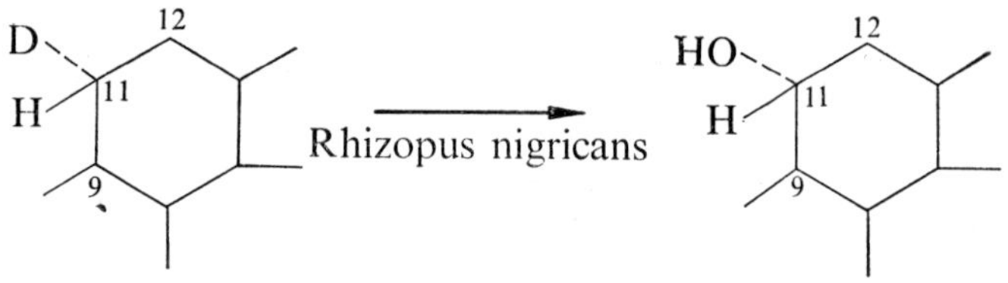

However 11α- hydroxylation of the [11α-D] compound gives the 11α-hydroxy-5β-pregnanedione with the loss of exactly one atom of deuterium:

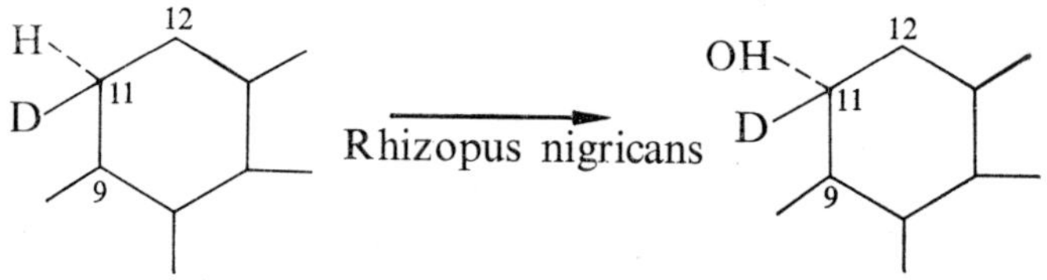

CONJUGATION

Steroids may circulate and are excreted mainly as glucosiduronates and sulphates, usually conjugated at the 3-hydroxyl group and sometimes at hydroxyl groups in other positions (Fig. 11.11).

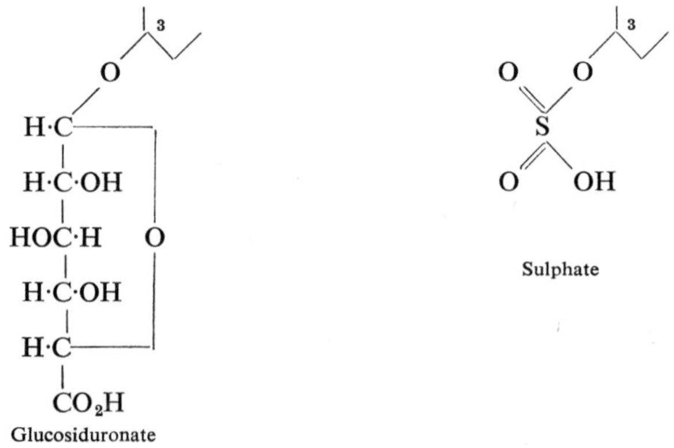

Glucosiduronate　　　　　　Sulphate

FIG. 11.11

The formation of glucosiduronates occurs primarily in the liver where it is believed that uridine diphosphoglucuronic acid (UDPGA) plays a part (70, 111, 118). A hexose molecule is transferred from UDPGA to an alcohol or phenol acceptor and the reaction is probably:

$$UDPGA + R—OH \rightarrow UDP + R—O—GA$$

where R—OH is the acceptor and R—O—GA the conjugate. Although glucuronic acid is joined to UDPGA by an α-linkage an inversion apparently occurs when it is transferred since a β-glucosiduronate results.

The formation of glucosiduronates is an efficient and irreversible process which is probably a means for the inactivation and excretion of the steroid. In contrast, the formation of sulphates is relatively inefficient and the renal clearance is low, and there is probably a fair amount of hydrolysis back to the free steroid. Thus oestrone-3-sulphate is quite active, probably because it is hydrolysed to free oestrone and oestradiol-17β. In this case and in others the activity of the conjugate is, therefore, more prolonged than that of the free steroid itself.

There is fairly good evidence that other conjugates such as phosphates occur in urine and blood (93–95) but their biological significance is not clear.

METABOLISM

The metabolites of individual steroids will be described in succeeding chapters. The Δ^4-3-one group, however, occurs so commonly in biologically active steroids that its metabolism will be mentioned here.

Urinary metabolites lack the Δ^4-3-one group since it is reduced in the liver. This step is probably the rate-limiting factor in the metabolic inactivation of hormones containing this group (126). Preparations of rat liver enzyme, dependent on $NADPH_2$ as hydrogen donor reduce Δ^4-3-oxosteroids giving 5α-H and 5β-H steroids. It is important to note that the reduction of the 3-oxo group does not occur until after the reduction of the double bond, when it then occurs rapidly.

The proportion of 5α to 5β steroids formed depends largely on the structure of the rest of the steroid, and some general conclusions were formulated by Dorfman (see 30). The ratio is 1:1 from C_{19} steroids without an oxygen function at carbon 11 and 4:1 from 11-oxygenated C_{19} steroids, while the 5β form predominates from C_{21} steroids. In man the 3α-ols make up the larger proportion of saturated metabolites of Δ^4-3-oxosteroids but in the rat the 3β-ols predominate.

Stereochemical factors and biological activity

This subject has been reviewed extensively recently (27). Important factors relating to activity are:

(a) OPTICAL ISOMERISM

By synthesis of the corticosteroids, cortisone and aldosterone, it has been shown that the D-compounds possess full biological activity, DL-compounds possess half the activity and L-compounds are inactive (97, 107, 132). Androgenic activity of the C_{19} steroids is confined to the natural optical isomers while all 8 possible stereo isomers of oestrone have been synthesized and again only the natural enantiomorphs possess full activity (71).

In contrast, it has been reported that L-equilenin has a low but definite activity (3).

(b) *Cis-trans* ISOMERISM

The *trans* structure seems essential for the possession of full activity of most steroid hormones which are usually Δ^4-3-ones or $5\alpha(H)$ steroids. A number of other types of activity, e.g. pyrogenic or anaesthetic, have been reported for the $5\beta(H)$ structures (73, 81).

17α-progesterone and 17α-deoxycorticosterone which differ from the

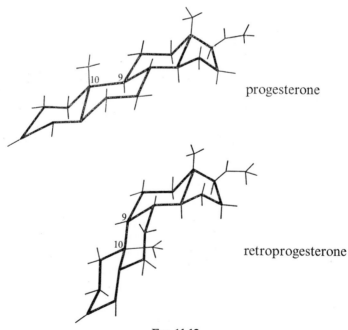

progesterone

retroprogesterone

FIG. 11.12

natural compounds at one centre of symmetry are inactive. Furthermore, changes in only one substituent may lead to inactive isomers. Thus 17-epitestosterone (17α-OH, 17β-H) is less active even than androstenedione; 17-epioestradiol is very weakly active; 11-epicortisol and 11-epicorticosterone are inert. However, in the androgen series both the 3α- and 3β-ols are active.

The activity of 9,10 isomeric steroids related to progesterone is remarkable. The normal structure of progesterone is 9α,10β; a group of synthetic steroids made from lumisterol (135, 136) with 9β,10α have been termed *retrosteroids*. They are extremely active as progestogens and show little or no masculinizing effects. In contrast to natural progesterone they are active orally (99, 108, 124). Useful derivatives are 6-dehydro-, 17α-acetoxy- and 6-dehydro-17α-acetoxyretroprogesterone. The contrast in structure between progesterone and retroprogesterone is seen in Fig. 11.12.

(c) OTHER STRUCTURAL CHANGES

Enlargement or contraction of various rings has been studied extensively. D-homo steroids have comparable or even much greater activity than their parents, e.g. in the cases of testosterone, androstenedione and androsterone. However D-homo deoxycorticosterone has no salt-retaining properties.

Contraction of ring A in testosterone, progesterone or cortisone abolishes activity.

A marked change in biological activity is caused by the removal of the 19-CH_3 group, i.e. in the 19-nor steroids. In the cases of progesterone, corticosterone and deoxycorticosterone the 19-nor compounds are more active than the parent steroids. The analogous 18-nor compounds, however, are inactive or only weakly active.

The introduction of double bonds or of halogens may alter considerably the activity of certain corticosteroids and many such compounds have been synthesized for therapeutic use. A 1,2 double bond increases glucocorticoid activity while generally reducing progestational, androgenic and sodium-retaining activities. 6,7 unsaturation of the 11-oxygenated steroids may have the reverse effect.

There are numerous fluorine derivations of the corticosteroids which are highly active. While substitution of 21-OH by fluorine increases both glucocorticosteroid and sodium-retaining activities, substitution by chlorine or bromine abolishes both.

Conclusions

This information, and a great deal more which is outside the scope of this survey (e.g. see 26) undoubtedly illustrates the importance of stereochemical factors on biological activity. It is not easy to draw any general conclusions, however, and it is still true that the mechanisms by which any steroid hormone acts at the cellular level have yet to be elucidated.

R

MODE OF ACTION

There have been many different theories concerning the mode of action of steroids (e.g. 26, 64, 65, 140). A fairly simple explanation of the specificity of hormonal action is in the classical idea of a *receptor*, a chemically reactive group in the cell where the first interaction with the steroid occurs. This would explain the importance of stereochemical factors. Bush (26) concludes from the use of molecular models that changes in the configuration of rings c and d have a greater effect on all types of biological activity than changes in rings A and B. This suggests that the closest and most specific attachment of the steroid to the receptor site would therefore be over the surface around carbon atoms 11, 12, 13, 16, 17 and 18 and in C_{21} steroids, 20 and 21.

However, experimental evidence in support of this theory is hard to obtain since the cell membrane, a likely site for receptors, is difficult to study chemically. It is not surprising, therefore, that other theories have been developed, notably that the steroid enters in some way into an enzyme system either by regulating its activity or by controlling its synthesis (63). Certainly the *in vivo* administration of certain steroids leads to changes in the concentration of enzymes, but it must be remembered that these may be the results of effects on metabolism rather than on direct synthesis of enzymes.

The possible effect of steroids on the permeability of cellular and intracellular membranes has been considered as a likely mode of action. There is a fair amount of evidence to support this concept in the case of protein and polypeptide hormones. Willmer (141) has considered that the arrangement of lipid molecules of different types in cellular membranes might be altered by the incorporation of steroid molecules into the membrane. The suggestion that sodium-retaining corticosteroids might act as lipid-soluble carriers for metal ions (138) is considered by Bush to be untenable (26). He points out that there is no good evidence that the ketol side chain can form the sort of chelates postulated, or that their stability or solubility would be sufficient to function as a carrier.

Finally a hormone-gene theory is now popular. The idea originated from Karlson's work on insect hormones (74) and is supported by the work of Williams-Ashman *et al.* (140) who showed that sex hormones stimulated synthesis of protein in the prostate, seminal vesicles and uterus, and that this synthesis was mediated through increases in messenger RNA. It could be that cellular receptors are in fact macromolecules, probably proteins, possessing areas of complementary structure to the steroid hormones.

Hydrolysis and extraction of steroids

The conjugates are completely hydrolysed by boiling with mineral acid but such treatment may lead to the formation of artifacts. To avoid this, many other methods have been devised.

Enzymic methods are available using preparations of β-glucuronidase and sulphatase. β-glucuronidase has been obtained from bacteria (110), beef liver, limpets (*Patella vulgata* (50)), snails (*Helix Pomatia* (25, p. 370)) and from the preputial gland of rats (114) which is a particularly rich source. Methods of extraction and purification usually consist of fractional precipitation from salt solutions and acetone. The product is standardized by measuring the release of phenolphthalein from its glucuronide.

The pH optimum of β-glucuronidase varies with its source, e.g. it is 4·7 for the limpet, 5·5 for liver and 6·2 for the bacterial preparation (131). Hydrolysis of conjugates is usually carried out at 37° but may need to be prolonged. The best yields are usually obtained when the conjugates are first extracted from urine, probably because there are many substances in urine which inhibit the activity of β-glucuronidase.

Preparations of sulphatase suitable for the hydrolysis of steroid sulphates are obtained from similar sources (66, 103, 104, 106, 117). The sulphatase from *Patella vulgata* has been purified by precipitation in a solution of 30–70 per cent saturated ammonium sulphate, and 33–50 per cent v/v aqueous-acetone at −9°. The enzyme is highly specific for 3β-sulphates of the 5α- and Δ^5-steroids and has no action on the isomeric 3α-sulphates. Inhibitors which occur in urine include Cl^-, SO_4^{2-}, BO_3^{3-} and $H_2PO_4^-$.

Enzymic methods were originally introduced to avoid the formation of artifacts during hydrolysis. However, there is some evidence that they may be formed (131). Thus 3,5-cyclo-androstenolone derived from dehydroepiandrosterone has been detected after enzymic hydrolysis. The production of artifacts may be due, not so much to the direct action of the enzyme, but because hydrolysis may need to go on for up to five days at 37° by which time the artifact may be formed even in the absence of the enzyme.

Slow hydrolysis of the sulphates, but not of the glucosiduronates, occurs at room temperature at pH 1. Hydrolysis may also occur in solvents such as ether or ethyl acetate (*solvolysis*, 24). This is a two-phase process whereby the sulphate is extracted by the solvent from acidified urine containing added NaCl, and is then hydrolysed in the solvent in the presence of acid (usually $2N-H_2SO_4$) at temperatures up to 37° (24, 105, 109). Sulphate conjugates may also be split by treatment with dioxan and trichloroacetic acid (38).

Burstein *et al.* (23) reported that glucosiduronates could be hydrolysed in dry ethyl acetate or tetrahydrofuran in the presence of perchloric acid. This has been reinvestigated by De Paoli *et al.* (43) who confirmed the earlier findings. Since sulphates are hydrolysed at the same time, this method promises to be a useful one for the extraction and hydrolysis of both types of conjugate, since it avoids the troublesome artifacts produced by acid hydrolysis, and takes far less time than the enzyme methods.

The conjugated steroids themselves may be extracted directly into a solvent such as n-butanol, or into a mixture of ether and ethanol from urine acidified to pH 1–2 and partially saturated with ammonium sulphate (53, 59, 79, 147). Ion-exchange methods have also been described, both by column chromatography (27) and by partitioning with liquid exchangers. Recently there have been many reports on the extraction of conjugated steroids by means of gel filtration with Sephadex gels. The G-25 grade retards the conjugated oestrogens and they may be concentrated considerably by this technique (9).

Methods of separation

The steroids differ considerably in polarity. This depends largely on the dipole moment which is determined by the asymmetry of electron-sharing by the constituent atoms, especially in ketonic and alcoholic groups. In solvents there may be an additional effect due to intra-molecular association (H$^+$ bonding). Therefore it is not surprising that nearly all methods of separation make use of these differences in polarity and depend on partitioning between solvents, either by countercurrent distributions or by liquid-liquid partition chromatography. In order to decide on the best procedure for the separation of steroids in a given instance, a knowledge of the *partition coefficients* of these steroids in a variety of solvents is required. An extensive series of partition coefficients has been published recently (55).

Liquid-liquid partitioning as in *countercurrent distributions* pioneered by Craig (42) has been used, particularly for the oestrogens and corticosteroids, both for the separation of mixtures and for checking purity. Efficient automatic countercurrent machines are now available which require very little attention but the method remains rather long compared with other methods and requires large volumes of solvents. It is uncomplicated, however, by any adsorptive effects and is capable of handling relatively large amounts of material. Since equilibrium is obtained at each distribution, the behaviour of the steroid in a given system depends entirely on its partition coefficient. Theoretical distributions can therefore be calculated, and the number of distributions required to achieve a given separation estimated. Thus two steroids can be separated by a 24-transfer countercurrent distribution if the ratio of their partition coefficients is greater than 3, assuming that these coefficients are within the useful working range of the system which in this case would be between 0·1 and 20. Formulae for these calculations have been summarized by Diczfalusy (45). An extension to the method is *steady-state distribution*, in which the liquid phases move in opposite directions; theoretical aspects and useful data for this technique have been published by Alderweireldt (2).

Paper chromatography has been the most widely used of all methods. Hundreds of modifications of two methods, one of Zaffaroni (145) and the other of Bush (25) have been described. In the first of these the stationary phase is a solvent such as propylene glycol or formamide while the moving phase may be toluene or benzene. Very little time is required for equilibration but the development of the chromatogram may take 24 hours. In addition the removal of the solvent from the paper before staining presents difficulties. However, the method is ideal for the separation of closely related steroids which are difficult to separate in other systems and the papers may be allowed to over-run in order to separate slow-moving compounds, or the moving phase may be changed.

The method of Bush employs solvents such as aqueous methanol for the stationary phase with a variety of solvents such as benzene, petroleum ether or hexane for development. The best results are obtained when systems are allowed to equilibrate for some hours, but the actual running times are quite short and the stationary phase is easily removed from the paper before staining. The chromatograms may be run at elevated temperatures such as 37° for those steroids which are not very soluble at room temperature.

For the identification of steroids or of mixtures of steroids it is best to use several systems, preferably of both the Zaffaroni and Bush types in addition to several colour reactions. Table 11.3 gives a selection of these systems suitable for the separation of different steroids.

Useful information concerning the molecular structure of steroids is obtained by consideration of the R_M values. This function, for paper chromatography, is defined as:

$$R_M = \log\left(\frac{1}{R_F} - 1\right)$$

where R_F refers to the velocity of the steroid under consideration to the velocity of the mobile phase (8). The latter is calculated on paper chromatograms as the ratio of the distance moved by the centre of the steroid zone to that moved by the front.

R_M is a function of the free energy of the steroid which in turn is made up of the free energy contributions of the various groups of which the steroid is composed. Thus the components contribute additively to the chromatographic mobility of the steroid.

The application of these concepts to the structural analysis of steroids has been reviewed by Bush (25) and the term ΔR_{M_g} has been introduced to denote the change in R_M resulting from the introduction of a group, g, into the molecule. Bush has tabulated a useful collection of ΔR_{M_g} values for several polar groups substituted in numerous positions of the steroid molecule.

Similar solvents may be usefully employed for partition *column chromatography*. Celite is a very suitable inert supporting medium for the stationary phase and provided the column material is packed evenly and firmly excellent separations are possible. Thus for the separation of progesterone from related steroids in extracts of plasma Butt *et al.* (29) employed a column containing 2g Celite with 80 per cent v/v methanol as stationary phase of dimensions

TABLE 11.3

Systems for Steroid Identification

Steroid	Solvent System	Reference
Progesterone	Light petroleum–methanol–water (100 : 95 : 5)	
	Decalin–methanol–water (100 : 85 : 15)	
	Ligroin–propylene glycol	(a)
Androgens		
(a) 11-oxygenated	Petroleum ether–toluene–methanol–water (200 : 100 : 170 : 30)	
	Petroleum ether–benzene–methanol–water (200 : 100 : 160 : 40)	
	Petroleum ether–toluene–methanol–water (100 : 100 : 140 : 60)	
	Decalin–xylene–methanol–water (200 : 100 : 170 : 30)	
	Ligroin–propylene glycol	(a)
	Methyl cyclohexane–formamide	(b)
	Methyl cyclohexane–dimethyl formamide	(c)
(b) 11-deoxy	Petroleum ether–methanol–water (100 : 96 : 4)	
	Petroleum ether–decalin–methanol–water (100 : 100 : 170 : 30)	
	Decalin–methanol–water (100 : 95 : 5)	
	Petroleum ether–methanol–water (100 : 85 : 15)	
Oestrogens	Methyl cyclohexane–propylene glycol	(d)
	Ligroin–absolute methanol	(e, f)
	Toluene–acetic acid	(g)
Methyl ethers	Decalin–acetic acid–water (100 : 90 : 10)	
Corticosteroids	Benzene–methanol–water (100 : 50 : 50)	
	Toluene–ethylene dichloride–methanol–water (50 : 50 : 50 : 50)	
	Chloroform–formamide	
	Toluene–propylene glycol	

References: (a) SAVARD, K. *Recent Prog. Horm. Res.* **9,** 185 (1954).
(b) AXELROD, L. R. *J. biol. Chem.* **205,** 173 (1953).
(c) SACHS, L. *Acta endocr. Copenh.* **38,** 534 (1961).
(d) AXELROD, L. R. *J. biol. Chem.* **201,** 59 (1953).
(e) MITCHELL, F. L. *Nature, Lond.* **170,** 621 (1952).
(f) MITCHELL, F. L. and DAVIES, R. E. *Biochem. J.* **56,** 690 (1954).
(g) BOSCOTT, R. J. *Biochem. J.* **51,** xiv (1952).

All other systems are described by Bush or Zaffaroni. Reference (a) gives extensive information on the rates of flow of steroids in the ligroin-propylene glycol and other systems.

The proportions of solvents are by volume in all cases.

6 × 0·6 cm. It was calculated that each centimetre length of column contained 10–13 theoretical plates. Gradient systems have increased considerably the versatility of single columns (Fig. 11.13). Reversed phase columns prepared by treating the Celite with silane are useful in some instances.

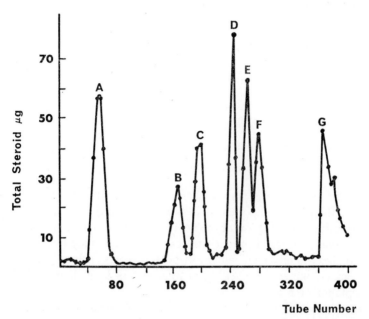

FIG. 11.13. Partition chromatography on column of Celite using gradient elution

A = androstenedione, B = deoxycorticosterone, C = 17-hydroxyprogesterone, D = 11β-hydroxyandrostenedione, E = 16α-hydroxyprogesterone, F = 17α,21-dihydroxypregn-4-ene-3,20-dione (Reichstein's cpd.S), G = cortisol.

Reprinted by permission from Villee, D. B. *J. clin. Endocr.* **22,** 726 (1963).

Excellent separations are obtained in a relatively short time by *thin layer chromatography* on alumina or silica gel. Solvents appear to have been chosen in rather an arbitrary fashion; they may be arranged in order of increasing power to elute substances from thin layers, e.g.:

> petroleum ether, carbon tetrachloride,
> benzene, chloroform, ether, ethyl acetate,
> acetone, alcohol and water.

Mixtures of two or more solvents of different polarities may give a better separation than a single solvent. It is usually necessary to experiment with several mixtures before the most satisfactory system is found; this may be accomplished quite quickly on microscope slides. A very useful general solvent is n-butyl acetate (115).

Generally steroids have the same relative polarities in thin layer chromatography as in partition paper chromatography but atypical behaviour has been noted in some systems, compounds with ketone groups being retained more than the corresponding alcohols (91). The table shows the R_F values for androstenedione and testosterone in four solvent systems:

TABLE 11.4

	Androstenedione	Testosterone
Acetone/chloroform (1/9 v/v)	0·84	0·65
Butyl acetate	0·66	0·64
Ethyl ether	0·47	0·56
Butanol/n-hexane (3 : 7 v/v)	0·35	0·65

R_F values in thin layer chromatography of androstenedione and testosterone (Ref. 91).

It will be seen that the atypical behaviour is maximal in the last system, i.e. where the polar component is in high concentration, and is least in the first where the concentration of the polar component is low. Atypical separations of polar steroids such as cortisol and cortisone may be achieved with t-butanol/hexane mixtures, while less polar steroids such as pregnanedione and pregnanolone are best separated by means of long chain alcohols such as n-heptanol or n-octanol.

Iodine is a useful locating agent since it forms loose addition compounds (6). Charring with sulphuric acid provides a very sensitive method for the detection of steroids, but they are destroyed in the process. Numerous reagents which are more specific have been described, and some will be mentioned in succeeding chapters (89, 90).

Separations by *adsorption chromatography* are sometimes extremely rapid and reproducible, provided that the adsorbent is properly standardized. Useful adsorbents are alumina, silica gel and magnesium trisilicate (Florisil). The technique is best suited to the separation of steroids into groups, e.g. 11-deoxy and 11-oxy, -diols and -triols etc., but in some cases it may be used for the separation of individual steroids, e.g. the methyl ethers of oestrone and oestradiol-17β. The method of chromatography is often useful when used in combination with the formation of derivatives. Thus pregnanediol is easily separated from -ols and -triols on alumina, and after acetylation the diacetate may be purified on a second column. These steps have been used in a routine method for the determination of pregnanediol (76) and the product shows a high degree of purity.

Gas chromatography promises to become one of the most important techniques in steroid chemistry. Columns are usually packed with a liquid phase of silicone polymer which is stable to 300°, or with a polyester; examples of these are given in Table 11.5. A coating of 1–5 per cent is made on a suitably inert support such as Celite which itself has been acid-washed and treated with dichlorodimethylsilane. Working temperatures of 200–225° are suitable for most steroids.

TABLE 11.5

Some liquid phases used in the gas chromatography of steroids

Type	Designations	Remarks
Silicone polymers:		
linear methyl siloxane methyl *p*-chlorophenyl siloxane	SE-30, XE-60, SF-96 F-60	Non-selective: separations are dependent largely on molecular size and shape. There is selective retention of C—C unsaturated steroids in the methyl phenyl siloxane polymers
linear polysiloxane with methyl and fluoro-alkyl groups	FS-1265(QF-1)	Selective: retention of alcohols, ketones and esters but not C—C unsaturated groups
Polyesters:		
neopentyl glycol adipate neopentyl glycol succinate polyester-siloxane co-polymers	NPGA NPGS EGSS-7	Selective: retention of aldehydes, ketones, esters and C—C unsaturated groups. Polysiloxanes with cyanoethyl groups have properties intermediate between polyesters and the QF-1 type polymers

Separations are fairly easily achieved for steroids of different molecular weights or of $5\alpha/5\beta$ epimers. Those differing only in the configuration of a hydroxyl group, however, are difficult to separate, but derivatives often help to accentuate the stereochemical differences. Acetates, propionates, trifluoroacetates, trimethyl silyl ethers and methyl ethers are examples of derivatives that are commonly used.

The observed retention time can be regarded approximately as the algebraic sum of the contributions from the unsubstituted nucleus and the substituents (36). A 'group retention factor' can be defined for a substituent as the ratio of the retentions of the substituted and unsubstituted steroid. It has been shown that the relative retention time (r) of a steroid can be expressed as:

$$\log r = \Sigma \Delta R_{M_g} + \log r_N$$

where ΔR_{M_g} is the change in $\log r$ resulting from the introduction of group g into the steroid nucleus N (34 and cf. paper chromatography, p. 245).

On SE-30 columns virtually the same factor is found for 3α- and 3β-hydroxyl groups irrespective of the configuration at $C_{(5)}$. On the more polar QF-1 the factors for 3α- and 3β-hydroxyl groups, however, are markedly different and are typical of axial and equatorial groups. 3α-hydroxy steroids differing only in configuration at $C_{(5)}$ are not resolved on QF-1 columns, however, because the difference in ΔR_{Mg} contributions of axial and equatorial hydroxyl groups is compensated by differences in the log r_N of the 5α- and 5β-steroid hydrocarbons; resolution of these epimers can be obtained by formation of derivatives such as acetates or trimethyl silyl ethers (34). On SE-30 the factor observed for the 3-oxo group is only slightly higher than for 3α- and 3β-hydroxyl groups. QF-1 on the other hand selectively retains carboxyl compounds and the factor is correspondingly large.

Retention factors for oxo groups decrease with increasing steric hindrance. Thus the 11-oxo factor on SE-30 is 1·3 compared with 2·3 for the 3-oxo group. Unsaturated ketones are more strongly retained and the order of elution is 11-, 20-, 3- and Δ^4-3-one.

A detector of high sensitivity is required in most steroid analyses. One of the first described was the argon ionization detector. Two other types, the flame ionization and the electron capture, have now become established as being particularly useful for steroid analyses. When the flame detector is used the response is linear over a very wide range and steroids may be detected at the nanogram level. The electron-capture detector is specific for certain molecular structures; it is extremely sensitive to halogen atoms which are often easily introduced into steroids.

SEPARATION OF KETONES

The very useful reagent, trimethyl ammonium acetyl hydrazide chloride, $(CH_3)_3N^+CH_2CONH\cdot NH_2$, was introduced by Girard and Sandelusco (60) and is known as Girard Reagent T. (Reagent P is sometimes used: it is pyridinium acetyl hydrazide chloride, $C_5H_5\cdot N^+CH_2CONH\cdot NH_2$). An extensive review of applications of the reagent has been published (137).

It forms water-soluble hydrazones when heated with ketones in glacial acetic acid, or in 10 per cent acetic acid in ethanol or methanol for 20–30 minutes. An acidic ion-exchange resin (IRC 50) has been suggested as the acid catalyst (123) but does not appear to have been widely used. It would certainly avoid the formation of acetates which have been reported to result from the use of acetic acid (122, 137).

The hydrazones are stable at pH 6·5–7 but are readily hydrolysed in acid. Thus, after formation of the ketonic hydrazone, the solution is diluted with aqueous buffer at neutral pH and washed with organic solvent to remove the non-ketonic steroids. The solution is then acidified to pH 1 and after hydrolysis for 1–2 hours the free ketone may be re-extracted into solvent.

Girard hydrazones are formed with ketones at carbon 17 or 20 and with

Δ^4-3-ones, but not with 11-ones. The hydrazones form coloured salts with suitable anions such as bromo-thymol blue. The product is then soluble in organic solvents (e.g. ethylene dichloride). Quantitative measurements based on the colour of the extracted salts are possible with compounds of the androstane and pregnane series which contain one or two carboxyl groups and altogether not more than three polar oxygen functions (87). The method has been adapted for the detection of oxosteroids on paper chromatograms.

SEPARATION OF α AND β ISOMERS

3α- and 3β-hydroxysteroids may be separated by means of digitonin, the 3β-steroids forming digitonides which precipitate from aqueous ethanol. They may, therefore, be separated from the 3α-steroids which do not react and remain in solution.

The digitonides are hydrolysed by pyridine, giving the 3β-hydroxysteroid back again in good yield (28).

Chemical reactions

There are numerous chemical reactions suitable for the quantitative measurement of steroids or for their detection on paper or thin layer chromatograms. These will be described for the different types of steroid in the succeeding chapters. The Δ^4-3-one group, however, is common to so many of the active steroids that some of its reactions will be discussed here.

Reactions of Δ^4-3-oxosteroids

1. Maximum absorption at about 240 mμ.
2. Fluorescence in alkali.
3. Formation of hydrazones.

Quantitative estimations in solution are usually carried out by the ultraviolet method. It has the advantage that the material is not lost in the process, and by the use of micro-cells can be made fairly sensitive (about 0·1 μg per ml is detectable). The fluorescence reaction has been adapted for quantitative work by using the reagent 0·1–0·3 M-t-butoxide (1, 127) and with some steroids 0·01 μg may be detected.

The phenylhydrazones may be measured by their absorption at 340–360 mμ and the Girard hydrazones are suitable for the polarographic method of estimation (see page 231).

The detection of Δ^4-3-ones on paper chromatograms is possible by ultraviolet absorption or by the extremely sensitive method of soda fluorescence. After treatment with 10 per cent NaOH in 60 per cent v/v methanol the paper is heated at 70–100° for fifteen minutes and the yellow fluorescence produced may be observed in u.v. light (25, 26).

These methods have also been adapted for thin layer chromatograms (83).

Under ultraviolet light, dark spots appear on a purple background; the sensitivity is improved by spraying the plate with 0·0005 per cent ethanolic fluorescein (32). The soda fluorescence method cannot be applied to thin layer chromatograms but a characteristic absorption at 260 mµ is given after spraying with t-butanolic sodium or aluminium butoxide (1, 83).

The hydrazone formed by reaction with slightly acidified iso-nicotinic acid hydrazide (57) gives a specific yellow colour (max. 380 mµ) clearly visible in ultraviolet light as a yellow fluorescence. Δ^{1-4}-3-ones react only very slowly and other ketones do not give this colour (113, 128, 134).

Another highly sensitive reaction is with phenylenediamine and phthalic acid (14) when an orange-brown colour results.

IMMUNOLOGICAL STUDIES WITH STEROIDS

There have been some interesting developments in this field in the last few years. Certain steroids can be linked to proteins (usually bovine serum albumin, BSA) and the protein-steroid complex used as antigen (82, 92). The two original methods described were the Schotten-Baumann and the mixed-anhydride methods. In the first, testosterone 17-chlorocarbonate was conjugated to protein at $C_{(17)}$ (Fig. 11.14).

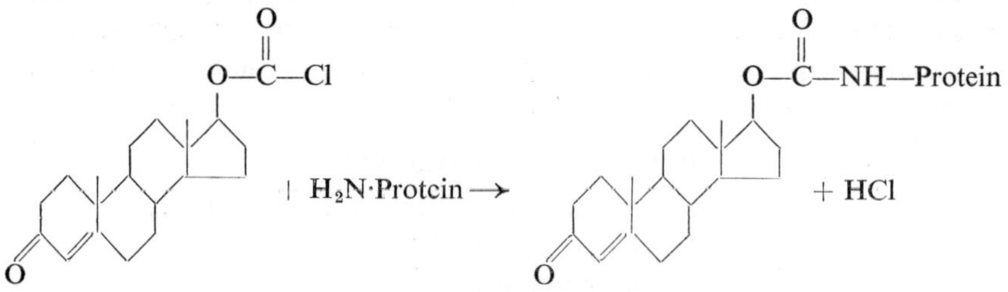

FIG. 11.14

In the second the oxime formed by reacting testosterone with (O-carboxymethyl) hydroxylamine was used, giving by the steps shown a conjugate at $C_{(3)}$ (Fig. 11.15).

The hemisuccinates could be used instead of the oxime in the latter method.

Similar methods were used for oestrone, progesterone, corticosterone, deoxycorticosterone and aldosterone. The conjugates were reported to contain 20–25 residues of the steroid per molecule of BSA.

When injected into rabbits antibodies are produced to the steroid conjugates and also to BSA. By suitable absorption of the antiserum with BSA it is possible to obtain specific antibodies to the steroid-BSA conjugates. These antibodies are capable of neutralizing the biological activity of the corresponding steroid hormones (62, 92).

The immunological method does not appear to have been applied to the

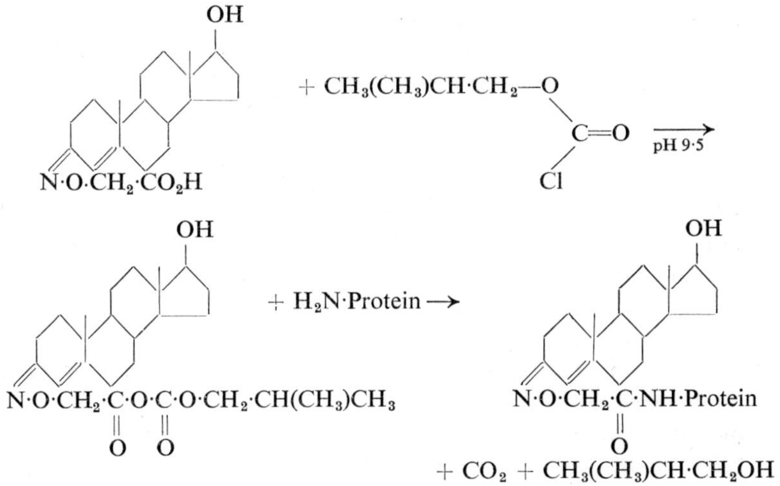

$$+ \ CH_3(CH_3)CH \cdot CH_2 \text{—} O$$
$$C=O \xrightarrow{\ pH \ 9 \cdot 5\ }$$
$$Cl$$

N·O·CH$_2$·CO$_2$H

$+ \ H_2N \cdot Protein \rightarrow$

N·O·CH$_2$·C·O·C·O·CH$_2$·CH(CH$_3$)CH$_3$
O O

N·O·CH$_2$·C·NH·Protein
O

$+ \ CO_2 + CH_3(CH_3)CH \cdot CH_2OH$

FIG. 11.15

qualitative or quantitative investigation of urinary or plasma steroids. Immunological methods are so sensitive and specific (see page 33) that they would be ideal for detecting the small amounts of some of the steroids in biological fluids. Presumably, at present the methods of conjugating proteins and steroids are rather too difficult for the method to be feasible.

REFERENCES

1 ABELSON, D. and BONDY, P. K. *Archs Biochem. Biophys.* **57**, 208 (1955).
2 ALDERWEIRELDT, F. C. *Analyt. Chem.* **33**, 1920 (1961).
3 BACHMANN, W. E., COLE, W. and WILDS, A. L. *J. Amer. chem. Soc.* **62**, 824 (1940).
4 BARNETT, J., HENLY, A. A. and MORRIS, C. J. O. R. *Biochem. J.* **40**, 445 (1946).
5 BARNETT, J. and MORRIS, C. J. O. R. *Biochem. J.* **40**, 450 (1946).
6 BARRETT, G. C. *Nature, Lond.* **194**, 1171 (1962).
7 BARTON, D. H. R. *J. chem. Soc.* 1027 (1953).
8 BATE-SMITH, E. C. and WESTALL, R. G. *Biochim. biophys. Acta* **4**, 427 (1950).
9 BELING, C. G. *Acta endocr. Copenh.* Suppl. 79 (1963).
10 BERNSTEIN, S. and LENHARD, R. H. *J. org. Chem.* **19**, 1269 (1954).
11 BERNSTEIN, S., LENHARD, R. H. and WILLIAMS, J. H. *J. org. Chem.* **18**, 1166 (1953).
12 BLECHER, M. and WHITE, A. *J. biol. Chem.* **235**, 282 (1960).
13 BLOCH, K. *Vitams and Horm.* **15**, 119 (1957).
14 BODÁNSZKY, A. and KOLLONITISCH, J. *Nature, Lond.* **175**, 729 (1955).

15 BOWEN, E. J. *Q. Rev. chem. Soc.* **1,** 1 (1947).

16 BRAUNSBERG, H. and OSBORN, S. B. *Analytica chim. Acta* **6,** 84 (1962).

17 BRAUNSBERG, H., OSBORN, S. B. and STERN, M. I. *J. Endocr.* **11,** 177 (1954).

18 BROOKS, R. V., DUPRÉ, J., GOGATE, A. N., MILLS, I. H. and PRUNTY, F. T. G. *J. clin. Endocr.* **23,** 725 (1963).

19 BROWSTEIN, S. *Chem. Rev.* **59,** 463 (1959).

20 BUDZIKIEWICZ, H. and DJERASSI, C. *J. Amer. chem. Soc.* **84,** 1430 (1962).

21 BUDZIKIEWICZ, H., DJERASSI, C. and WILLIAMS, D. In *Structural Elucidation of Natural Products by Mass Spectrometry*, Vol. II, Holden-Day, San Francisco (1964).

22 BUNNENBERG, E., DJERASSI, C., MISLOW, K. and MOSCOWITZ, A. *J. Amer. chem. Soc.* **84,** 2823 (1962).

23 BURSTEIN, S., JACOBSON, G. and LIEBERMAN, S. *J. Amer. chem. Soc.* **82,** 1226 (1960).

24 BURSTEIN, S. and LIEBERMAN, S. *J. biol. Chem.* **233,** 331 (1958).

25 BUSH, I. E. In *The Chromatography of Steroids* p. 224, Pergamon Press, Oxford (1961).

26 BUSH, I. E. *Pharmac. Rev.* **14,** 317 (1962).

27 BUSH, I. E. and GALE, M. *Biochem. J.* **67,** 29P (1957).

28 BUTT, W. R., HENLY, A. A. and MORRIS, C. J. O. R. *Biochem. J.* **42,** 447 (1948).

29 BUTT, W. R., MORRIS, P., MORRIS, C. J. O. R. and WILLIAMS, D. C. *Biochem. J.* **49,** 434 (1951).

30 CALLOW, R. K. *Rep. Prog. Chem.* **53,** 305 (1956).

31 CALLOW, R. K. and KENNARD, O. *J. Pharm. Pharmac.* **13,** 723 (1961).

32 ČERNÝ, V. *Third Conf. Inst. Chem.* Prague, **21,** 12 (1951).

33 CHAMBERLAIN, N. F. *Analyt. Chem.* **31,** 56 (1959).

34 CHAMBERLAIN, J., KNIGHTS, B. A. and THOMAS, G. H. *J. Endocr.* **26,** 367 (1963).

35 CHARNEY, W., WEBER, L. and OLIVETO, E. *Archs Biochem. Biophys.* **79,** 402 (1959).

36 CLAYTON, R. B. *Nature, Lond.* **190,** 1071 (1961).

37 CLAYTON, R. B. *Q. Rev. chem. Soc.* **19,** 168 (1965).

38 COHEN, S. L. and ONESSON, I. B. *J. biol. Chem.* **204,** 245 (1953).

39 COLLINS, D. J., HOBBS, J. J. and STERNHALL, S. *Tetrahedron Lett.* 197 (1963).

40 COREY, E. J., GREGORION, G. A. and PETERSON, D. H. *J. Amer. chem. Soc.* **80,** 2338 (1958).

41 CORNFORTH, J. W., GORE, I. Y. and POPJÁK, G. *Biochem. J.* **65,** 94 (1957).

42 CRAIG, L. C. *J. biol. Chem.* **155,** 519 (1944).

43 DE PAOLI, J. C., NISHIZAWA, E. and EIK-NES, K. B. *J. clin. Endocr.* **23,** 81 (1963).

44 DICKSON, D. H. W., PAGE, J. E. and ROGERS, D. *J. chem. Soc.* 443 (1955).
45 DICZFALUSY, E. *Acta endocr. Copenh.* **10**, 373 (1952).
46 DJERASSI, C. In *Optical Rotatory Dispersion: Applications to Organic Chemistry* McGraw-Hill, New York (1960).
47 DJERASSI, C. *Pure appl. Chem.* **2**, 475 (1961).
48 DJERASSI, C., FINCH, N. and MAULI, R. *J. Amer. chem. Soc.* **81**, 4997 (1959).
49 DJERASSI, C., RINIKER, R. and RINIKER, B. *J. Amer. chem. Soc.* **78**, 6362 (1956).
50 DODGSON, K. S. and SPENCER, B. *Biochem. J.* **55**, 315 (1953).
51 DORFMAN, L. *Chem. Rev.* **53**, 47 (1953).
52 DUSZA, J. P., HELLER, M. and BERNSTEIN, S. In *Physical Properties of Steroid Hormones* (edited by L. L. Engel), p. 69, Pergamon Press, Oxford (1963).
53 EDWARDS, R. W. H., KELLIE, A. E. and WADE, A. P. *Mem. Soc. Endocr.* **2**, 53 (1953).
54 ELLINGTON, P. S. and MEAKINS, G. D. *J. chem. Soc.* 697 (1960).
55 ENGEL, L. L. and CARTER, P. In *Physical Properties of Steroid Hormones* (edited by L. L. Engel), p. 1, Pergamon Press, Oxford (1963).
56 EPPSTEIN, S. H., MEISTER, P. D., MURRAY, H. C. and PETERSON, D. H. *Vitams Horm.* **14**, 359 (1956).
57 ERCOLI, A., DE GUISEPPE, L. and DE RUGGIERI, P. *Farm. Sci. tec.* Pavia, **7**, 170 (1952).
58 FISHMAN, J. and DJERASSI, C. *Experientia* **12**, 325 (1956).
59 FOGGITT, F. and KELLIE, A. E. *Biochem. J.* **91**, 209 (1964).
60 GIRARD, A. and SANDELUSCO, G. *Helv. chim. Acta* **19**, 1095 (1936).
61 GLENN, E. M., MILLER, W. L. and SCHLAGEL, C. A. *Recent Prog. Horm. Res.* **19**, 107 (1963).
62 GOODFRIEND, L. and SEHON, A. *Can. J. Biochem. Physiol.* **39**, 961 (1961).
63 GREEN, D. E. *Adv. Enzymol.* **1**, 177 (1941).
64 HECHTER, O. *Vitams Horm.* **13**, 293 (1955).
65 HECHTER, O. and LESTER, G. *Recent Prog. Horm. Res.* **16**, 139 (1960).
66 HENRY, R., THEVENET, M. and JARRIGE, P. *Bull. Soc. Chim. biol.* **34**, 897 (1952).
67 HERZOG, H. L., GENTLES, M. J., BASCH, A., COSCARELLI, W., ZEITZ, M. E. A. and CHARNEY, W. *J. org. Chem.* **25**, 2177 (1960).
68 HEUSGHEM, C. and LEJEUNE, G. *Annls Endocr.* **13**, 479 (1952).
69 HURLOCK, B. and TALALAY, P. *Archs Biochem. Biophys.* **80**, 468 (1959).
70 ISSELBACHER, K. J. *Recent Prog. Horm. Res.* **12**, 134 (1956).
71 JOHNSON, W. S., DAVID, I. A., DEHM, H. C., HIGHET, R. J., WARNHOFF, E. W., WOOD, W. D. and JONES, E. T. *J. Amer. chem. Soc.* **80**, 661 (1958.)

72 JONES, R. N. and SANDORFY, C. in *Technique of Organic Chemistry* (edited by A. Weissberger) Vol. IX, p. 247, Wiley-Interscience, New York (1956).

73 KAPPAS, A., SOYBEL, W., GLICKMAN, P. and FUKUSHIMA, D. K. *Archs intern. Med.* **105,** 701 (1960).

74 KARLSON, P. *Perspect. Biol. Med.* **6,** 203 (1963).

75 KITA, D. A., SARDINAS, J. L. and SHULL, G. M. *Nature, Lond.* **190,** 627 (1961).

76 KLOPPER, A., MICHIE, E. A. and BROWN, J. B. *J. Endocr.* **12,** 209 (1955).

77 KLYNE, W. *Jl R. Inst. Chem.* **84,** 50 (1960).

78 KLYNE, W. in *Advances in Organic Chemistry*, Vol. 1 (edited by R. A. Raphael, E. C. Taylor, and H. Wynberg), p. 239, Wiley-Interscience, New York (1960).

79 KORNEL, L. *Metabolism* **8,** 432 (1959).

80 LANGER, L. J. and ENGEL, L. L. *J. biol. Chem.* **233,** 583 (1958).

81 LERMAN, L. H. *Br. med. J.* **2,** 129 (1956).

82 LIEBERMAN, S., ERLANGER, R. F., BEISER, S. M. and AGATE, F. J. *Recent Prog. Horm. Res.* **15,** 165 (1959).

83 LISBOA, B. P. *Acta endocr. Copenh.* **43,** 47 (1963).

84 LITTLE, H. N. and BLOCH, K. *J. biol. Chem.* **183,** 33 (1950).

85 MARCUS, P. I. and TALALAY, P. *J. biol. Chem.* **218,** 661 (1956).

86 MCANALLY, J. S. and HAUSMAN, E. R. *J. Lab. clin. Med.* **44,** 647 (1954).

87 MENINI, E. and NORYMBERSKI, J. K. *Biochem. J.* **93,** 11 (1964).

88 MOORE, J. A. and HEFTMANN, E. In *The Adrenocortical Hormones: Their Origin, Chemistry, Physiology and Pharmacology*, Part 1 (edited by H. W. Deane), p. 186, Springer-Verlag, Berlin (1962).

89 NEHER, R. *Chromat. Rev.* **1,** 99 (1959).

90 NEHER, R. In *Physical Properties of Steroid Hormones* (edited by L. L. Engel), p. 37, Pergamon Press, Oxford (1963).

91 NIENSTEDT, W. *Biochem. J.* **92,** 8P (1964).

92 NERI, R. O., TOLKSDORF, S., BEISER, S. N., ERLANGER, B. F., AGATE, F. J. and LIEBERMAN, S. *Endocrinology* **74,** 593 (1964).

93 OERTEL, G. W. *Clin. Chim. Acta* **8,** 154 (1963).

94 OERTEL, G. W. and EIK-NES, K. B. *Acta endocr. Copenh.* **30,** 93 (1959).

95 OERTEL, G. W., KAISER, E. and BRUHL, P. *Biochem. Z.* **336,** 154 (1962).

96 PAGE, J. E. *Chemy Ind.* 58 (1957).

97 POOS, G. I., LUKES, R. M., ARTH, G. E. and SARETT, L. H. *J. Amer. chem. Soc.* **76,** 5031 (1954).

98 REED, R. I. *J. chem. Soc.* 3432 (1958).

99 REERINK, E. H., SCHOLER, H. F. L., WESTERHOF, P., QUERIDO, A., KASSENAAR, A. A. H., DICZFALUSY, E. and TILLINGER, K.-G. *Nature, Lond.* **186,** 168 (1960).

100 RIONDEL, A., TAIT, J. F., TAIT, S. A. S., GUT, M. and LITTLE, B. *J. clin. Endocr.* **25,** 229 (1965).
101 ROBERTS, G. *Analyt. Chem.* **29,** 911 (1957).
102 ROBERTS, G. in *Infrared Absorption Spectra of Steroids; An Atlas* (edited by K. Dobriner *et al.*). Vol. II, Wiley-Interscience, New York (1958).
103 ROY, A. B. *Biochim. biophys. Acta* **15,** 300 (1954).
104 ROY, A. B. *Biochem. J.* **62,** 41 (1956).
105 RYAN, M. T. *Acta endocr. Copenh.* **46,** 170 (1964).
106 SAVARD, K., BAGNOLI, E. and DORFMAN, R. I. *Fedn. Proc.* **13,** 289 (1954).
107 SCHMIDLIN, J. VON, ARMER, G., BILLETER, J.-R. and WETTSTEIN, A. *Experientia* **11,** 365 (1955).
108 SCHOLER, H. F. L. *Acta endocr. Copenh.* **35,** 188 (1960).
109 SEGAL, L., SEGAL, B. and NES, W. R. *J. biol. Chem.* **235,** 3108 (1960).
110 SMITH, E. E. B. and MILLS, G. T. *Biochem. J.* **47,** xlix (1950).
111 SMITH, E. E. B. and MILLS, G. T. *Biochim. biophys. Acta* **13,** 386 (1954).
112 SMITH, L. L. and BERNSTEIN, S. In *Physical Properties of Steroid Hormones* (edited by L. L. Engel), p. 321, Pergamon Press, Oxford (1963).
113 SMITH, L. L. and FOELL, T. *Analyt. Chem.* **31,** 102 (1959).
114 STERN, M. I. *Nature, Lond.* **192,** 359 (1961).
115 STEVENS, P. J. *Proc. Ass. clin. Biochem.* **2,** 156 (1963).
116 STIMSON, M. M. and O'DONNELL, M. J. *J. Amer. chem. Soc.* **74,** 1805 (1952).
117 STITCH, S. R. and HALKERSTON, I. D. K. *Nature, Lond.* **172,** 398 (1953).
118 STOREY, I. D. E. and DUTTON, G. J. *Biochem. J.* **59,** 279 (1955).
119 STOUDT, T. H. *Adv. appl. Microbiol.* **2,** 183 (1960).
120 TAIT, J. F. *J. clin. Endocr.* **23,** 1285 (1963).
121 TALALAY, P. *Physiol. Rev.* **37,** 362 (1957).
122 TAYLOR, W. *Nature, Lond.* **182,** 1735 (1958).
123 TEITELBAUM, C. L. *J. org. Chem.* **23,** 646 (1958).
124 TILLINGER, K.-G. and DICZFALUSY, E. *Acta endocr. Copenh.* **35,** 197 (1960).
125 TOMKINS, G. M. *J. biol. Chem.* **218,** 437 (1956).
126 TOMKINS, G. M. *Recent Prog. Horm. Res.* **12,** 125 (1956).
127 TOUCHSTONE, J. C. and MURAWEC, T. *Fedn. Proc.* **19,** 236 (1960).
128 UMBERGER, E. J. *Analyt. Chem.* **27,** 768 (1955).
129 VAN DE WIELE, R. L., MACDONALD, P. C., GURPIDE, E. and LIEBERMAN, S. *Recent Prog. Horm. Res.* **19,** 275 (1963).
130 VELLUZ, L. and LEGRAND, M. *Angew. Chem.* **73,** 603 (1961).
131 VESTERGAARD, P. *Acta endocr. Copenh.* Suppl. 64, 50 (1962).
132 VISCHER, E., SCHMIDLIN, J. and WETTSTEIN, A. *Experientia* **12,** 50 (1956).
133 VISCHER, E. and WETTSTEIN, A. *Adv. Enzymol.* **20,** 237 (1958).
134 WEISCHELBAUM, T. E. and MARGRAF, H. W. *J. clin. Endocr.* **17,** 959 (1957).

s

135 WESTERHOF, P. and REERINK, E. H. *Recl Trav. chim. Pays-Bas Belg.* **79**, 771 (1960).

136 WESTERHOF, P. and REERINK, E. H. *Rec. Trav. Chim. Pays-Bas Belg.* **79**, 794 (1960).

137 WHEELER, O. H. *Chem. Rev.* **62**, 205 (1962).

138 WILBRANDT, W. *J. Pharmacol.* **11**, 65 (1959).

139 WILLIAMS, D. H., WILSON, J. M., BUDZIKIEWICZ, H. and DJERASSI, C. *J. Amer. chem. Soc.* **85**, 2091 (1963).

140 WILLIAMS-ASHMAN, H. G., LIAO, S., HANCOCK, R. L., JURKOWITZ, L. and SILVERMAN, D. A. *Recent Prog. Horm. Res.* **20**, 247 (1964).

141 WILLMER, E. N. *Biol. Rev.* **36**, 368 (1961).

142 WILLSTRUCK, T. A., MALHOTRA, S. K. and RINGOLD, H. J. *J. Amer. chem. Soc.* **85**, 1699 (1963).

143 WOLFE, J. K., HERSHBERG, E. B. and FIESER, L. F. *J. biol. Chem.* **136**, 653 (1940).

144 ZAFFARONI, A. *J. Amer. chem. Soc.* **72**, 3828 (1950).

145 ZAFFARONI, A. *Recent Prog. Horm. Res.* **8**, 51 (1953).

146 ZDERIC, J. A., BOWERS, A., CARPIO, H. and DJERASSI, C. *J. Amer. chem. Soc.* **80**, 2596 (1958).

147 ZUMOFF, B. and BRADLOW, H. L. *J. clin. Endocr.* **23**, 799 (1963).

148 ZÜRCHER, R. F. *Helv. chim. Acta* **44**, 1380 (1961).

149 ZÜRCHER, R. F. *Helv. chim. Acta.* **46**, 2054 (1963).

12

PROGESTERONE

Progesterone is secreted by the corpus luteum of the ovary and is responsible for preparing the endometrium for pregnancy. In conjunction with oestrogens it produces the secretory hypertrophy of the endometrium suitable for nidation of the fertilized ovum. Corner and Allen prepared extracts from the corpora lutea of swine and in 1929 developed a relatively simple assay for progestational activity (21). By 1934 several reports had appeared of the isolation of the crystalline hormone with structural studies and confirmation of structure by synthesis (12–14). It is now known that other natural sources are the placenta, the adrenal cortex and the testis (22, 65, 73).

In 1947 Hooker and Forbes improved enormously the sensitivity of the earlier methods of assay and were able to demonstrate progestational activity in peripheral blood (43). They used an intra-uterine injection method in mice and were able to detect as little as 0.0002 μg of the hormone. Although it was subsequently shown that this assay was not entirely specific for progesterone (115), the results obtained by using it stimulated a great deal of chemical work and led to the development of methods for its determination in plasma.

Synthesis

The biosynthesis of progesterone has been demonstrated to occur from small molecules such as acetate. There is an enormous literature on the subject and it is only possible to quote here from some of the more recent publications.

The *in vitro* biosynthesis from ^{14}C-labelled acetate has been demonstrated using bovine (97) or human (37, 45) corpora lutea. Luteinizing hormone, but neither follicle stimulating hormone nor prolactin increases the incorporation of ^{14}C (59, 81). The quantity of progesterone formed is increased also by $NADPH_2$ but the incorporation of ^{14}C is not (81). Thus the trophic hormone, but not $NADPH_2$, stimulates the synthesis from small molecules.

259

Further information on this comes from experiments using other labelled precursors, cholesterol and pregnenolone (60). Now neither luteinizing hormone nor other gonadotrophins increase the production of labelled progesterone, but the addition of $NADPH_2$ in experiments with cholesterol does so. Thus it seems that luteinizing hormone acts mainly on the precursors of cholesterol and Hellig and Savard (in 60) report that it does, in fact, increase the incorporation of acetate into squalene. $NADPH_2$, however, increases the production of progesterone mainly through its action on cholesterol (Fig. 12.1).

Acetate

↓ ←——— LH

Squalene

↓

Cholesterol

↓ ←——— $NADPH_2$

Pregnenolone

↓

Progesterone

FIG. 12.1. Biosynthesis of progesterone

Progesterone was first synthesized from other naturally occurring steroids such as cholesterol, stigmasterol, sapogenins and bile acids (for review of methods see 68). It may also be obtained from urinary steroids such as pregnanediol and dehydroepiandrosterone. Butenandt and Schmidt (8) oxidized pregnanediol with chromic oxide to the dione which was then brominated at

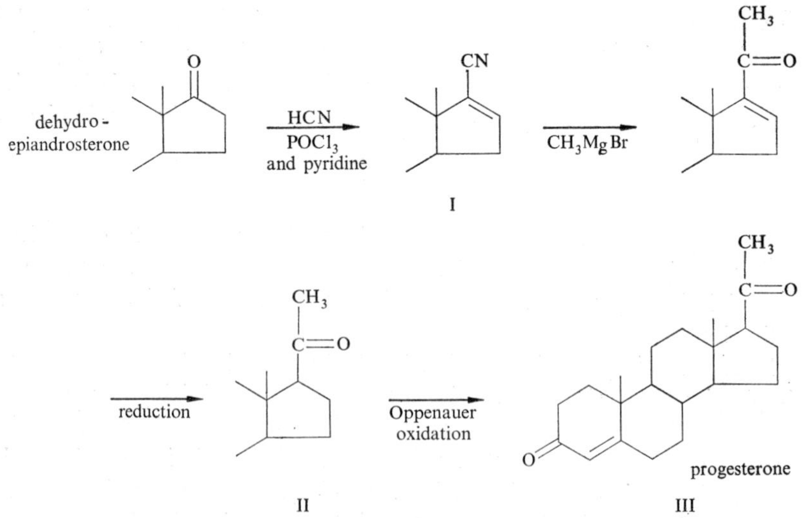

FIG. 12.2

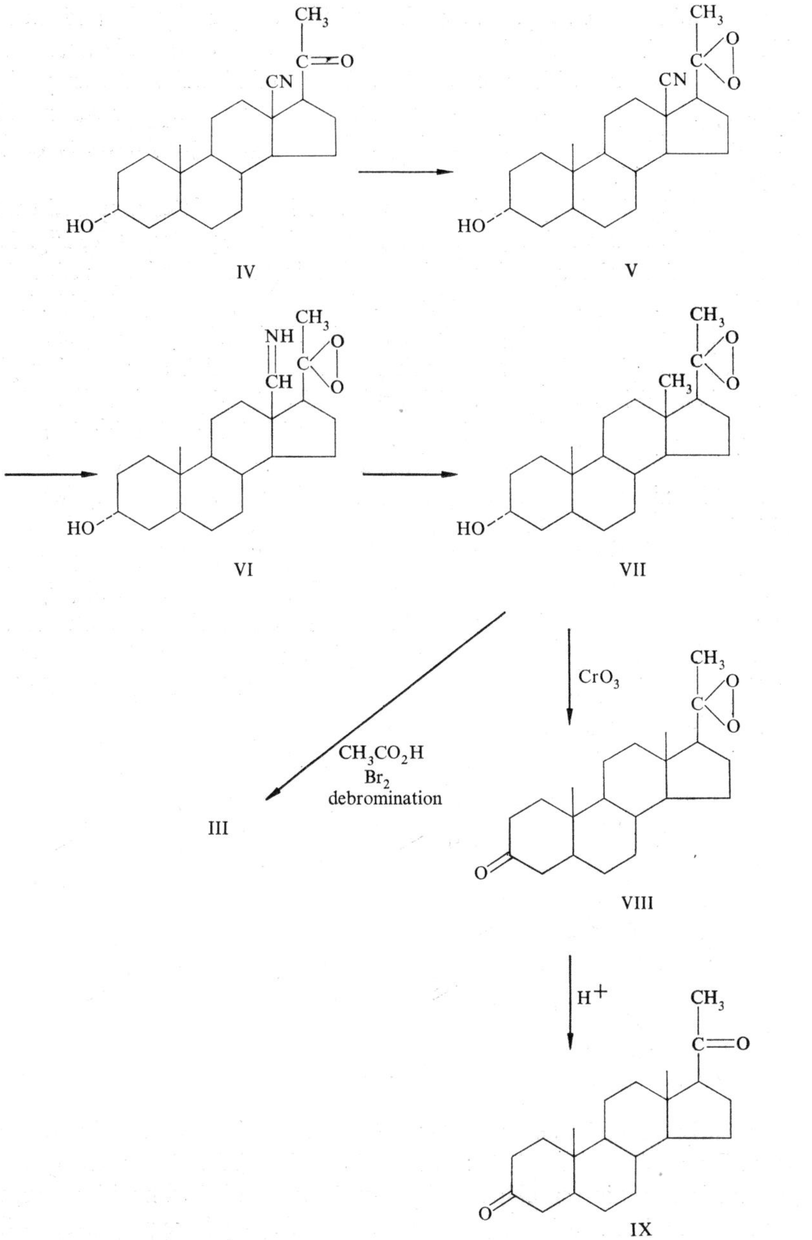

FIG. 12.3

$C_{(4)}$ and treated with pyridine to eliminate hydrogen bromide and give progesterone. There are several routes from dehydroepiandrosterone including that of Butenandt and Schmidt-Thomé (10, 11) from the acetate. The unsaturated nitrile (I, Fig. 12.2) is formed via the cyanohydrin and then the side chain is introduced with CH_3MgBr. Reduction of the Δ^{16} unsaturated bond by treatment with an ethanolic solution of NaOH and Raney nickel gives 3β-hydroxypregn-5-en-20-one (II). A modified Oppenauer reaction with aluminium isopropoxide and cyclohexane gives progesterone (III) in 40 per cent yield.

A relatively simple synthesis makes use of intermediates prepared during the synthesis of conessine (46, 58). The cyanohydroxyketone (IV, Fig. 12.3) is converted to the cyanoketal (V), which is then selectively reduced by refluxing for 5 hours with excess $LiAlH_4$ in tetrahydrofuran giving VI. Treatment with excess hydrazine hydrate and KOH in triethylene glycol for 17 hours at 130° gives the corresponding hydrazone which on reduction gives VII. This ketal is hydrolysed and brominated at $C_{(4)}$ by acetic acid and bromine. DL-progesterone is obtained by debromination on heating in acetone containing trimethylbenzylammonium mesitoate.

If VII is oxidized by CrO_3 in pyridine to the ketone VIII, hydrolysis in weak acid gives DL-pregnanedione (IX).

Progesterone is widely used for metabolic studies and for this purpose it has been labelled both with ^{14}C and with ^{3}H. The enol lactone X (Fig. 12.4) is a useful intermediate for the introduction of ^{14}C into ring A. Treatment with ^{14}C-labelled CH_3MgI or phenylacetate gives progesterone labelled at $C_{(3)}$ or $C_{(4)}$ (28, 35, 101). ^{14}C has also been introduced into the side-chain of progesterone at $C_{(21)}$.

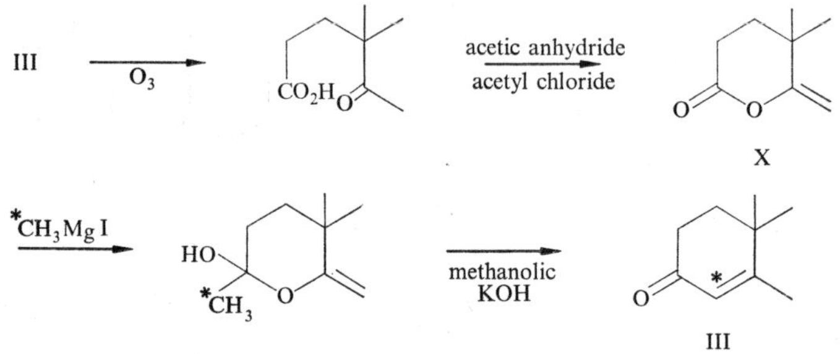

FIG. 12.4

An early method was reported for the preparation of deuterium-labelled progesterone from methyl (11:12^{2}H) lithocholate (52). More recently, useful preparations of high specific activity have been labelled with tritium (36, 69). In the method of Pearlman (69) the acetate of 3β-hydroxypregna-5,16-dien-20-one (XI, Fig. 12.5) is tritiated in the presence of a 10 per cent Pd-charcoal catalyst. After refluxing in methanolic KOH, [16-^{3}H]pregnenolone (XII) is extracted in ether and is converted into [16-^{3}H]progesterone by Oppenauer oxidation carried out in toluene, cyclohexanone and aluminium isopropoxide.

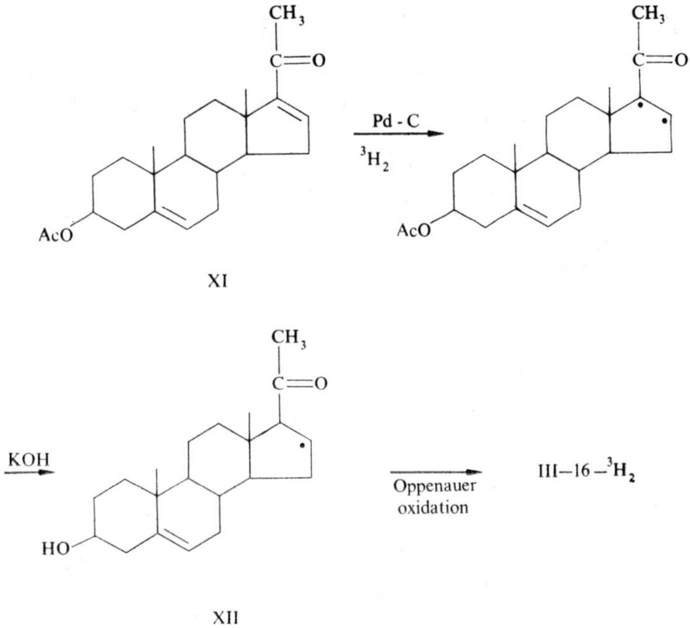

FIG. 12.5

[7-³M]progesterone has also been prepared (36). 7α-bromo-pregnenolone acetate was reduced with carrier-free tritium. The pregnenolone formed was subjected to an Oppenauer oxidation (aluminium isopropoxide in cyclohexanone) to give progesterone with a specific activity of 31 mc/mg.

Methods of extraction and separation

EXTRACTION

Progesterone is usually extracted from biological fluids or tissues by ether or a mixture of ethanol and ether (3:1 v/v.) There is good evidence that the best recoveries from plasma are obtained when it is first treated with alkali, after which ether (39, 73, 74, 85), ether and methylene chloride, 4:1 v/v, (93) or ethyl acetate and benzene (32) may be used for the extraction. The alkali keeps most of the lipids in the plasma when the steroid is extracted, and prevents troublesome emulsions.

PURIFICATION

A partition between hexane or petroleum ether and 70 per cent methanol is a useful preliminary step to provide cleaner extracts for chromatography. Alternatively progesterone remains soluble in 70 per cent methanol at −15° while less polar material comes out of solution (15).

In most systems of paper chromatography, progesterone has a fairly high R_F value. Bush (6) has therefore recommended a combination of the systems light petroleum–methanol–water (100:95:5 by vol., R_F 0·48) or decalin–methanol–water (100:85:15 by vol., R_F 0·57) followed by light petroleum–acetic acid–water (10:9:1 by vol., R_F 0·2). The last system allows considerable over-running of the chromatogram with improved resolution.

Some interesting alterations in R_F values occur in reversed phase systems. Thus with benzene as the stationary phase the R_F values for progesterone increase from 0·1 to 0·68 with change of moving phase from 50 to 70 per cent methanol (24), and clear separation from 17α-hydroxyprogesterone, androstenedione and testosterone is obtained.

Progesterone resists acetylation but contaminating material can often be removed by re-chromatography after the mixture has been acetylated.

A system of column partition chromatography with 40–70 per cent aqueous methanol on Celite as the stationary phase, and hexane or petroleum ether as the moving phase, gives clear separation of progesterone from androstenedione and testosterone (15). Many developments of this method have been described, notably those using gradient elution (105, 109). With 80 per cent methanol on the column and elution commencing with trimethylpentane, a gradient of ethylene dichloride may be introduced so that many closely related steroids occurring in blood or arising from *in vitro* experiments may be separated.

Recently the method of thin layer chromatography has proved useful,

TABLE 12.1

Partition coefficients $\left(\dfrac{conc.\ in\ upper\ phase}{conc.\ in\ lower\ phase}\right)$ *of progesterone and related steroids between petroleum ether (P.E.) or n-hexane (H) and aqueous methanol (M) or ethanol (E)*

	Solvents				
	P.E 70%M	H 70%M	H 40%M	P.E 34·5%E	H 38·8%E
Progesterone	0·33	0·51	2·55	3·55	3·35
Androstenedione	0·07	0·17	—	—	0·56
Testosterone	0·05	—	—	0·28	0·16
Dehydroepiandrosterone	0·03	—	—	—	0·14
Deoxycorticosterone	0·03	0·05	0·38	0·21	—
References	(a)	15	15	22	(b)

(a) PEARLMAN, W. H. *Recent Prog. Horm. Res.* **9**, 22 (1954).
(b) ZANDER, J. In *Methods in Hormone Research* Vol. 1 (edited by R. I. Dorfman), p. 91, Academic Press, New York (1962).

often as a preliminary to gas liquid chromatography. Thus Collins and Sommerville (19) used chromatography in two dimensions on thin layers of Kieselgel. The solvents were benzene–ethyl acetate (3:2 v/v) followed by ether–dimethyl formamide (99:1 v/v) and progesterone was well separated from 20α- or 20β-hydroxypregn-4-en-3-one and androstenedione.

Many systems of countercurrent distribution have been described (22, 45, 98, 109). The partition coefficients for progesterone and some related steroids between suitable solvents are given in Table 12.1.

Methods of detection and estimation

Progesterone may be detected on paper chromatograms by the methods described for Δ^4-3-oxosteroids in Chapter 11 (p. 251). Among other non-specific reactions are:

(a) Phosphomolybdic acid in 5 per cent alcohol which gives a blue colour on a yellow-green background after heating at 90° for 5–10 minutes. Sensitivity 2·0 $\mu g/cm^2$.

(b) Antimony trichloride (63, 92). The paper is pre-treated with chlorine gas and then dipped in the saturated reagent in acetic anhydride. After 4 minutes at 90° a yellow colour develops with a yellow-orange fluorescence. The method of choice is probably the soda-fluorescence reaction of Bush (6).

Quantitative determinations of progesterone may also be made by any of the methods described for Δ^4-3-oxosteroids. The ultraviolet absorption at 240 $m\mu$ has been employed in many methods (38, 77, 85, 116). A list of derivatives showing maximum absorptions at various other wavelengths is given in Table 12.2.

TABLE 12.2

Absorption maxima of some derivatives of progesterone

Derivative	E max (mμ)	Reference
2,4-dinitrophenylhydrazone	380	(a)
Semicarbazone	267	74
Thiosemicarbazone	245, 301	74
Isonicotinic acid hydrazone	380	(b)
Bisthiosemicarbazone	302	(c)

(a) Hinsberg, K., Pelzer, H. and Senken, A. *Biochem. Z.* **328,** 117 (1956).
(b) Umberger, E. J. *Analyt. Chem.* **27,** 768 (1955).
(c) Sommerville, I. F., Pickett, M. T., Collins, W. P. and Denyer, D. C. *Acta endocr. Copenh.* **43,** 101 (1963).

Improved sensitivity is obtained by using the fluorescence reaction in alkali by employing 0·1–0·3N-t-butoxide (1) but even greater sensitivity is given by the method of Touchstone and Murawec (100). These workers showed that if progesterone is treated with 2N-KOH at 60° and subsequently with 88 per cent H_2SO_4 the fluorescence was enhanced fourfold over the normal H_2SO_4 fluorescence. A similar increase in fluorescence was noted with 17α-hydroxy-progesterone. This method has been applied to extracts of peripheral blood and the results on samples from pregnant women were similar to those obtained by ultraviolet absorption (88).

Even greater sensitivity is obtained in the fluorescence method of Heap (40). Progesterone is converted to 20β-hydroxypregn-4-en-3-one by a 20 β-hydroxysteroid dehydrogenase prepared from *Streptomyces hydrogenans*. After purification by paper chromatography the 20β-hydroxypregn-4-en-3-one is measured by the fluorescence developed at 60° with H_2SO_4–80 per cent ethanol (2:1 v/v). The excitation wavelength is 365 mμ and the fluorescence intensity is measured at 520 mμ. This method is capable of measuring 3 ng of 20β-hydroxypregn-4-en-3-one derived from progesterone as compared with the 500 ng required for u.v. spectrophotometry. Its sensitivity is therefore of the same order as the double-isotope derivative method (Table 11.2, p. 234) and the latest gas chromatographic methods (e.g. 29).

In H_2SO_4, progesterone shows maximum absorption in the region of 280–290 mμ (114). A development of this reaction using a mixture of ethanol and H_2SO_4 provides a sensitive method for quantitative work (66, 67). A mixture of ethyl acetate and H_2SO_4 has also been proposed (25). Although 0·06 μg progesterone may be detected by this method at the time of writing it has only been described for pure steroids. Chromogens with maximum absorptions at slightly different wavelengths are given with dehydroepiandrosterone and oestrogens.

The detection of progesterone by gas liquid chromatography is possible on several types of column. It is well separated from other likely constituents of plasma using columns of cyclohexane-dimethanol succinate on Gas Chrom, P. (19). At 210° the retention time for progesterone is 72 minutes.

Oral contraceptives

The oral contraceptive 'pills' have been strikingly successful in controlling fertility; their mode of action is still incompletely understood. The 'pills' usually consist of a synthetic progestogen with a small amount of oestrogen. When taken cyclically, anovulatory artificial menstrual cycles result; the small amount of oestrogen helps to control the duration of the cycle and the menstrual flow. Besides affecting the process of ovulation, it has been suggested that the 'pills' may also affect fertilization, the transport of ova, the development of the blastocyst and implantation.

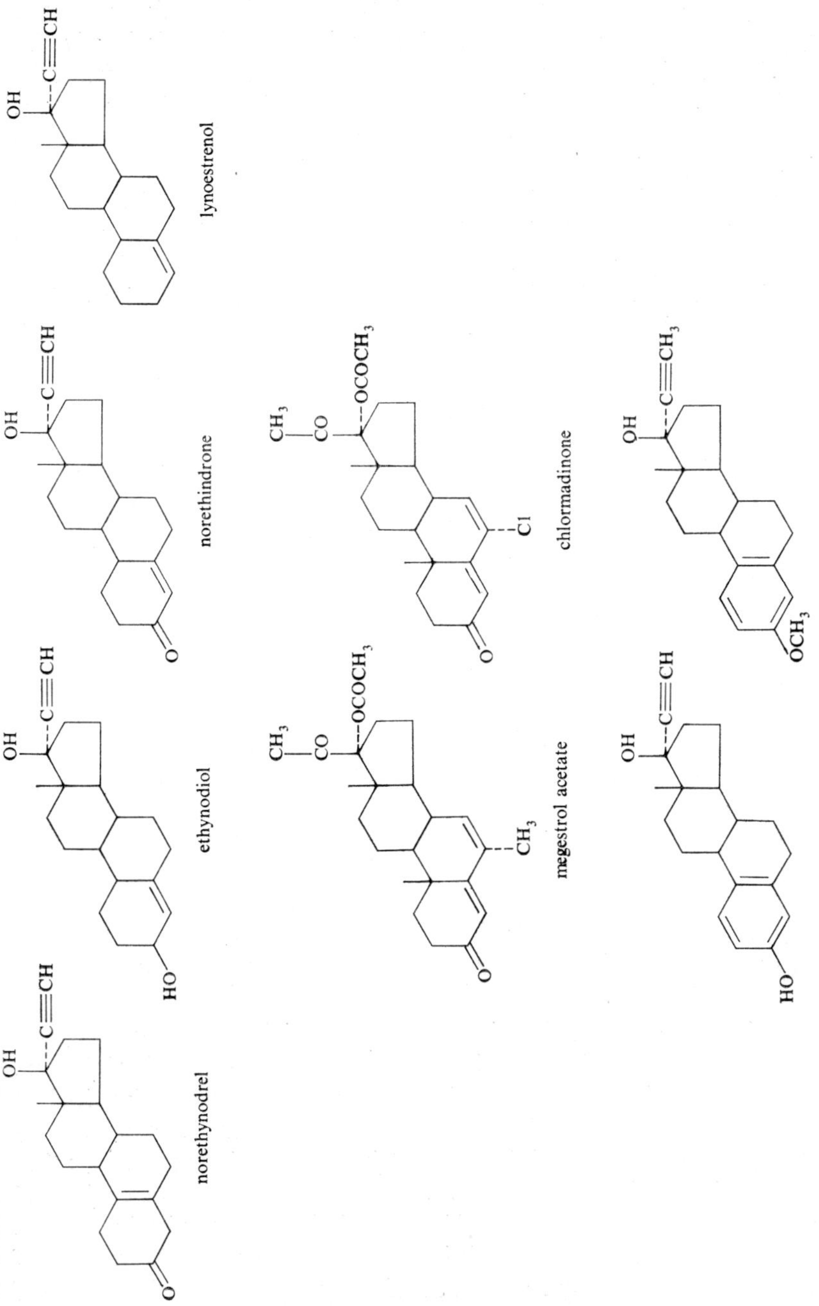

FIG. 12.6. Some synthetic steroids used as oral contraceptives

Although it has been known for many years that the corpus luteum of pregnancy inhibits ovulation, contraceptives based on the use of progesterone only became available much later, since the hormone itself is inactive by mouth. The first breakthrough came with the discovery that the removal of the methyl group at $C_{(19)}$ greatly increased the oral effectiveness of the hormone. There followed intensive studies of other synthetic steroids so that the undesirable androgenic, oestrogenic or other side effects noted with some combinations of steroids should be eliminated. Eventually several acceptable compounds were synthesized, particularly those derived from 19-nortestosterone and 17α-hydroxyprogesterone. Some of the best known of these are shown in Fig. 12.6, and their proprietary names when mixed with various oestrogens are given in Table 12.3.

TABLE 12.3

Some oral contraceptive preparations

Proprietary name	Gestogen component	Oestrogenic component
Conovid	Norethynodrel	Mestranol
Enovid	Norethynodrel	Mestranol
Previson	Norethynodrel	Mestranol
Feminor sequential	Norethynodrel	Mestranol
Ortho-novin	Norethisterone	Mestranol
Anovlar	Norethisterone	Ethinyloestradiol
Gynovlar	Norethisterone	Ethinyloestradiol
Norlestrin	Norethisterone	Ethinyloestradiol
Norlutin A	Norethisterone	Ethinyloestradiol
Lyndiol	Lynoestrenol	Mestranol
Metrulen	Ethynodiol diacetate	Mestranol
Ovulen	Ethynodiol diacetate	Mestranol
Volidan	Megestrol	Ethinyloestradiol

There is no adequate explanation for the oral activity of these compounds. Since some are more active following oral administration than after injection, it is conceivable that some metabolites formed by the liver are involved. It is known that 19-nor derivatives of testosterone give more 5α reduced metabolites than testosterone and these are conjugated largely as sulphates; they are present in the circulation longer, therefore, than if they were conjugated as glucosiduronates. Moreover, 10β-hydroxy derivatives may be formed and these appear to have some synergistic effect with oestrogens. More work of this nature may eventually lead to a satisfactory explanation of the mode of action.

METABOLISM

The metabolism of progesterone has been studied extensively using the hormone labelled with ¹⁴C or tritium. It is well established that in the liver the double bond in ring A is first reduced, after which the 3-oxo group is rapidly reduced to give 3α-hydroxypregnan-20-one. Reduction of the 20-one group follows, and the resulting pregnanediol is conjugated with glucuronic acid and excreted in the urine. Studies with labelled progesterone, however, have shown that although up to 50 per cent of the injected radioactivity is accounted for in the urine only 10–15 per cent is pregnanediol (70, 79, 80). We shall return to a further discussion of the metabolism of progesterone after the section on this important metabolite, pregnanediol.

Pregnanediol

Pregnanediol has been detected in urine, blood, faeces (48, 93) and the bile of patients given large doses of progesterone by mouth (78). It was isolated as a crystalline solid by Marrian (57) and its formula was worked out and its synthesis achieved by Butenandt (7, 8, 51).

Many methods have been described for its measurement in urine, the early ones depending on gravimetric techniques. The most satisfactory method is that of Klopper, Michie and Brown (49) which depends on the separation of the diol fraction on a column of alumina, formation of the di-acetate, further chromatography on alumina and finally colorimetric determination using the H_2SO_4 chromogen. The purity of the di-acetate obtained by this method has been demonstrated by infra-red analysis (49).

EXTRACTION

Pregnanediol glucosiduronate may be extracted from urine by n-butanol and purified by repeated precipitation from acetone (102). Hydrolysis of the conjugate occurs in hot acid or by means of β-glucuronidase, and the free pregnanediol may be extracted into toluene. There is some evidence that the hydrolysis is not complete with β-glucuronidase and that some pregnanediol may be excreted as other conjugates, probably sulphates (84).

PURIFICATION

Adsorption chromatography on alumina has already been mentioned above. Silica gel has been used in its place for the purification of the free steroid and its di-acetate (30).

Paper chromatography based on the Bush systems gives useful separations of pregnanediol from closely related steroids. Eberlein and Bongiovanni (23) used methanol–water–iso-octane–toluene (400:100:225:275 by vol.) in which the R_F value for pregnanediol is 0·5. It may be located by phosphomolybdic acid in ethanol giving a blue stain after heating at 80° for five minutes.

Rapid separations may be achieved on glass fibre paper (95) or preferably by thin layer chromatography (84, 94). In the solvents cyclohexane–acetone (100:3 v/v) on glass fibre paper impregnated with potassium silicate pregnanediol moves with an R_F value of 0·47, well separated from allopregnanediol with R_F 0·64. The system $CHCl_3$–acetone (4·7:1 v/v) on silica gel is another useful system for thin layer chromatography.

GAS LIQUID CHROMATOGRAPHY

Pregnanediol may be separated from its isomer, 5β-pregnane-$3\alpha,20\beta$-diol, on columns of QF-1 at 250° (17, 18, 50). The 5α-isomer, allopregnanediol separates as the acetate on QF-1 or as the trimethylsilyl ether on NPGA.

QUANTITATIVE DETERMINATION

Pregnanediol is chemically inert and there are no specific chemical reactions. It is usually measured by formation of its H_2SO_4 chromogen. The H_2SO_4 spectrum of pregnanediol is not identical to that of its acetate, as might be expected if the acetate groups exerted no influence on the formation of the coloured complex (47). The rate at which the yellow colour develops with each is also different. Oxidizing agents decrease and reducing agents increase the colour intensity. It is recommended that for quantitative work the colour should be developed in H_2SO_4 containing sodium sulphite.

Other metabolic products of progesterone

(1) 20-HYDROXYPREGN-4-EN-3-ONES

Elsewhere in the body, the metabolism of progesterone may proceed differently with reduction of the 20-oxo group first. Dehydrogenases of the 20-hydroxysteroids have been identified in many tissues (64, 111) and have been purified (16, 83).

The conversion *in vitro* to 20α-hydroxypregn-4-en-3-one (20α-OH) has been shown to occur in experiments with human placentae (55), luteal tissue (26, 45), uterine fibroblasts (96) and with foetal liver (103). Tissue from normal human ovaries (2) or from an ovarian arrhenoblastoma (82) when incubated with labelled progesterone gave rise to both 20α-OH and 20β-hydroxypregn-4-en-3-one (20β-OH), while a granulosa-theca cell tumour of the ovary gave 20α-OH as the major metabolite (33).

Metabolism to 20α-OH has been demonstrated repeatedly in studies with rodents. Thus it occurred in experiments with mouse fibroblasts (72) and with muscle and adipose tissue as well as with ovaries from the rat (96, 110, 112, 113). Muscle and adipose tissue gave rise to 20α-OH with no evidence of reduction in ring A. This does occur, however, with uterine tissue, particularly when taken from rats at oestrous. Kidney tissue, including human kidney, also contains a 3α-reductase system and produces no 20-hydroxy compounds.

Examination of the steroids in tissues, as distinct from the incubation of tissues, has also given evidence of this metabolic pathway. The 20α-OH epimer has been extracted from human placentae and ovaries (115) and from the corpus luteum of ewes and mares (87, 88, 89). The placenta of the mare, however, contains mainly 20β-OH while in the urine both 5α-pregnane-3β, 20-diol epimers are excreted with a preponderance of the 20β (4). Short has suggested a 'two cell type' theory to account for the synthesis of ovarian steroids in the mare. No 20α-OH is found in the follicular fluid but there is plenty in the corpus luteum. Conversely 17α-hydroxyprogesterone and oestrogens are found in the follicular fluid but not in the corpus luteum. Short suggests, therefore, that the *theca interna* cells which line the follicles are responsible for the production of oestrogens and the luteinized *granulosa cells* for progesterone (see also p. 281). It is interesting that both types of cell occur in the human corpus luteum and oestrogens are detected both in the corpus luteum and in the urine during the luteal phase of the cycle.

Bovine corpora lutea produce 20β-OH (31) and the same epimer has been found in a granulosa cell tumour of the ovary in a heifer (91).

Both compounds have been detected in human blood (86, 115) and Hilliard *et al.* (41) consider 20α-OH to be the principal progestogen in rabbit blood; it is also excreted by the rabbit (20).

The life of progesterone in circulating blood is short (71). Injected [¹⁴C]progesterone was converted rapidly to 20α-OH in a pregnant ewe (5, 90) and within five minutes the concentration of 20α-OH was almost as high as that of progesterone. Hooker and Forbes (44), using a bioassay which at the time was considered to be specific for progesterone, showed that the biological activity of progesterone disappeared rapidly from plasma kept at room temperature. By the use of a chemical method, however, no loss was reported after incubation of progesterone with ovine blood at 37° for one hour (24) but a definite breakdown was recognized when blood was used, although the reaction was slow (half-life approx. 7 hrs) (85). In this instance the progesterone was converted to 20β-OH.

Chemical properties of the 20-hydroxypregn-4-en-3-ones

The first synthesis of 20α-OH was achieved by Butenandt and Schmidt (9). Both isomers may readily be prepared from progesterone (99). A methanolic solution of progesterone is treated with pyrrolidine and gives the 3-*N*-pyrrolidine enamine. After reduction with LiAlH₄ the pyrrolidino group is removed by hydrolysis. LiAlH₄ is not stereo-specific in the reduction of 20-ketones but the reduction favours the formation of the β-ol. This is generally the case except where there is a steric effect of substituents in ring D.

The separation of the two isomers is relatively easy, since the 20β-OH is less polar than the 20α-OH. This is because the 20β-ol group is enclosed by neighbouring groups ($C_{(21)}$ methyl, axial $C_{(18)}$ methyl and the equatorial 12β-H atom) to a greater extent than the 20α-ol. In system A of Bush the 20α-OH has an R_F of 1·41 and the 20β-OH has an R_F of 1·88 with respect to deoxycorticosterone. Many other systems of paper chromatography based on the systems of Bush and Zaffaroni have been used (e.g. 115). The 20β-OH epimer may be confused with androstenedione in some systems of paper chromatography, but since this latter substance resists acetylation the two compounds may be differentiated by reaction with acetic anhydride and pyridine followed by a second chromatography.

Partition chromatography on Celite columns with 90 per cent methanol as stationary phase has been used by Villee and Loring (103). After removal of progesterone in trimethylpentane the more polar steroids are eluted with a gradient of dichloroethane. A reverse-phase system was used by Huang and Pearlman (45) with the system of 70 per cent methanol–toluene. Further purification may be achieved by countercurrent distribution in 70 per cent methanol–CCl_4 in which system K for 20α-OH is 0·62.

20α-OH may be identified on paper by development of a blue colour with iodine whereas 20β-OH gives a brown colour. Both give infra-red absorption peaks at 1655 and 1616 cm^{-1} and absorb maximally in the ultraviolet at 240 mμ, characteristic of Δ^4-3-oxosteroids. They do not react with blue tetrazolium or give the characteristic Zimmermann chromogen. On oxidation with chromium trioxide they give progesterone.

Finally both isomers are biologically active. In the Clauberg test in rabbits 20α-OH is between 30 and 50 per cent and 20β-OH is between 10 and 20 per cent as active as progesterone (115). In the Hooker-Forbes test 20β-OH appears to be more active than progesterone, the minimum effective dose being 0·0001 μg (progesterone 0·0002 μg) while the 20 α-OH epimer is about half as active as progesterone. In the human the 20β epimer has been found to be nearly half as active as progesterone as a progestational agent (53).

(2) 16-HYDROXYLATION

16α-hydroxyprogesterone has been isolated from hog adrenal homogenates (61, 62, 76), human ovaries and umbilical blood (117) and human foetal homogenates (106). It has been recognized after incubations of [^{14}C]progesterone with adrenocortical tissue from patients with Cushing's syndrome, adrenal hyperplasia and adrenal tumours (104, 105, 107, 109) and with human foetal adrenals (106), ovarian tissue (108), placentae (56) and testis (34). Villee et al. (105) found that there was a 5·5 per cent conversion to 16α-hydroxyprogesterone from [^{14}C]progesterone incubated with adrenal hyperplastic tissue and that this increased to 21 per cent in the presence of NADPH$_2$ and corticotrophin.

Metabolites have been isolated from the urine of patients with congenital

adrenal hyperplasia (62) and during pregnancy (42, 54). These include 5α-
and 5β-pregnane-3α,16α-diol-20-one, 5α- and 5β-pregnane-3α,16α,20α-triol
and 5α-pregnane-3β,16α,20α-triol.

16α-hydroxyprogesterone has been prepared from progesterone microbiologically with *actinomycete* culture (27). Similar methods have been used
to prepare 16α-hydroxyl derivatives of corticosteroids and androgens.

This compound may be separated from other steroids by the usual methods
of paper chromatography (34, 56, 108), column chromatography (106) and
countercurrent distribution (56, 106). A selection of suitable solvent systems
is given in Table 12.4.

TABLE 12.4

Solvent systems for 16α-hydroxyprogesterone

For paper chromatography

System	R_F	Reference
n-hexane–benzene (1 : 1 v/v)/formamide	0·07	108
Ligroin–toluene (1 : 1 v/v)/70% methanol	0·16	56
Trimethylpentane–toluene (1 : 1 v/v)/80% methanol	0·28	56
Benzene/formamide	0·29	108
Benzene–chloroform (1 : 1 v/v)/formamide	0·45	108
Petroleum ether–benzene (1 : 1 v/v)/70% methanol	0·46	34
Light petroleum–benzene (3 : 7 v/v)/50% methanol	0·77	56

For countercurrent distributions

System	K	Reference
70% methanol/carbon tetrachloride–chloroform (6 : 4 v/v)	1·05	56
70% methanol/carbon tetrachloride–chloroform (9 : 1 v/v)	2·3	104

When treated with acetic acid and H_2SO_4 (108) or by the base, aluminium
t-butoxide (75) it is dehydrated giving 16-dehydro-progesterone. This
steroid may be separated by chromatography in ligroin–propylene glycol
($R_F = 0·82$) (56). It is unchanged by treatment with periodic acid, but is
oxidized by Kiliani reagent to 16-oxoprogesterone (34). This gives a violet
colour with $FeCl_3$ in acid and may be separated by chromatography in
petroleum ether–benzene (1:1 by vol.)/70 per cent methanol in which it has
an R_F of 0·9.

An extensive review of the chemistry and biological activity of 16-hydroxyl-
ated steroids has appeared (3). Some are oestrogenic and others have sodium
diuretic properties: examples of these will be found in later chapters.

T

METABOLISM TO OESTROGENS, ANDROGENS AND CORTICOSTEROIDS

The major metabolic pathway from acetate is through cholesterol and pregnenolone to progesterone which then serves as a key substance for the synthesis of androgens, oestrogens and corticosteroids. These will be described in the three following chapters.

REFERENCES

1 ABELSON, D. and BONDY, P. K. *Archs. Biochem. Biophys.* **57**, 208 (1955).
2 AXELROD, L. R. and GOLDZIEHER, J. W. *J. clin. Endocr.* **22**, 431 (1962).
3 BERNSTEIN, S. *Recent Prog. Horm. Res.* **14**, 1 (1958).
4 BROOKS, R. V., KLYNE, W., MILLER, E. and PATERSON, J. Y. F. *Biochem. J.* **51**, 694 (1952).
5 BRUSH, M. G. *J. Endocr.* **26**, 65 (1963).
6 BUSH, I. E. In *Chromatography of Steroids*, Pergamon Press, Oxford (1961).
7 BUTENANDT, A. *Ber. dt. chem. Ges.* **63**, 659 (1930).
8 BUTENANDT, A. and SCHMIDT, J. *Ber. dt. chem. Ges.* **67**, 1901 (1934).
9 BUTENANDT, A. and SCHMIDT, J. *Ber. dt. chem. Ges.* **67**, 2092 (1934).
10 BUTENANDT, A. and SCHMIDT-THOMÉ, J. *Ber. dt. chem. Ges.* **71**, 1487 (1938).
11 BUTENANDT, A. and SCHMIDT-THOMÉ, J. *Ber. dt. chem. Ges.* **72**, 182 (1939).
12 BUTENANDT, A. and WESTPHAL, U. *Ber. dt. chem. Ges.* **67**, 2085 (1934).
13 BUTENANDT, A., WESTPHAL, U. and COBLER, H. *Ber. dt. chem. Ges.* **67**, 1611 (1934).
14 BUTENANDT, A., WESTPHAL, U., COBLER, H. and FERNHOLZ, E. *Ber. dt. chem. Ges.* **67**, 1855 (1934).
15 BUTT, W. R., MORRIS, P., MORRIS, C. J. O. R. and WILLIAMS, D. C. *Biochem. J.* **49**, 434 (1951).
16 CARVAGAL, F. *J. org. Chem.* **24**, 695 (1959).
17 CHAMBERLAIN, J., KNIGHTS, B. A. and THOMAS, G. H. *J. Endocr.* **28**, 235 (1964).
18 CHAMBERLAIN, J., KNIGHTS, B. A. and THOMAS, G. H. *J. Endocr.* **26**, 367 (1963).
19 COLLINS, W. P. and SOMMERVILLE, I. F. *Nature, Lond.* **203**, 836 (1964).
20 COOKE, A. M., ROGERS, A. W. and THOMAS, G. H. *J. Endocr.* **27**, 299 (1963).
21 CORNER, G. W. and ALLEN, W. M. *Amer. J. Physiol.* **88**, 326 (1929).
22 DICZFALUSY, E. *Acta endocr. Copenh.* **10**, 373 (1952).
23 EBERLEIN, W. E. and BONGIOVANNI, A. M. *J. clin. Endocr.* **18**, 300 (1958).
24 EDGAR, D. G. *Biochem. J.* **54**, 50 (1953).
25 EMSUN, K. and ARAS, K. *Acta endocr. Copenh.* **46**, 507 (1964).
26 FORLEO, R. and COLLINS, W. P. *Acta endocr. Copenh.* **46**, 265 (1964).

27 FRIED, J., THOMA, R. W., PERLMAN, D., HERZ, J. E. and BORMAN, A. *Recent Prog. Horm. Res.* **11**, 149 (1955).
28 FUJIMOTO, G. I. and PRAGER, J. *J. Amer. chem. Soc.* **75**, 3259 (1953).
29 FUTTERWEIT, W., McNIVEN, N. L. and DORFMAN, R. I. *Biochim. biophys. Acta* **71**, 474 (1963).
30 GOLDZIEHER, J. W. and NAKAMURA, Y. *Acta endocr. Copenh.* **41**, 371 (1962).
31 GORSKI, J., DOMINGUEZ, O. V., SAMUELS, L. T. and ERB, R. E. *Endocrinology* **62**, 234 (1958).
32 GORSKI, J., ERB, R. E., DICKINSON, W. and BUTLER, H. *J. Dairy Sci.* **41**, 1380 (1958).
33 GRIFFITHS, K., GRANT, J. K. and SYMINGTON, T. *J. Endocr.* **30**, 247 (1964).
34 GRIFFITHS, K., GRANT, J. K. and WHYTE, W. G., *J. clin. Endocr.* **23**, 1044 (1963).
35 GUT, M. *Helv. chim. Acta* **36**, 906 (1953).
36 GUT, M. and USKOKOVIĆ, M. *Naturwissenschaften* **47**, 40 (1960).
37 HAMMERSTEIN, J., RICE, B. F. and SAVARD, K. *J. clin. Endocr.* **24**, 597 (1964).
38 HASKINS, A. L. *Proc. Soc. exp. Biol. Med.* **73**, 439 (1950).
39 HASKINS, A. L. *Amer. J. Obstet. Gynec.* **67**, 330 (1954).
40 HEAP, R. B. *J. Endocr.* **30**, 293 (1964).
41 HILLIARD, J., ARCHIBALD, D. and SAWYER, C. H. *Endocrinology* **72**, 59 (1963).
42 HIRSCHMANN, H., HIRSCHMANN, F. B. and ZALA, A. P., *J. biol. Chem.* **236**, 3141 (1961).
43 HOOKER, C. W. and FORBES, T. R. *Endocrinology* **41**, 158 (1947).
44 HOOKER, C. W. and FORBES, T. R. *Endocrinology* **44**, 61 (1949).
45 HUANG, W. Y. and PEARLMAN, W. H. *J. biol. Chem.* **238**, 1308 (1963).
46 JOHNSON, W. S., KEANA, J. F. W. and MARSHALL, J. A. *Tetrahedron Lett.* 193 (1963).
47 KLOPPER, A. I. *J. Endocr.* **13**, 291 (1956).
48 KLOPPER, A. I. and MACNAUGHTON, M. C. *J. Endocr.* **18**, 319 (1959).
49 KLOPPER, A. I., MICHIE, E. A. and BROWN, J. B. *J. Endocr.* **12**, 209 (1955).
50 KNIGHTS, B. A. and THOMAS, G. H. *J. Endocr.* **24**, iii (1962).
51 KOBER, S. *Biochem. Z.* **239**, 20 (1931).
52 KOECHLIN, B. A., KRITCHEVSKY, T. H. and GALLAGHER, T. F. *J. biol. Chem.* **184**, 393 (1950).
53 LAURITZEN, C. *Acta endocr. Copenh.* **44**, 225 (1963).
54 LIEBERMAN, S., PRAETZ, B., HUMPHRIES, P. and DOBRINER, K. *J. biol. Chem.* **204**, 491 (1953).
55 LITTLE, B., DI MARTINIS, J. and NYHOLM, B. *Acta endocr. Copenh.* **30**, 530 (1959).

56 LITTLE, B., SHAW, A. and PURDY, R. *Acta endocr. Copenh.* **43,** 510 (1963).

57 MARRIAN, G. F. *Biochem. J.* **23,** 1090 (1929).

58 MARSHALL, I. A. and JOHNSON, W. S. *J. Amer. chem. Soc.* **84,** 1485 (1962).

59 MASON, N. R. and SAVARD, K. *Endocrinology* **74,** 664 (1964).

60 MASON, N. R. and SAVARD, K. *Endocrinology* **75,** 215 (1964).

61 NEHER, R., DESAULLES, P., VISCHER, E., WIELAND, P. and WETTSTEIN, A. *Helv. chim. Acta* **41,** 1667 (1958).

62 NEHER, R., MEYSTRE, C. and WETTSTEIN, A. *Helv. chim. Acta.* **42,** 132 (1959).

63 NEHER, R. and WETTSTEIN, A. *Helv. chim. Acta* **35,** 276 (1952).

64 NEHER, R. and WETTSTEIN, A. *Helv. chim. Acta.* **43,** 1171 (1960).

65 NEHER, R. and WETTSTEIN, A. *Helv. chim. Acta* **43,** 1628 (1960).

66 OERTEL, G. W. and EIK-NES, K. B. *Analyt. Chem.* **31,** 98 (1959).

67 OERTEL, G. W., WEISS, S. P. and EIK-NES, K. B. *J. clin. Endocr.* **19,** 213 (1959).

68 PEARLMAN, W. H. In *The Hormones* Vol. 1 (edited by G. Pincus and K. V. Thimann), p. 407, Academic Press, New York (1948).

69 PEARLMAN, W. H. *Biochem. J.* **66,** 17 (1957).

70 PEARLMAN, W. H. *Biochem. J.* **67,** 1 (1957).

71 PEARLMAN, W. H. *Ciba Fdn Colloq. Endocr.* **11,** 233 (1957).

72 PEARLMAN, W. H. *Can. J. Biochem. Physiol.* **38,** 393 (1960).

73 PEARLMAN, W. H. and CERCEO, E. *J. biol. Chem.* **198,** 79 (1952).

74 PEARLMAN, W. H. and CERCEO, E. *J. biol. Chem.* **203,** 127 (1953).

75 PERLMAN, D., TITUS, E. and FRIED, J. *J. Amer. chem. Soc.* **74,** 2126 (1952).

76 RAO, B. G. and HEARD, R. D. H. *Archs. Biochem. Biophys.* **66,** 504 (1957).

77 REYNOLDS, S. R. M. and GINSBURG, N. *Endocrinology* **31,** 147 (1942).

78 RODGERS, J. and MCLELLAN, F. *J. clin. Endocr.* **11,** 246 (1951).

79 ROMANOFF, L. P., MORRIS, C. W., WELCH, P., GRACE, M. P. and PINCUS, G. *J. clin. Endocr.* **23,** 283 (1963).

80 SANDBERG, A. A. and SLAUNWHITE, W. R. *J. clin. Endocr.* **18,** 253 (1958).

81 SAVARD, K. and CASEY, P. J. *Endocrinology* **74,** 599 (1964).

82 SAVARD, K., GUT, M., DORFMAN, R. I., GABRILOVE, J. L. and SOFFER, L. J. *J. clin. Endocr.* **21,** 165 (1961).

83 SCHMIDT-THOMÉ, J. and HUBENER, H. J. *Angew. Chem.* **73,** 44 (1961).

84 SHEN, N.-H. C., KATZMAN, M. B., FRANCIS, F. E. and KINSELLA, R. A. *J. Lab. clin. Med.* **61,** 174 (1963).

85 SHORT, R. V. *J. Endocr.* **16,** 415 (1958).

86 SHORT, R. V. *J. Endocr.* **20,** xv (1960).

87 SHORT, R. V. *J. Endocr.* **24,** 59 (1962).

88 SHORT, R. V. and LEVETT I. *J. Endocr.* **25,** 239 (1962).

89 SHORT, R. V. and MOORE, N. W. *J. Endocr.* **19,** 288 (1959).

90 SHORT, R. V. and POWELL, J. G. *J. Endocr.* **25,** 369 (1962).

91 SHORT, R. V., SHORTER, D. R. and LINZELL, J. L. *J. Endocr.* **27,** 327 (1963).

92 SHULL, G. M., SARDINAS, J. L. and NUBEL, R. C. *Archs. Biochem. Biophys.* **37,** 186 (1952).

93 SOMMERVILLE, I. F. and DESHPANDE, G. N. *J. clin. Endocr.* **18,** 1223 (1958).

94 STARKA, L. and RIEDLOVA, J. *Endokrinologie* **43,** 201 (1962).

95 STAUB, M. C., GAITAN, E. and DINGMAN, J. F. *J. clin. Endocr.* **22,** 87 (1962).

96 SWEAT, M. L. *Biochim. biophys. Acta* **28,** 591 (1958).

97 SWEAT, M. L., BERLINER, D. L., BRYSON, M. J., NABORS, C., HASKELL, J. and HOLMSTROM, E. G. *Biochim. biophys. Acta* **40,** 289 (1960).

98 TAYLOR, W. *Biochem. J.* **56,** 463 (1954).

99 THOMAS, G. H. *Biochem. J.* **83,** 450 (1962).

100 TOUCHSTONE, J. C. and MURAWEC, C. T. *Fedn. Proc.* **19,** 236 (1960).

101 TURNER, R. B. *J. Amer. chem. Soc.* **72,** 579 (1950).

102 VENNING, E. H. and BROWN, J. S. L. *Proc. Soc. exp. Biol. Med.* **34,** 792 (1936).

103 VILLEE, C. A. and LORING, J. M. *Endocrinology* **72,** 824 (1963).

104 VILLEE, D. B. *J. clin. Endocr.* **24,** 442 (1964).

105 VILLEE, D. B., DIMOLINE, A. R., ENGEL, L. L., VILLEE, C. A. and RAKER, J. *J. clin. Endocr.* **22,** 726 (1962).

106 VILLEE, D. B., ENGEL, L. L., LORING, J. M. and VILLEE, C. A. *Endocrinology* **69,** 354 (1961).

107 WARD, P. J. and GRANT, J. K. *J. Endocr.* **26,** 139 (1963).

108 WARREN, J. C. and SALHANICK, H. A. *J. clin. Endocr.* **21,** 1376 (1961).

109 WELINSKY, I. and ENGEL, L. L. *J. biol. Chem.* **238,** 1302 (1963).

110 WIEST, W. G. *J. biol. Chem.* **234,** 3115 (1959).

111 WIEST, W. G. *Acta endocr. Copenh.* Suppl. 51, 965 (1960).

112 WIEST, W. G. *Endocrinology* **73,** 310 (1963).

113 WIEST, W. G. and WILCOX, R. B. *J. biol. Chem.* **236,** 2425 (1961).

114 ZAFFARONI, A. *J. Amer. chem. Soc.* **72,** 3828 (1950).

115 ZANDER, J., FORBES, T. R., VON MUNSTERMANN, A. M. and NEHER, R. *J. clin. Endocr.* **18,** 337 (1958).

116 ZANDER, J. and SIMMER, H. *Klin. Wschr.* **32,** 529 (1954).

117 ZANDER, J., THYSSEN, J. and VON MUNSTERMANN, A. M. *J. clin. Endocr.* **22,** 861 (1962).

13

OESTROGENS

The oestrogens, in combination with other hormones, are responsible for the development and maintenance of the female sexual organs. They are produced in the gonads, the placenta and the adrenal cortex. The main site of formation in the female is normally the ovary, but during pregnancy the amount formed by the placenta gradually increases until in late pregnancy it may produce up to a thousand times as much as the ovary.

The three main oestrogens in the human are oestrone, oestradiol-17β, and oestriol, the most potent of these as judged by bioassays being oestradiol-17β. Oestrone, equilin and some equilenin are found in the mare. Early workers (see 128) observed that both equilin and equilenin increased in late pregnancy in the mare at a time when total oestrogens actually dropped. By the fourth to fifth months the amount of equilin excreted is equal to and sometimes more than the amount of oestrone (128). Several other oestrogens have been detected or isolated from urine or tissues of the human and other species and some of these are listed in Table 13.1.

Biosynthesis

There are numerous studies showing that oestrogens may arise from acetate, cholesterol, progesterone and androgens.

In vitro studies have shown that oestrone and oestradiol-17β are produced from ^{14}C-labelled *acetate* in the ovaries of many species including the human (70, 112, 117, 124, 147, 162), dog (116), cat (117) and pig (157), and in the testes of the human, dog, cat (117) and stallion (111). Injection of labelled acetate to the pregnant mare leads to the excretion of radioactive oestrone, equilin and equilenin (73).

Labelled pregnenolone may act as a precursor to oestrone and oestradiol-17β in the ovaries of the human (6, 121) and the pig (166) and the same oestrogens have repeatedly been shown to arise from progesterone in the

278

TABLE 13.1

Some oestrogens isolated from biological fluids and tissues

Source	Trivial name	References
Human urine	16α-hydroxyoestrone	(a)
	16β-hydroxyoestrone	(b)
	16 oxo-oestrone	(c)
	2-methoxyoestrone	(d), (e), (f)
	2-hydroxyoestrone	55
	6-hydroxyoestrone	(g)
	18-hydroxyoestrone	(h)
	16-oxo-oestradiol-17β	90, (b)
	2-methoxyoestradiol-17β	(f)
	16-epioestriol	(i)
	2-methoxyoestriol	(j)
	17-epioestriol	(k)
	16, 17-epioestriol	(l)
Pregnant mare urine	Dihydroequilenin-17α	(m)
	Dihydroequilenin-17β	(n)
	Dihydroequilin-17α	(o)
	3β-hydroxyoestra-5,7,9-trien-17-one	(p)
	3-deoxyequilenin	(q)
Mare follicular fluid	6α-hydroxyoestradiol-17β	(r)
Mouse ovaries	17-epioestriol	155
Tissues and fluids from cow, sheep and goat	17α-oestradiol	(s), (t)

(a) MARRIAN, G. F., LOKE, K. H., WATSON, E. J. D. and PANATTONI, M. *Biochem. J.* **66,** 60 (1957).
(b) LAYNE, D. S. and MARRIAN, G. F. *Biochem. J.* **70,** 244 (1958).
(c) MARLOW, H. W. *J. biol. Chem.* **183,** 167 (1950).
(d) KRAYCHY, S. and GALLAGHER, T. F. *J. Amer. chem. Soc.* **79,** 754 (1957).
(e) LOKE, K. H. and MARRIAN, G. F. *Biochim. biophys. Acta* **27,** 213 (1958).
(f) FRANDSEN, V. A. *Acta endocr. Copenh.* **31,** 603 (1959).
(g) LOKE, K. H., WATSON, E. J. D. and MARRIAN, G. F. *Biochim. biophys. Acta* **26,** 230 (1957).
(h) LOKE, K. H., MARRIAN, G. F. and WATSON, E. J. D. *Biochem. J.* **71,** 43 (1959).
(i) MARRIAN, G. F. and BAULD, W. S. *Biochem. J.* **59,** 136 (1955).
(j) FISHMAN, J. and GALLAGHER, T. F. *Archs. Biochem. Biophys.* **77,** 511 (1958).
(k) BREUER, H. *Nature, Lond.* **185,** 613 (1960).
(l) BREUER, H. and PANGELS, G. *Biochim. biophys. Acta* **36,** 572 (1959).
(m) SCHWENK, E. and HILDEBRANDT, F. *Naturwissenschaften* **20,** 658 (1932).
(n) WINTERSTEINER, O., SCHWENK, E., HIRSCHMANN, H. and WHITMAN, B. *J. Amer. chem. Soc.* **58,** 2652 (1936).
(o) WINTERSTEINER, O. and HIRSCHMANN, H. *J. biol. Chem.* **119,** cvii (1937).
(p) HEARD, R. D. H. and HOFFMAN, M. M. *J. biol. Chem.* **135,** 801 (1940).
(q) PRELOG, V. and FÜHRER, I. *Helv. chim. Acta* **28,** 583 (1945).
(r) BUSH, I. E., KLYNE, W. and SHORT, R. V. *J. Endocr.* **20,** i (1960).
(s) ROMMEL, P. *Acta endocr. Copenh.* **45,** 605 (1964).
(t) VELLE, W. *Gen. Comp. Endocr.* **3,** 621 (1963).

ovaries of many species (6, 58, 121, 125). The ovaries of mice produce 17-epioestriol and a compound which is probably 16-oxoestriol (155).

Androstenedione and testosterone act as precursors of oestrogens in the presence of tissues from placentae (8, 120), ovaries (9, 66, 74, 98, 163), corpora lutea (77, 147), testes and adrenal cortex (8). The intermediate, 19-hydroxyandrostenedione, is also an effective substrate (94).

The biosynthetic pathway to the oestrogens has thus been established as indicated in Fig. 13.1. Pathways not involving progesterone may be of some slight significance in the ovary (124, 160). In a careful study of equine follicular

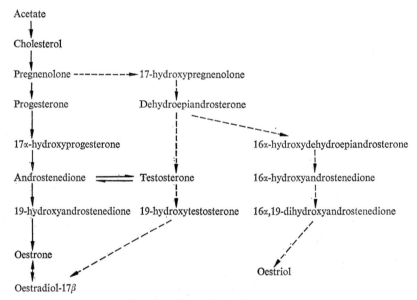

FIG. 13.1. Biosynthesis of oestrogens

fluid neither pregnenolone nor 17α-hydroxypregnenolone could be detected, but a small amount of dehydroepiandrosterone (DHA) was recognized (133). This suggests that there may be an alternative pathway with DHA serving as an intermediate in the conversion of pregnenolone to androstenedione. It has also been found that a granulosa-theca cell tumour of the ovary could not utilize progesterone as a precursor for oestrogens although androstenedione did give rise to some oestrogen (66).

The biosynthesis of oestrogens in the ovary occurs in the cells lining the follicles which must possess the enzymes necessary for 17-hydroxylation, $C_{(21)}$ side-chain cleavage and aromatization of ring A. The cells of the corpus luteum are mainly responsible for the production of progesterone and in the mare (134) are, in fact, incapable of producing oestrogen. Short (134) has found all the steroids on the main pathway to oestrogen (Fig. 13.1) present in fluid from follicular cysts of the mare, but only progesterone and 20α-hydroxy-pregn-4-en-3-one in corpora lutea. His 'two cell type' theory to explain this has already been mentioned (p. 271). There is evidence, however, that some of the enzymes necessary for the synthesis of oestrogen are present in the granulosa cells of the corpus luteum. Thus luteinized granulosa cells of the mare may aromatize ring A of C_{19} steroids (96), and tissue from a granulosa cell tumour containing no thecal cells, converted testosterone to oestrogen (98).

Enhanced production of oestrogens is noted when gonadotrophins are included in the incubation media. Thus with human corpora lutea the amount of [14C]acetate incorporated into oestrogens is increased by human luteinizing hormone or chorionic gonadotrophin, but it is interesting to note that no such effect is demonstrated when ovine luteinizing hormone or ovine prolactin is used (118). Ovine luteinizing hormone, however, is effective with bovine corpora lutea, but only a small effect is observed with ovine follicle stimulating hormone, and this is probably due to its slight contamination with luteinizing hormone (99).

The *in vivo* effects of gonadotrophins on the production of oestrogens is well established. Patients with polycystic ovaries produce excess androgen, notably androstenedione, due to a failure of the follicle to aromatize ring A of this steroid. Under the influence of human follicle stimulating hormone and chorionic gonadotrophin the follicles mature and eventually rupture. Large amounts of oestrogen may appear in the follicular cyst fluid and in the urine (38).

The mechanism of the aromatization step has been investigated using the 1α, 2α[3H]- and 4[14C]-derivatives of androstenedione and testosterone (7). After hydroxylation at $C_{(19)}$ (Fig. 13.2) the simplest mechanism for aromatization is the simultaneous elimination of this group together with a hydrogen from $C_{(1)}$ forming a 3-oxo-1(10),4-diene which then aromatizes spontaneously.

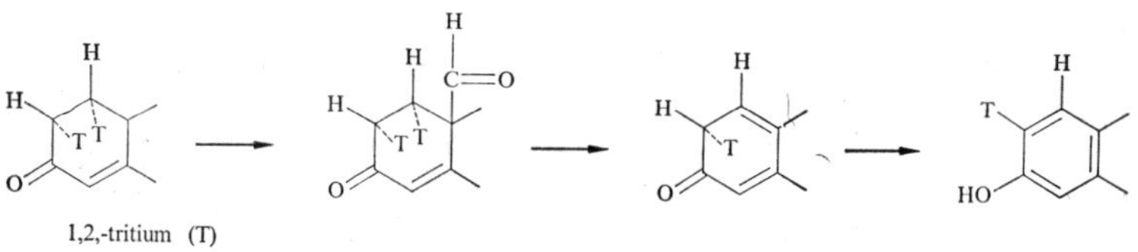

1,2,-tritium (T)

FIG. 13.2

If the hydrogen atom at 1β is eliminated in the formation of the diene, no tritium is removed and the $^3H/^{14}C$ ratio remains unchanged, whereas removal of the 1α-tritium reduces the ratio by half. The latter is found to occur experimentally. Such preferential removal of the α (axial) rather than the β (equatorial) constituent from $C_{(1)}$ at the same time that the $C_{(19)}$ (β-axial) group is being removed is consistent with theoretical considerations which favour diaxial transelimination. Acetylation of the final product does not alter the $^3H/^{14}C$ ratio which indicates that the 2β-axial H and not the 2α-equatorial tritium forms the hydroxyl group at $C_{(3)}$.

Diczfalusy and his colleagues have made a very careful and extensive study of the biosynthesis of oestrogens during pregnancy. *In vivo* and *in vitro* experiments have shown that unconjugated C_{19} steroids such as DHA, androstenedione and testosterone undergo extensive conversion to oestrogens; conjugated DHA-sulphate is aromatized to a smaller degree. In experiments involving perfusion of placentae the products are oestrone and oestradiol-17β but not oestriol; the latter, however, is formed in an intact foetal-placental unit. It is considered that oestrone and oestradiol-17β formed in the placenta are transferred to the foetus where a part of the oestrone is 16α-hydroxylated and then returned to the placenta where conversion to oestriol occurs. An interesting theory is put forward that the placenta thus acts as an efficient barrier to protect the foetus from the undesirable effects of maternal androgens (18, 19, 20).

Other reports suggest that DHA-sulphate is more efficiently converted to oestrogens by pregnant women than either DHA itself, testosterone or androstenedione. This may be a function of the marked difference in plasma half-life of the conjugated and the free steroids (15, 135). DHA-sulphate may act as a reserve, from which the free steroid gradually becomes available.

Oestrone may be produced as a sulphate in the *adrenal cortex* (142). Labelled oestrone incubated with bovine adrenal tissue was shown to give variable amounts of a water-soluble radioactive metabolite which was probably oestrone sulphate.

There is some evidence for the conversion of cortisol to 11-hydroxylated oestrogens but the mechanism remains obscure. Administration of $[^{14}C]$cortisone acetate to adrenalectomized and oophorectomized women with carcinoma of the breast resulted in the excretion of 11β-hydroxy-17β-oestradiol, 11β-hydroxyoestrone and 16-epioestriol. (33). The conversion of cortisone to 11β-hydroxyoestrone occurs *in vitro* with slices of human breast tissue (34) and the conversion of C_{19} steroids of adrenal origin to oestrogens probably takes place in extra-adrenal tissue such as liver or spleen.

The interconversion of oestrone, oestradiol-17β and oestriol has been studied extensively by *in vitro* experiments involving liver and kidney slices (122, 152). The enzymes involved are present also in other organs including the ovary, placenta, intestine and mammary gland and in the red cells (123). The presence of a 17β-dehydrogenase has been demonstrated in human red cells, and for the conversion of oestrone to oestradiol-17β it is NADP-dependent and couples with glucose-6-phosphate dehydrogenase (108). The presence of both 17β- and 17α-dehydrogenases is reported in bovine kidney cells (152). Figure 13.3 summarizes the conversions that are considered to occur in the metabolism of oestradiol-17β and oestrone.

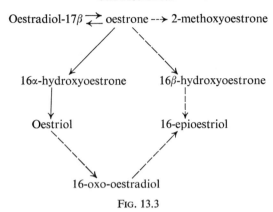

Oestradiol-17β $\rightleftarrows$ oestrone $\dashrightarrow$ 2-methoxyoestrone

16α-hydroxyoestrone   16β-hydroxyoestrone

Oestriol   16-epioestriol

16-oxo-oestradiol

FIG. 13.3

It is still not clear whether oestriol is the last stage in the inactivation process of the circulating oestrogens. Certainly not all the labelled oestradiol-17β administered can be accounted for in the phenolic fractions from urine; this may indicate that perhaps ring A is opened and the metabolites are difficult to identify (16, 81).

Synthesis

A convenient synthesis for oestrone and equilenin has been described, and is similar to that for testosterone mentioned on page 304.

In another synthesis for oestrone, also suitable for derivatives of equilenin, compounds (1; R=O) and (1; R=β-O-tetrahydropyranyl,α-H) are refluxed in benzene and potassium t-butoxide and then treated with m-methoxyphenylethyl bromide to give II (Fig. 13.4) (36). This compound undergoes cyclization in polyphosphoric acid at 60° to the methyl ether of bisdehydro-oestrone (III) which is reduced to give the oestrone derivative IV (141). If the compound II is dehydrated with SeO_2 in boiling t-butanol containing pyridine the product is equilenin methyl ether (V).

Another route to (III) is by alkylation of 2-methyl cyclopentane-1,3-dione with 6-methoxy-1-vinyl-1-tetralol (VI) in Triton B which gives the diketone (VII). Gentle warming in methanol containing dilute HCl gives (III) in good yield (3, 37).

Oestrogens labelled with ^{14}C or ^3H are available for metabolic studies or for use in methods of determination. An interesting doubly-labelled derivative, [6,7-^{3}H]oestrone-[^{35}S]sulphate has been synthesized (87). [6,7-^{3}H]oestrone is easily prepared by the catalytic reduction of oestra-1,3,5(10),6-tetraene-3-ol-17-one with tritium. Sulphurylation with labelled chlorosulphonic acid or with SO_3 would constitute a radioactive hazard. However, labelled pyridine sulphate is formed from pyridine and labelled H_2SO_4, and in the presence of a 10 per cent molar excess of acetic anhydride reacts with oestrone to give

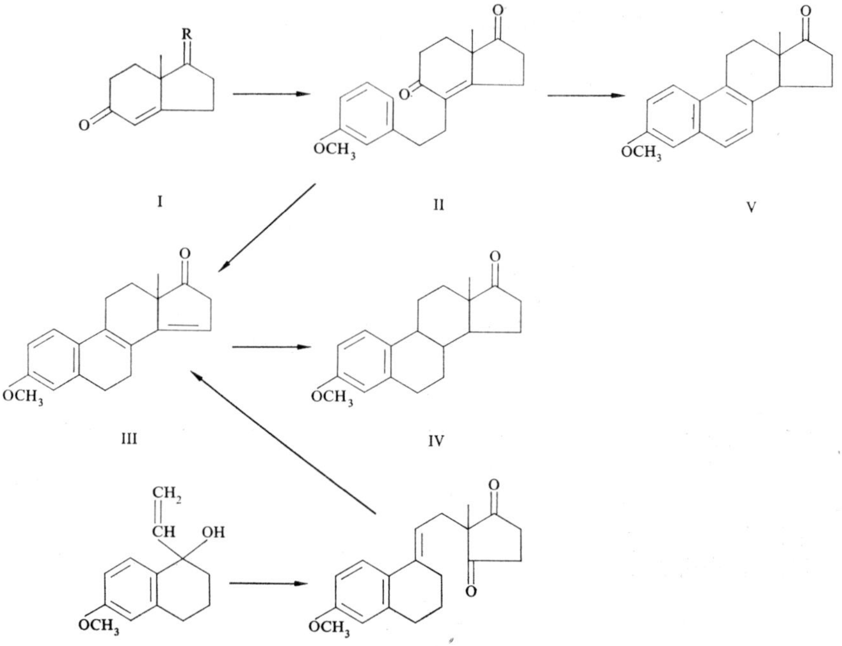

Fig. 13.4

pyridinium oestrone sulphate from which the sodium salt of oestrone sulphate is readily obtained by the addition of NaOH.

Metabolism

Much information about the metabolism of oestrogens in the human has been obtained by the use of natural and labelled oestrogens (for a review see 29).

Placental oestriol is extensively sulphurylated by the foetus (40, 42, 88, 104, 105). Oestriol-3-sulphate has been isolated and identified in human meconium (102), and the products from the intra-amniotic administration of oestrogens have been shown to be 17β-oestradiol-3-sulphate, oestriol-3-sulphate and probably 2-methoxy-17β-oestradiol and oestrone sulphate (43, 46, 104, 105). Following the intra-amniotic injection of labelled oestriol and oestrone sulphate there is a striking difference in the nature of the steroids extracted from the foetus and the placenta. In the former the oestrogens are conjugated whereas in the placenta they are in an ether-soluble, non-conjugated form even when oestrone sulphate has been injected. In untreated foetuses two conjugated forms are detected, oestriol 3-sulphate and oestriol 16 (? 17) glucosiduronate. [16-^{14}C]oestriol injected into the umbilical vein of a new-born anencephalic monster was shown to be quickly conjugated, mostly to the 3-sulphate and partly to the 3-sulphate-16 (? 17)-glucosiduronate. In this case no oestriol 16 (? 17) glucosiduronate was detected (41).

Although the physiological significance of the extensive sulphurylation is not known it is possible that the ability to sulphurylate 3β-hydroxy-steroids may have an important influence on regulating the amount of 3β-hydroxy-C_{19} steroid available for placental conversion to oestrogen (20, 115).

In the foetus and in children up to about two years of age, oestrogens are rapidly metabolized in a rather different way from that in adults. The products are mainly conjugated oestriol and other highly polar compounds such as 2-hydroxy- and 2-methoxy-oestrogens. The 2-hydroxylation appears to be as important as 16-hydroxylation (55) and it is probable that 2-hydroxylated oestradiol may be more active in stimulating certain tissue growth in the foetus and young children than in acting as an oestrogen (42).

The 2-hydroxylated derivatives were probably missed in much of the early work since they are easily destroyed by quite mild acid hydrolysis. Even condensation with Girard's Reagent T which is used for separating 2-hydroxy oestrone from oestradiol- 17β may lead to very poor recoveries (53). Further study of the compound has been facilitated by the synthesis of labelled 2-hydroxyoestrone (56). It should be noted that 16α-hydroxyoestrone, a steroid of quantitative importance, and 16-oxo-oestradiol-17β may also be largely destroyed during quite mild acid hydrolysis or during treatment with Girard's Reagent T.

[16-^{14}C]oestriol given to pregnant women is detected in the circulation as the free steroid, as 3-sulphate and as 3-sulphate 16 (? 17) glucosiduronate. Free oestriol and the 3-sulphate are present in urine, but most of the injected steroid is excreted as the 16 (? 17) glucosiduronate and as a more polar glucosiduronate (di- or tri-) and a little as 3-sulphate 16 (? 17) glucosiduronate (161).

Oestriol 16α-glucosiduronate has also been detected in pregnancy urine (71) and oestrone glucosiduronate in the human intestinal tract (44).

It should be noted that oestriol differs from most other steroids in conjugating at the 16α- rather than the 3α-position (110). Evidence available from competitive experiments suggests that the 16α-transferase is a separate entity from the 3α-transferase (138).

Methods of extraction

(a) URINE AND PLASMA

Oestrogens may not only be free and conjugated, as just discussed, but they may also be bound to protein. Experimentally it has been shown that they bind to bovine serum albumin, to bovine γ-globulin and to human serum albumin (146). Clinical work calls for methods of hydrolysing the conjugated and bound oestrogens without destroying them appreciably. Hot-acid hydrolysis is usually used and an authoritative study on this has appeared (30). Maximum yields of oestrone, oestradiol-17β and oestriol are obtained using 15 vol. per cent HCl for 60 minutes at 100°. In some cases, however, when other oestrogens are being investigated, or in the presence of bile (2, 146), enzymic hydrolysis is better. Preparations of β-glucuronidase and of phenol sulphatase (17, 30, 32, 107, 140) are used, usually at 37° for 96 hours at pH 4·7. Alternatively the conjugates themselves may be extracted by solvents as described elsewhere (35, 45, 130, 137, 153), or conveniently by gel filtration (18). In the latter method urine is passed through a column of G-25 Sephadex and the oestrogen conjugates are eluted in water in two main peaks, the first containing oestrone-3-glucosiduronate, oestradiol-3, 17-diglucosiduronate and oestriol-3-glucosiduronate, and the second oestradiol-17-glucosiduronate, oestriol-16(? 17)-glucosiduronate and the sulphate conjugates.

Another interesting method employs a liquid anion exchange resin (84), Amberlite LA-2, a high molecular weight secondary amine. The resin in ethyl acetate extracts the conjugates from urine at pH 2–3 and they may then be back-extracted with dilute ammonia. Recoveries of 90 per cent are reported by this method.

Ether is usually used for the subsequent extraction of the free steroids. Neutral steroids are then easily separated since the oestrogens are soluble in alkali. The more polar oestrogens such as oestriol may later be separated from the others by partitioning between water and organic solvents such as benzene (109).

Further purification has been achieved in some methods by saponification (13, 31). The oestrogens are stable in boiling dilute NaOH, and at the same time the amount of interfering material in urinary extracts is reduced.

Oestrogens are also bound to red cell proteins from which they may be extracted by a mixture of methylal and methanol (107, 127, 156).

(b) Tissue

Free, conjugated and protein-bound oestrogens occur in placental tissue. Direct extraction in solvents, or extraction after acid hydrolysis may be used, but protein-bound oestrogen is best extracted in strong NaOH. Then the free oestrogens may be re-extracted into solvents after acidification of the alkaline extract (39, 109). Similar methods have been used for the extraction of oestrogens from rat liver (122) and many human tissues (123).

Methods of separation

(a) PAPER CHROMATOGRAPHY

A variety of moving phases have been used with formamide, as the stationary phase, including O-dichlorobenzene, methylene chloride or cyclohexane (5), chloroform (90), or monochlorobenzene (26). In the last solvent the three main oestrogens and 16α-hydroxyoestrone, 16-oxo-oestradiol and 16-epioestriol may be separated. Aqueous methanol (70–80 per cent by volume) as the stationary phase may be used with solvents such as benzene–light petroleum (139), iso-octane–toluene, 1:3 v/v, or benzene–light petroleum, 2:3 v/v (107).

Derivatives such as the acetates also separated well in modified systems of Bush (82). They may be hydrolysed on the paper by dioxan in an atmosphere of HCl (129).

(b) THIN LAYER CHROMATOGRAPHY

An authoritative paper on this technique has appeared (93). By using silica gel and several solvent systems (44, 92) in two dimensions, it is possible to identify up to 32 oestrogens.

(c) COUNTERCURRENT DISTRIBUTIONS

This method of fractionation has been developed extensively for the oestrogens by Engel (49, 51) and Diczfalusy (45) and others (53, 62, 72, 158, 159). Examples of partition coefficients are given in Table 13.2. It will be seen that this technique is useful for the separation of the methyl ethers as well as the free steroids. The conjugated oestrogens may be purified by partitioning between water and quinoline (137) and many other solvents (89, 101).

(d) PARTITION CHROMATOGRAPHY ON COLUMNS

A practical method has been devised for the urinary oestrogens (12) which has also been applied successfully to plasma (114), using Celite as the supporting material for the stationary phase. With 0·8N-NaOH as the stationary phase oestrone is eluted first in benzene followed by oestradiol in a mixture of ethylene dichloride–benzene (3:1 v/v). Oestriol is purified on a second column in the system 70 per cent methanol–ethylene dichloride. An efficient version of this method has been described (121) using 90 per cent methanol as stationary phase and gradient elution in trimethyl pentane–ethylene dichloride.

The aqueous phase of t-butanol–n-butanol–2N-NH$_4$OH (125:375:500 v/v) has been used as the stationary phase on Sephadex G-25. The organic phase elutes conjugated oestrone first, followed by oestradiol-17β and oestriol (17).

(e) ADSORPTION CHROMATOGRAPHY

Very rapid separations of the free oestrogens or their methyl ethers may be obtained on columns of alumina. Provided the adsorbent is properly

TABLE 13.2

$$\text{Partition coefficients} \left(\frac{\text{concentration in upper phase}}{\text{concentration in lower phase}}\right) \text{for oestrogens}$$

Reference	[1]	[1]	[2]	[3]
		Solvent System		
	(a)	(b)	(c)	(d)
Oestrone	4·2	0·33	0·37	10·0
Oestradiol-17β	2·9	2·10	1·59	5·2
Oestriol	0·35	—	—	0·35
6-oxo-oestrone	3·3	1·05	—	—
7-oxo-oestrone	6·3	0·44	—	—
16-oxo-oestrone	1·9	1·71	—	—
6-oxo-oestradiol	2·4	—	—	—
16-oxo-oestradiol	0·94	—	—	—
Oestradiol-17α	2·5	—	—	—
16-epioestriol	—	—	—	1·6[5]
2-methoxyoestradiol	2·64[2]	—	0·19	—
2-methoxyoestriol	0·38[4]	—	0·85	—
Equilenin	4·2	0·55	—	—
Dihydroequilenin	2·5	2·9	—	—
Equilin	3·6	0·25	—	—

Reference	[6]	[7]	[7]	[7]
		Solvent System		
	(e)	(f)	(g)	(h)
Oestrone-3-methyl ether	0·85	—	—	—
Oestradiol-17β-3-methyl ether	0·27	—	—	—
Oestriol-3-methyl ether	—	0·20	0·85	2·5
Epioestriol-3-methyl ether	0·08[5]	—	—	—

Solvent Systems
(a) Ethyl acetate–cyclohexane (1 : 1 v/v)/ethanol–water (1 : 1 v/v)
(b) Methanol–water (1 : 1 v/v)/carbon tetrachloride
(c) Methanol–water (7 : 3 v/v)/ethyl acetate–carbon tetrachloride (1 : 9 v/v)
(d) Ethyl acetate–cyclohexane (2 : 3 v/v)/ethanol–water (2 : 3 v/v)
(e) 2-Hexane/methanol–water (9 : 1 v/v)
(f) Methanol–water (1 : 9 v/v)/carbon tetrachloride
(g) Methanol–water (2 : 3 v/v)/carbon tetrachloride
(h) Methanol–water (7 : 3 v/v)/carbon tetrachloride

References
[1] SLAUNWHITE, W. R., ENGEL, L. L., OLMSTED, P. C. and CARTER, P. *J. biol. Chem.* **191**, 627 (1951).
[2] FRANDSEN, V. A. *Acta endocr. Copenh.* **31**, 603 (1959).
[3] ENGEL, L. L., SLAUNWHITE, W. R., CARTER, P. and NATHANSON, I. T. *J. biol. Chem.* **185**, 255 (1950).
[4] FISHMAN, J. and GALLAGHER, T. F. *Archs. Biochem. Biophys.* **77**, 511 (1958).
[5] DICZFALUSY, E. and HALLA, M. *Acta endocr. Copenh.* **27**, 303 (1958).
[6] DICZFALUSY, E. *Acta endocr. Copenh.* **15**, 317 (1954).
[7] DICZFALUSY, E. *Acta endocr. Copenh.* **22**, 203 (1956).

standardized, reproducible results can be obtained and such columns are used in the most reliable of the routine methods for oestrogens (28, 48).

Numerous other adsorbents have been used but none possess any real advantage over the commonly used materials—alumina, silica gel (16, 68, 83, 88, 90, 91, 103, 127) or magnesium silicate (Florisil: 139).

(f) ION-EXCHANGE

Column chromatography has been described for the oestrogens using Dowex 2 (50) or Amberlite IRC-50 (131). Conjugated oestrogens may also be separated on Deacidite FF using ethanol buffered at pH 6·7 (69).

Liquid resins may be incorporated on Celite and used for the separation of both free and conjugated oestrogens (84, 85). The best separations using Amberlite LA-1 have been achieved by gradient elution in formic acid between pH 3·10 and 5·04.

(g) GAS LIQUID CHROMATOGRAPHY

Derivations of the oestrogens are usually preferred for gas chromatography since there is some loss of free oestrogens on the column and they have long retention times. The acetates are suitable derivatives (4, 54, 164, 165) and are easily prepared. The trimethyl silyl ethers separate well on 1 per cent silicone SE-30 columns or on 0·75 per cent NGS and they have reasonably short retention times (95, 100).

(h) ELECTROPHORESIS

High-voltage electrophoresis will separate the free and conjugated oestrogens (61). Electrophoresis at pH values between 4·5 and 8·9 have been used as a means to identify oestriol sulphates and glucosiduronates extracted from blood and urine (151).

(i) OTHER METHODS

16-epioestriol may be separated from oestriol by converting it to the acetonide. This is a selective reaction for *cis*-glycols (Fig. 13.5).

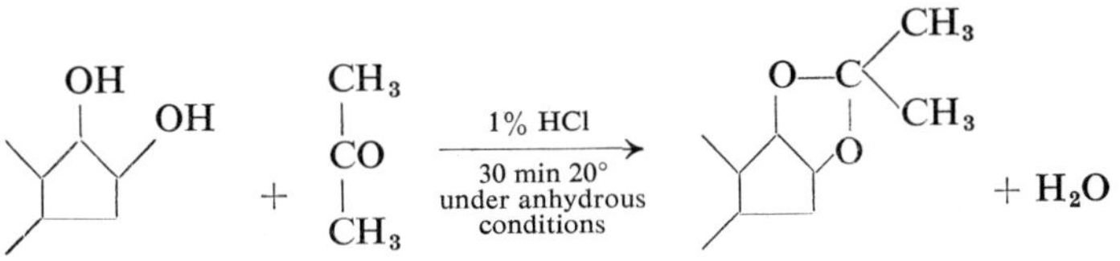

FIG. 13.5

Detection

Extensive lists of reagents used for the detection of oestrogens on paper or thin layer chromatograms have been published (5, 92, 132). These include

U

reagents for phenolic groups such as the Folin and Ciocalteau reagent, reaction with diazo compounds and exposure to ammonia or nitrogen dioxide (22).

There are a number of more specific reagents such as phloroglucinol in NaOH at 80° which gives colours only with 2-hydroxylated oestrogens and 7-oxo-oestrone (92) and vanadic acid which reacts rapidly with 2-hydroxylated oestrogens and more slowly with 16-oxo-oestrone, 7-oxo-oestrone and 2-methoxy compounds (92). Then there are several reagents which give a variety of colours with different oestrogens, including p-toluene sulphonic acid, phosphoric acid in ethanol, $SbCl_3$ and $ZnCl_2$ in glacial acetic acid.

The conjugated oestrogens are often detected by the naphthoresorcinol reagent (57, 59, 60) or by rhodizonic acid (129). Anisaldehyde-H_2SO_4 reagent gives a characteristic emerald green colour with oestradiol-17β and derivatives and a pale violet colour with oestriol (44).

Quantitative estimations

COLORIMETRIC METHODS

The Kober reaction (27) is the best known colorimetric method for the oestrogens. The method consists of two stages: the initial formation of a yellow compound with a green fluorescence on heating with H_2SO_4 and a reducing agent such as a phenol, followed by its conversion into a pink non-fluorescent complex on reheating it with more dilute H_2SO_4. The reaction has been very carefully studied and the optimum conditions established (11, 27). Hydroquinone is recommended as the reducing agent instead of phenol and separate reagents are used for individual oestrogens, 65 per cent v/v H_2SO_4 for oestrone and oestradiol-17β and 76 per cent v/v H_2SO_4 for oestriol. Absorptions are read at three wavelengths so that corrections can be made for interference from non-specific materials. It must be remembered that only a few micrograms of each oestrogen are excreted per 24 hours by normal females so that the problem of removing interfering materials which give colours with strong H_2SO_4 is a difficult one.

A useful modification for reducing this non-specific absorption and thus increasing the sensitivity is that of Ittrich (78) in which the pink colour formed by the oestrogens in the acid reagent is diluted and extracted by 2 per cent w/v p-nitrophenol in chloroform or tetrachloroethane (126) while coloured impurities remain behind. A satisfactory development of this method is to dilute the acid solution with trichloroacetic acid after which the pink colour may be extracted in chloroform (24). Corrected readings are about three times as great as those derived from measurements on the original Kober colour.

In an investigation of the groups responsible for this reaction maximum colour development was noted in compounds with a carbonyl group at $C_{(17)}$

adjacent to an active methylene group as in oestrone and equilenin. A definite colour was also given by 3-methoxy-16-oxo-oestradiol-17α (97).

FLUORIMETRIC METHODS

The oestrogens fluoresce on heating with strong phosphoric acid (52) or H_2SO_4 (1, 10, 14, 25, 63, 80, 136). Phosphoric acid does not form chromogenic substances or fluorescent products with other steroids and impurities as readily as H_2SO_4 but the intensity of fluorescence is less.

There are various methods of reducing the non-specific fluorescence when using H_2SO_4 such as the addition of H_2O_2 (75) or the extraction of the fluorescent compound as in the Ittrich modification of the Kober reaction. Suitable solvents are 2 per cent w/v p-nitrophenol in acetylene tetrachloride or tetrabromide containing 1 per cent v/v ethanol (79, 119, 144, 145). The limit of sensitivity in this method is about 0·025 μg oestrogen: incident light of wavelength 540 mμ is used and the fluorescence is measured at 550–560 mμ. A two to threefold increase in sensitivity has been claimed when $POCl_3$ is included in the H_2SO_4 reagent (150). It has been found that 2-methoxy-oestrone has the same order of fluorescent activity by this method as the other oestrogens; in contrast, it has only poor intensity with H_2SO_4 or phosphoric acid alone.

An interesting differentiation of oestradiol-17α from oestradiol-17β was noted by Boscott (21) who reported that the 17α, but not the 17β, fluoresced after heating with 90 per cent formic acid.

Full details of the fluorescence spectra of the oestrogens have been published by Goldzieher (64).

ENZYMIC REACTIONS

Several hydroxysteroid dehydrogenases have been purified sufficiently for use in estimations of the oestrogens (65, 149). These are pyridine nucleotide-linked enzymes which catalyse the reversible oxidations of hydroxyl groups in steroid hormones (see p. 236). In the course of the reaction NAD(NADP) is reduced to $NADH_2(NADPH_2)$, the rate of reduction being a function of the concentration of the steroid reduced.

Thus:

Steroid alcohol $+$ NAD $\rightleftarrows$ steroid ketone $+$ $NADH_2$ $+$ H^+.

The amount of $NADH_2$ formed is related to the amount of steroid alcohol oxidized and may be measured by its characteristic absorption peak at 340 mμ.

There has been some controversy over the mode of action of the placental dehydrogenases (148, 154), but it is clear that a 17β-hydroxysteroid dehydrogenase has been isolated and purified (65, 86, 148) which is highly specific for reactions involving 17β-hydroxy-steroids with aromatic ring A. It reacts with NAD or NADP at comparable rates.

Another enzyme useful for determinations of oestrogens is obtained from *Pseudomonas* adapted to grow in the presence of testosterone as the only source of carbon (149). It consists of two NAD-linked hydroxysteroid dehydrogenases. The α catalyses oxidation of 3α-hydroxysteroids; the β catalyses the oxidation of 3β-hydroxysteroids of the C_{19} and C_{21} series and 6β- and 17β-hydroxysteroids of the C_{18} and C_{19} series. A rather elaborate method has been described for the separation of the α and β enzymes (149); alternatively they may both be extracted at pH 7·5 at 4° and precipitated with acetone. Then careful extraction at pH 9·5 gives a rather crude mixture of the two; addition of p-hydroxymercuribenzoate, however, completely suppresses the action of the α enzyme (143).

Synthetic oestrogens

Dodds and his colleagues investigated many compounds related chemically to the natural oestrogens and in 1938 synthesized diethylstilboestrol (I, Fig. 13.6), a compound active orally and more potent than the natural com-

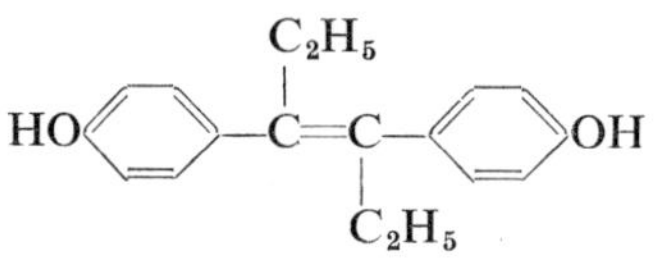

$$\underset{\underset{C_2H_5}{|}}{\overset{\overset{C_2H_5}{|}}{HO\!\!\diamondsuit\!\!-C\!\!=\!\!C\!\!-\!\!\diamondsuit\!\!OH}}\qquad \text{diethylstilboestrol}\qquad\qquad \text{I}$$

$$\underset{\underset{C_2H_5}{|}}{\overset{\overset{C_2H_5}{|}}{HO\!\!\diamondsuit\!\!-CH\!\!-\!\!CH\!\!-\!\!\diamondsuit\!\!OH}}\qquad \text{hexoestrol}\qquad\qquad \text{II}$$

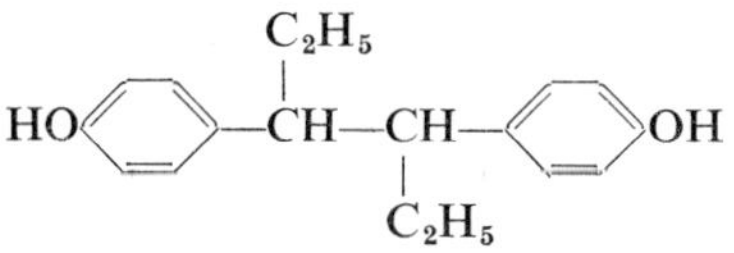

$$\underset{\underset{CHCH_3}{\|}}{\overset{\overset{CHCH_3}{[\|}}{HO\!\!\diamondsuit\!\!-C\!\!-\!\!C\!\!-\!\!\diamondsuit\!\!OH}}\qquad \text{dienoestrol}\qquad\qquad \text{III}$$

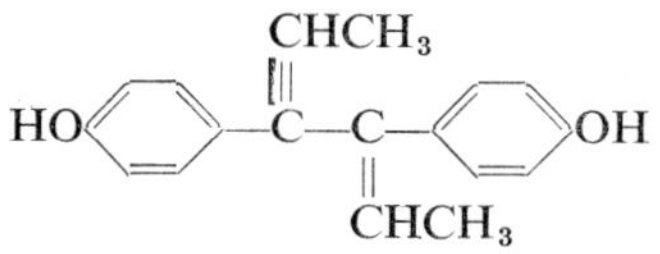

FIG. 13.6

pounds (47). Other related compounds were soon synthesized, notably hexoestrol (II) and dienoestrol (III) and many more that have not attained practical significance.

The original synthesis of diethylstilboestrol started with anisaldehyde which was converted in three steps to the key intermediate for this and other derivatives of stilboestrol, p-$CH_3OC_6H_4CH(C_2H_5)COC_6H_4OCH_3$-$p$ (α-ethyl deoxyanisoin). Methods of synthesis have been reviewed by Grundy (67).

These compounds possess all the biological properties of the natural oestrogens, are cheap to produce and above all are active orally. They have been widely used for the treatment of menstrual disorders, menopausal symptoms, carcinoma of the prostate etc.

A number of other non-steroidal compounds are potent oestrogens. Examples are the allenolic acids, e.g. horeau acid, Fig. 13.7, I, (Vallestril) (76), and the isoflavins, e.g. genistein (23), Fig. 13.7, II.

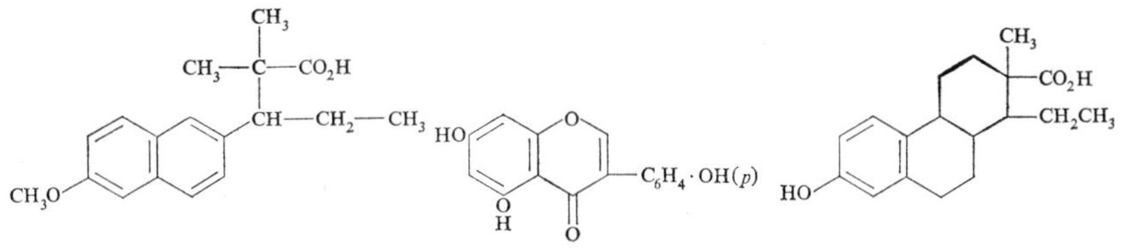

FIG. 13.7

A synthetic oestrogen closely related to the natural compounds is doisynolic acid (106), Fig. 13.7, III.

Modifications to the structure of natural steroids have produced many useful orally active compounds, three being shown in Fig. 13.8. 17α-ethinyl oestradiol, prepared by the action of acetylene on oestrone, is the most potent of all oestrogens.

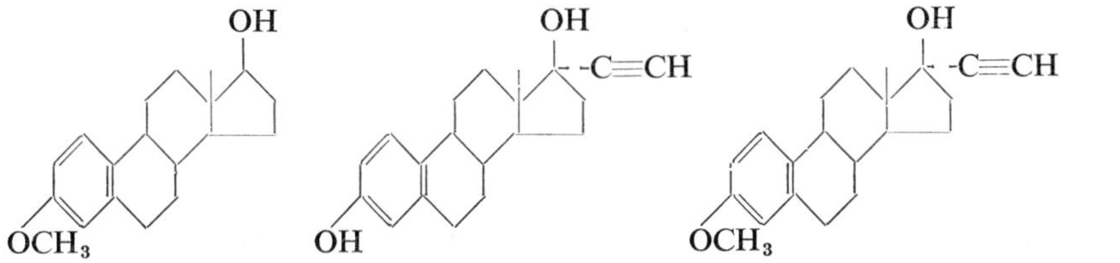

3-methoxyoestradiol   17α-ethinyloestradiol   3-methoxy-17α-ethinyloestradiol
                          (ethinyl-oestradiol)   (Mestranol)

FIG. 13.8

The interesting compound, 1-α-methyl-allylthiocarbamoyl-2-methyl-thio-carbamoyl hydrazine (ICI-33,828), possesses the oestrogenic property of blocking the release of pituitary gonadotrophin (113).

REFERENCES

1 AITKEN, E. H. and PREEDY, J. R. K. *J. Endocr.* **9,** 251 (1953).
2 ALDERCREUTZ, H. and SHAUMANN, K.-O. *Acta endocr. Copenh.* **46,** 230 (1964).
3 ANANCHENKO, S. N. and TORGOV, I. V. *Tetrahedron Lett.* 1553 (1963).
4 ANDERS, M. W. and MANNERING, G. J. *Analyt. Chem.* **34,** 730 (1962).
5 AXELROD, L. R. *J. biol. Chem.* **201,** 59 (1953).
6 AXELROD, L. R. and GOLDZIEHER, J. W. *J. clin. Endocr.* **22,** 431 (1962).

7 AXELROD, L. R. and GOLDZIEHER, J. W. *J. clin. Endocr.* **22,** 537 (1962).

8 BAGGETT, B., ENGEL, L. L., BALDERAS, L. and LANMAN, G. *Endocrinology* **64,** 600 (1959).

9 BAGGETT, B., ENGEL, L. L., SAVARD, K. and DORFMAN, R. I. *J. biol. Chem.* **221,** 931 (1956).

10 BARLOW, J. J. *Analyt. Biochem.* **6,** 435 (1963).

11 BAULD, W. S. *Biochem. J.* **56,** 426 (1954).

12 BAULD, W. S. *Biochem. J.* **59,** 294 (1955).

13 BAULD, W. S. *Biochem. J.* **63,** 488 (1956).

14 BAULD, W. S. *Can. J. Biochem. Physiol.* **38,** 213 (1960).

15 BAULIEU, E. E. and DRAY, F. *J. clin. Endocr.* **23,** 1298 (1963).

16 BEER, C. T. and GALLAGHER, T. F. *J. biol. Chem.* **214,** 335 and 351 (1955).

17 BELING, C. G. *Acta endocr. Copenh.* Suppl. 79 (1963).

18 BOLTÉ, E., MANCUSO, S., ERIKSSON, G., WIQVIST, N. and DICZFALUSY, E. *Acta endocr. Copenh.* **45,** 535 (1964).

19 BOLTÉ, E., MANCUSO, S., ERIKSSON, G., WIQVIST, N. and DICZFALUSY, E. *Acta endocr. Copenh.* **45,** 560 (1964).

20 BOLTÉ, E., MANCUSO, S., ERIKSSON, G., WIQVIST, N. and DICZFALUSY, E. *Acta endocr. Copenh.* **45,** 576 (1964).

21 BOSCOTT, R. J. *Nature, Lond.* **164,** 140 (1949).

22 BOUTE, J. *Annls. Endocr.* **14,** 518 (1953).

23 BRADBURY, R. W. and WHITE, D. E. *J. chem. Soc.* 3447 (1951).

24 BRADSHAW, L. *Nature, Lond.* **190,** 809 (1961).

25 BRAUNSBERG, H. *J. Endocr.* **8,** 11 (1952).

26 BREUER, H. and NOCKE, L. *Acta endocr. Copenh.* **29,** 489 (1958).

27 BROWN, J. B. *J. Endocr.* **8,** 196 (1952).

28 BROWN, J. B. *Biochem. J.* **60,** 185 (1955).

29 BROWN, J. B. *J. Obstet. Gynaec. Br. Emp.* **66,** 795 (1959).

30 BROWN, J. B. and BLAIR, H. A. F. *J. Endocr.* **17,** 411 (1958).

31 BROWN, J. B., BULBROOK, R. D. and GREENWOOD, F. C. *J. Endocr.* **16,** 49 (1957).

32 BUGGE, S., NILSEN, M., METCALF-GIBSON, A. and HOBKIRK, R. *Can. J. Biochem. Physiol.* **39,** 1501 (1961).

33 CHANG, E. and DAO, T. *J. clin. Endocr.* **21,** 624 (1961).

34 CHANG, E. and DAO, T. *Biochim. biophys. Acta* **57,** 609 (1962).

35 CREPY, O. *C. R. Soc. Biol. Paris,* **151,** 322 (1957).

36 CRISPIN, D. J. and WHITEHURST, J. S. *Proc. chem. Soc.* 356 (1962).

37 CRISPIN, D. J. and WHITEHURST, J. S. *Proc. chem. Soc.* 22 (1963).

38 CROOKE, A. C., BUTT, W. R., PALMER, R., MORRIS, R., EDWARDS, R. L., TAYLOR, C. W. and SHORT, R. V. *Bt. Med. J.* i, 1119 (1963).

39 DICZFALUSY, E. *Acta endocr. Copenh.* Suppl. 12 (1953).

40 DICZFALUSY, E. *Bull. Soc. belge Gynéc. Obstét.* **28,** 459 (1958).

41 DICZFALUSY, E., BARR, M. and LIND, J. *Acta endocr. Copenh.* **46**, 511 (1964).
42 DICZFALUSY, E., CASSMER, O., ALONSO, C. and DE MIQUEL, M. *Recent Prog. Horm. Res.* **17**, 147 (1961).
43 DICZFALUSY, E., CASSMER, O., ALONSO, C. and DE MIQUEL, M. *Acta endocr. Copenh.* **38**, 31 (1961).
44 DICZFALUSY, E., FRANKSSON, C., LISBOA, B. P. and MARTINSEN, B. *Acta endocr. Copenh.* **40**, 537 (1962).
45 DICZFALUSY, E. and LINDKVIST, P. *Acta endocr. Copenh.* **22**, 203 (1956).
46 DICZFALUSY, E., TILLINGER, K.-G., WIQVIST, N., LEVITZ, M., CONDON, G. P. and DANCIS, M. D. *J. clin. Endocr.* **23**, 503 (1963).
47 DODDS, E. C., GOLDBERG, L., LAWSON, W. and ROBINSON, R. *Nature, Lond.* **141**, 247 (1938).
48 EBERLEIN, W. R., BONGIOVANNI, A. M. and FRANCIS, C. M. *J. clin. Endocr.* **18**, 1274 (1958).
49 ENGEL, L. L., BAGGETT, B. and CARTER, P. *Endocrinology* **61**, 113 (1957).
50 ENGEL, L. L., CAMERON, C. B., STOFFYN, A., ALEXANDER, J. A., KLEIN, O. and TROFIMOW, N. D., *Analyt. Biochem.* **2**, 114 (1961).
51 ENGEL, L. L., SLAUNWHITE, W. R., CARTER, P. and NATHANSON, I. T. *J. biol. Chem.* **185**, 255 (1950).
52 FINKELSTEIN, M. *Acta endocr. Copenh.* **10**, 149 (1952).
53 FISHMAN, J. *J. clin. Endocr.* **23**, 207 (1963).
54 FISHMAN, J. R. and BROWN, J. B. *J. Chromat.* **8**, 21 (1962).
55 FISHMAN, J. R., COX, R. I. and GALLAGHER, T. F. *Archs. Biochem. Biophys.* **90**, 318 (1960).
56 FISHMAN, J., TOMASZ, M. and LEHMAN, R. *J. org. Chem.* **25**, 585 (1960).
57 FISHMAN, W. and GREEN, S. *J. biol. Chem.* **215**, 527 (1955).
58 FORLEO, R. and COLLINS, W. P. *Acta endocr. Copenh.* **46**, 265 (1964).
59 FRANDSEN, V. A. and STAKEMAN, G. *Acta endocr. Copenh.* **44**, 183 (1963).
60 FRANDSEN, V. A. and STAKEMAN, G. *Acta endocr. Copenh.* **44**, 196 (1963).
61 FUJII, K., MIZOTA, S., TAKAMA, T., MIYAMOTO, S. and OZAKI, T. *J. Biochem. Tokyo,* **51**, 167 (1962).
62 GALLAGHER, T. F., KRAYCHY, S., FISHMAN, J., BROWN, J. B. and MARRIAN, G. F. *J. biol. Chem.* **233**, 1093 (1958).
63 GOLDZIEHER, J. W. *Endocrinology* **53**, 527 (1953).
64 GOLDZIEHER, J. W. In *Physical Properties of Steroid Hormones* (edited by L. L. Engel), p. 288, Pergamon Press, Oxford (1963).
65 GORDON, E. E. and VILLEE, C. A. *Endocrinology* **58**, 150 (1956).
66 GRIFFITHS, K., GRANT, J. K. and SYMINGTON, T. *J. Endocr.* **30**, 247 (1964).
67 GRUNDY, J. *Chem. Rev.* **57**, 281 (1957).
68 HAGOPIAN, M. and LEVY, L. K. *Biochim. biophys. Acta* **30**, 641 (1958).
69 HAHNEL, R. *Clin. Chim. Acta* **7**, 768 (1962).

70 HAMMERSTEIN, J., RICE, B. F. and SAVARD, K. *J. clin. Endocr.* **24,** 597 (1964).
71 HASHIMOTO, Y. and NEEMAN, M. *J. biol. Chem.* **238,** 1273 (1963).
72 HAYNES, R. C., MIKHAIL, G., ERIKSSON, G., WIQVIST, N. and DICZFALUSY, E. *Acta endocr. Copenh.* **45,** 297 (1964).
73 HEARD, R. D. H., BLIGH, E. G., CANN, M. C., JELLINCK, P. H., O'DONNELL, V. J., RAO, B. G. and WEBB, J. L. *Recent Prog. Horm. Res.* **12,** 45 (1956).
74 HOLLANDER, N. and HOLLANDER, V. P. *J. biol. Chem.* **233,** 1097 (1958).
75 HONDA, K. *Acta med. biol. Niigata,* **10,** 323 (1963).
76 HOREAU, A. and JACQUES, J. *C. R. Acad. Sci. Paris* **224,** 862 (1947).
77 HUANG, W. Y. and Pearlman, W. H. *J. biol. Chem.* **237,** 1060 (1962).
78 ITTRICH, G. *Z. physiol. Chem.* **312,** 1 (1958).
79 ITTRICH, G. *Acta endocr. Copenh.* **35,** 34 (1960).
80 JAILER, J. W. *J. clin. Endocr.* **8,** 564 (1948).
81 JELLINCK, P. H. *Biochem. J.* **71,** 665 (1959).
82 KECSKÉS, L., MUTSCHLER, F., THAN, E. and FARKAS, I. *Acta endocr. Copenh.* **39,** 483 (1962).
83 KUSHINSKY, S. *Nature, Lond.* **182,** 874 (1958).
84 KUSHINSKY, S. and TANG, J. W. *Acta endocr. Copenh.* **43,** 345 (1963).
85 KUSHINSKY, S. and TANG, J. W. *Acta endocr. Copenh.* **43,** 361 (1963).
86 LANGER, L. J. and ENGEL, L. L. *J. biol. Chem.* **233,** 583 (1958).
87 LEVITZ, M. *Steroids* **1,** 117 (1963).
88 LEVITZ, M., CONDON, G. P. and DANCIS, J. *Endocrinology* **68,** 825 (1961).
89 LEVITZ, M., CONDON, G. P., MONEY, W. L. and DANCIS, J. *J. biol. Chem.* **235,** 973 (1960).
90 LEVITZ, M., SPITZER, J. R. and TWOMBLY, G. H. *J. biol. Chem.* **222,** 981 (1956).
91 LEVY, L. K. *Archs. Biochem. Biophys.* **50,** 206 (1954).
92 LISBOA, B. P. and DICZFALUSY, E. *Acta endocr. Copenh.* **40,** 60 (1962).
93 LISBOA, B. P. and DICZFALUSY, E. *Acta endocr. Copenh.* **43,** 545 (1963).
94 LONGCHAMPT, J. E., GUAL, C., EHRENSTEIN, M. and DORFMAN, R. I. *Endocrinology* **66,** 416 (1960).
95 LUUKKAINEN, T., VAN DEN HEUVEL, W. J. A. and HORNING, E. C. *Biochim. biophys. Acta* **62,** 153 (1962).
96 MAHAJAN, D. K. and SAMUELS, L. T. *Fedn. Proc.* **22,** 531 (1963).
97 MARLOW, H. W. *J. biol. Chem.* **183,** 167 (1950).
98 MARSH, J. M., SAVARD, K., BAGGETT, B., VAN WYK, J. J. and TALBOT, L. M. *J. clin. Endocr.* **22,** 1196 (1962).
99 MASON, N. R. and SAVARD, K. *Endocrinology* **74,** 664 (1964).
100 MCKERNS, K. W. and NORDSTRAND, E. *Biochim. biophys. Acta.* **82,** 198 (1964).
101 MENINI, E. and DICZFALUSY, E. *Endocrinology* **67,** 500 (1960).

102 MENINI, E. and DICZFALUSY, E. *Endocrinology* **68,** 492 (1961).
103 MEYER, A. S. *Biochim. biophys. Acta* **17,** 441 (1955).
104 MICKHAIL, G., WIQVIST, N. and DICZFALUSY, E. *Acta endocr. Copenh.* **42,** 519 (1962).
105 MICKHAIL, G., WIQVIST, N. and DICZFALUSY, E. *Acta endocr. Copenh.* **43,** 213 (1963).
106 MIESCHER, K. *Helv. chim. Acta* **27,** 1727 (1944).
107 MIGEON, C. J., WALL, P. E. and BERTRAND, J. *J. clin. Invest.* **38,** 619 (1959).
108 MIGEON, C. J., LESCURE, O. L., ZINKHAM, W. H. and SIDBURY, J. B. *J. clin. Invest.* **41,** 2025 (1962).
109 MITCHELL, F. L. and DAVIES, R. E. *Biochem. J.* **56,** 690 (1954).
110 NEEMAN, M. and HASHIMOTO, Y. *Tetrahedron Lett.* **5,** 183 (1961).
111 NYMAN, M. A., GEIGER, J. and GOLDZIEHER, J. W. *J. biol. Chem.* **234,** 16 (1959).
112 O'DONNELL, V. J. and McCAIG, J. G. *Biochem. J.* **71,** 9P (1959).
113 PAGET, G. E., WALPOLE, A. L. and RICHARDSON, D. N. *Nature, Lond.* **192,** 1191 (1961).
114 PREEDY, J. R. K. and AITKEN, E. H. *J. biol. Chem.* **236,** 1300 (1961).
115 PURDY, R. H., ENGEL, L. L. and ONCLEY, J. L. *J. biol. Chem.* **236,** 1043 (1961).
116 RABINOWITZ, J. C. and DOWBEN, R. M. *Biochim. biophys. Acta* **16,** 96 (1955).
117 RABINOWITZ, J. C. *Archs. Biochem. Biophys.* **64,** 285 (1956).
118 RICE, B. F., HAMMERSTEIN, J. and SAVARD, K. *J. clin. Endocr.* **24,** 606 (1964).
119 ROY, E. J. *J. Endocr.* **25,** 361 (1962).
120 RYAN, K. J. *J. biol. Chem.* **234,** 268 (1959).
121 RYAN, K. J. *Acta endocr. Copenh.* **44,** 81 (1963).
122 RYAN, K. J. and ENGEL, L. L. *Endocrinology* **52,** 277, (1953).
123 RYAN, K. J. and ENGEL, L. L. *Endocrinology* **52,** 287 (1953).
124 RYAN, K. J. and SMITH, O. W. *J. biol. Chem.* **236,** 705 (1961).
125 RYAN, K. J. and SMITH, O. W. *J. biol. Chem.* **236,** 710 (1961).
126 SALOKANGAS, R. A. A. and BULBROOK, R. D. *J. Endocr.* **22,** 47 (1961).
127 SANDBERG, A. A. and SLAUNWHITE, W. R. *J. clin. Invest.* **36,** 1266 (1957).
128 SAVARD, K. *Endocrinology* **68,** 411 (1961).
129 SCHNEIDER, J. J. and LEWBART, M. L. *J. biol. Chem.* **222,** 787 (1956).
130 SCHNEIDER, J. J. and LEWBART, M. L. *Recent Prog. Horm. Res.* **15,** 201 (1959).
131 SEKI, T. *Nature, Lond.* **181,** 768 (1958).
132 SHOPPEE, C. W. In *Chemistry of the Steroids* 2nd Edn. p. 107 (1964).
133 SHORT, R. V. *J. Endocr.* **23,** 277 (1961).
134 SHORT, R. V. *J. Endocr.* **24,** 59 (1962).

135 SIITERI, P. K. and MacDONALD, P. G. *Steroids* **2**, 713 (1963).

136 SLAUNWHITE, W. R., ENGEL, L. L., SCOTT, J. F. and HAM, C. L. *J. biol. Chem.* **201**, 65 (1953).

137 SLAUNWHITE, W. R., KARSAY, M. A. and SANDBERG, A. A. *J. clin. Endocr.* **24**, 638 (1964).

138 SLAUNWHITE, W. R., LICHTMAN, M. A. and SANDBERG, A. A. *J. clin. Endocr.* **24**, 638 (1964).

139 SLAUNWHITE, W. R. and SANDBERG, A. A. *Archs. Biochem. Biophys.* **63**, 478 (1956).

140 SLAUNWHITE, W. R. and SANDBERG, A. A. *Endocrinology* **67**, 815 (1960).

141 SMITH, K., HUGHES, G. A. and McLOUGHLIN, B. J. *Experientia* **19**, 177 (1963).

142 SNEDDON, A. and MARRIAN, G. F. *Biochem. J.* **86**, 385 (1963).

143 STEMPFEL, R. S. and SIDBURY, J. B. *J. clin. Endocr.* **24**, 367 (1964).

144 STOA, K. F. and THORSEN, T. *Acta endocr. Copenh.* **41**, 481 (1962).

145 STRICKLER, H. S., WILSON, G. A. and GRAUER, R. C. *Analyt. Biochem.* **2**, 486 (1961).

146 STRUCK, M. *Z. physiol. Chem.* **333**, 89 (1963).

147 SWEAT, M. L., BERLINER, D. L., BRYSON, M. J., NABORS, C., HASKELL, J. and HOLMSTROM, E. G. *Biochim. biophys. Acta* **40**, 289 (1960).

148 TALALAY, P., HURLOCK, B. and WILLIAMS-ASHMAN, H. G. *Proc. natn. Acad. Sci. U.S.A.* **44**, 862 (1958).

149 TALALAY, P. and MARCUS, P. I. *J. biol. Chem.* **218**, 675 (1956).

150 TOUCHSTONE, J. C., GREENE, J. W. and KUKOVETZ, W. R. *Analyt. Chem.* **31**, 1693 (1959).

151 TROEN, P., NILSSON, B., WIQVIST, N. and DICZFALUSY, E. *Acta endocr. Copenh.* **38**, 361 (1961).

152 VELLE, W. and ERICHSEN, S. *Acta endocr. Copenh.* **33**, 277 (1960).

153 VENNING, E. *J. biol. Chem.* **120**, 225 (1937).

154 VILLEE, C. A., HAGERMAN, D. D. and JOEL, P. B. *Recent Prog. Horm. Res.* **16**, 49 (1960).

155 VINSON, G. P., NORYMBERSKI, J. K. and CHESTER JONES, I. *J. Endocr.* **25**, 557 (1963).

156 WALL, P. E. and MIGEON, C. J. *J. clin. Invest.* **36**, 611 (1959).

157 WERTHESSEN, N. T., SCHWENK, E. and BAKER, C. *Science* **117**, 380 (1953).

158 WEST, C. D. *J. clin. Invest.* **37**, 341 (1958).

159 WEST, C. D., DAMOST, B. and PEARSON, O. H. *J. clin. Endocr.* **18**, 15 (1958).

160 WEST, C. D. and NAVILLE, A. H. *Biochemistry* **1**, 645 (1962).

161 WILSON, R., ERIKSSON, G. and DICZFALUSY, E. *Acta endocr. Copenh.* **46**, 525 (1964).

162 WOTIZ, H. H., DAVIS, J. W. and LEMON, H. M. *J. biol. Chem.* **216**, 677 (1955).

163 WOTIZ, H. H., DAVIS, J. W., LEMON, H. M. and GUT, M. *J. biol. Chem.* **222,** 487 (1956).

164 WOTIZ, H. H. and MARTIN, H. F. *J. biol. Chem.* **236,** 1312 (1961).

165 WOTIZ, H. H. and MARTIN, H. F. *Analyt. Biochem.* **3,** 97 (1962).

166 YORNADA, K. *J. Jap. obstet. gynaec. Soc.* **11,** 1355 (1959).

14

ANDROGENS

The androgens are those compounds which are capable of stimulating the male secondary sexual characteristics. They are measured by biological assay and there is an international standard, one unit being defined as the androgenic activity of 0·1 mg of androsterone. There seems to be no general rule correlating androgenic activity with structure; the most potent natural androgen, *testosterone*, contains the Δ^4-3-one structure, characteristic of so many active steroid hormones, and a 17-hydroxyl group. The urinary steroids *androsterone* and *dehydroepiandrosterone* (DHA) are much weaker androgens and contain neither of these groups but are 3-hydroxy-17-oxosteroids. Structure-activity relationships have been discussed at length by Bush (21).

Biosynthesis

The androgens are synthesized in the gonads under the influence of the gonadotrophins and in the adrenal cortex under the influence of corticotrophin.

In both organs the evidence for the conversion of progesterone and its precursors, acetate and cholesterol, to androgens is extensive (44, 75). Here it may be mentioned that first reports came from Slaunwight and Samuels (151) and Savard *et al.* (141) who incubated rat and human testes with labelled progesterone and detected radioactive androgens in the products. Similar results have been obtained in later work with normal and abnormal human ovaries (2, 58, 69, 82, 83, 116, 142, 169), adrenal tissue (81, 133, 168), testes (1, 67), bovine ovaries (154, 159) and ovine adrenals (107). The main biosynthetic pathways from progesterone established from these experiments are shown in Fig. 14.1 (a).

The same steroids have repeatedly been shown to be present in follicular fluid from the human ovary and from other species (48, 103, 148, 174). In this fluid the androgens may occur as intermediates in the synthesis of oestrogens (see Chapter 13), but in patients with polycystic ovaries (e.g. Stein-Leventhal syndrome) the concentration of 17α-hydroxyprogesterone and androstenedione is very high (63, 104, 149). This is due to a failure of the follicle to aromatize ring A which is essential for the production of the oestrogens.

There are other routes to the biosynthesis of androgens—five others are listed in a recent review (44). In some of these progesterone is not involved. Thus pathway (b) in Fig. 14.1 has been demonstrated both in the adrenal and the gonads, *in vivo* and *in vitro* (51, 80, 92, 102). The Δ^5-3-oxoisomerase which catalyses the conversion of DHA to androstenedione has been found in the adrenals of the rat and cow (55, 94), in rat liver and in human blood (160).

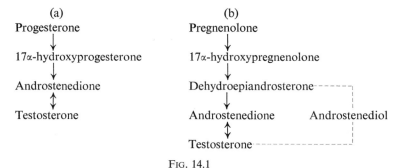

FIG. 14.1

The alternative pathway from DHA to testosterone through androstenediol was demonstrated by perfusion through the isolated liver of dogs (92), and in double isotope experiments with rabbit testes (132). The conversion of androstenediol to testosterone has also been observed in homogenates of human placentae and adrenocortical tumour tissue (7, 8).

DHA appears to be secreted partly as the sulphate (DHAS). In women with adrenal tumours, higher concentrations of DHAS have been found in the adrenal vein plasma than in the peripheral plasma; this suggests that DHAS rather than DHA is the primary secretory product of these adrenals (6). DHAS was also found in the tumour tissue itself. Studies on the secretion rate of adrenal androgens also lead to the conclusion that DHAS is secreted by the adrenal cortex of normal individuals (101, 163). Further work on the *in vitro* conversion of DHA to DHAS with adrenal tumour tissue (31, 167) has shown quite convincingly the existence of sulphurylating enzymes in this gland, although formerly it had been assumed that steroid sulphates in man were only synthesized in extra-adrenal tissue such as the liver. The preponderance of sulphurylating enzymes in the human foetus is discussed at greater length in the chapter on oestrogens (p. 284).

Androgens may also be formed from C_{21} compounds in tissues such as liver and muscle. Numerous *in vivo* and *in vitro* experiments with cortisol and related steroids have yielded 17-oxosteroids, some of which are androgenic (42). Important intermediates are 11β-hydroxyandrostenedione and adrenosterone, although these compounds may arise from the alternative route in the adrenal by the 11β-hydroxylation of androstenedione (171) (Fig. 14.2).

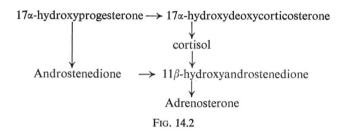

17α-hydroxyprogesterone → 17α-hydroxydeoxycorticosterone

cortisol

Androstenedione → 11β-hydroxyandrostenedione

Adrenosterone

FIG. 14.2

Chemistry

General methods

Methods for the separation of the androgens and precursors from tissues and biological fluids nearly always include paper chromatography of the Bush or Zaffaroni types, thin layer or gas chromatography. Since many of these steroids are relatively non-polar, stationary phases of 80–90 per cent methanol are commonly used in Bush-type chromatography. Similar systems are useful for countercurrent distributions (e.g. ethyl acetate–cyclohexane–methanol–water, 40:60:80:20 by vol.) or partition column chromatography.

Individual steroids

17α-HYDROXYPROGESTERONE AND ANDROSTENEDIONE

17α-hydroxyprogesterone is some 60 times as active as progesterone in the Hooker-Forbes test (175) but androstenedione is inert in this assay.

4-[14C]-labelled androstenedione has been widely used for metabolic studies. Preparations of high specific activity labelled with tritium are also useful. In a convenient method for introducing the label at $C_{(19)}$, 19-hydroxyandrostenedione is treated with p-toluene sulphonyl chloride to give the 19-tosyl derivative which cyclizes to 5β-19-cyclo-androstenedione (129). Reduction with lithium aluminium hydride in tetrahydrofuran gives a mixture of androstenediol and 5β-19-cyclo-androstenedione. Oxidation with CrO_3 then gives the desired product.

1,2-tritiated androstenedione has also been described. Tritiation of a Δ^1 bond in $\Delta^{1,4}$ steroids with palladium on charcoal yields 75–90 per cent tritiation in the 1α and 2α positions (3). [1,2-³H]androstenedione with specific activity of 3,600 μc/mg has been obtained by this method; such compounds are very stable and drastic chemical treatment does not alter the specific activity.

In the separation of these steroids from others in tissues and biological fluids, use may be made of the fact that they both resist acetylation. On reduction with $NaBH_4$, the products are $17\alpha,20\beta$-dihydroxypregn-4-ene-3-one and testosterone respectively. 17α-hydroxyprogesterone is converted to androstenedione by oxidation with CrO_3. Its side chain resists oxidation with bismuthate or periodate but after reduction with $NaBH_4$ subsequent oxidation gives the 17-oxosteroid.

Both steroids contain the Δ^4-3-one group and may therefore be recognized by their soda fluorescence or by their absorption at 240 mμ. The H_2SO_4 chromogens show two peaks in the absorption spectra at 288 and 430 mμ for 17α-hydroxyprogesterone and a maximum at 296 mμ for androstenedione.

Studies on the metabolism of 17α-hydroxyprogesterone show that it is one of the precursors of urinary pregnanetriol (see p. 345). Androstenedione may be excreted as 17-oxosteroids but it has been detected in the urine of patients with adrenal hyperplasia (97) and adrenal tumours (140).

TESTOSTERONE

Testosterone was first isolated from the testes of bulls (36). It is only comparatively recently with the aid of extremely sensitive methods of estimation that it has been found in human urine (25, 144), blood and in adrenal tissue (168).

It is produced in the interstitial, or Leydig cells of the testis under the influence of gonadotrophins. In addition to its androgenic effects, testosterone has powerful metabolic activity, and causes retention of nitrogen, potassium and phosphorus. It increases body weight particularly by growth of bone and muscle, but growth is arrested after an initial spurt due to closure of the epiphyses. This has led to a great deal of investigation into the preparation of derivatives in which androgenic effects have been dissociated from other biological effects. Thus certain derivatives have anabolic, progestational or anti-ovulatory properties and may suppress adrenocortical function. The 19-nor derivatives and their 17α-alkyl derivatives are more active as progestogens, but do have androgenic side-effects (158) while the 17α-alkylated derivatives suppress adrenocortical function (77). The oral activity of these steroids is enhanced by 3-enol esterification (109).

Kincl and Dorfman (89) have compared androgenicity with another function, the gonadotrophin-inhibiting power, of a large number of derivatives. Particularly powerful inhibitors are 6α-chloro-testosterone acetate (potency 375 compared with testosterone, 100), 6α-fluorotestosterone (350), 2-nitrilo-17α-methyl-5α-androst-2-en-17β-ol (350) and several others greater than 200. Particularly good separation of androgenicity and gonadotrophin-inhibiting power is found in compounds with substituents at $C_{(2)}$ such as formyl or hydroxymethyl which increase the gonadotrophin-inhibition at the expense of the androgenicity. An interesting difference in activity is noted with a formyl substituent at $C_{(2)}$ in the 10β-methyl derivative of 5α-androst-2-en-17β-ol which is 6 times as active as an antigonadotrophin as the same substituent in the corresponding 10β-hydrogen derivative.

Synthesis

Testosterone was originally synthesized from cholesterol by oxidation of the dibromo acetate derivative (22, 135). The resulting DHA acetate is then reduced to give Δ^5-androstene-3β, 17α-diol-3-monoacetate which is benzoylated and partially saponified to give Δ^5-androstene-3β,17β-diol-17-benzoate. Bromination of this compound followed by oxidation, de-bromination and saponification yields testosterone.

A recent method of synthesis is applicable also to cortisone and oestrone (165). The initial steps were described previously (172) and the catalytic step is of interest in giving stereospecifically the trans-ring junction (12, 152), (Fig. 14.3).

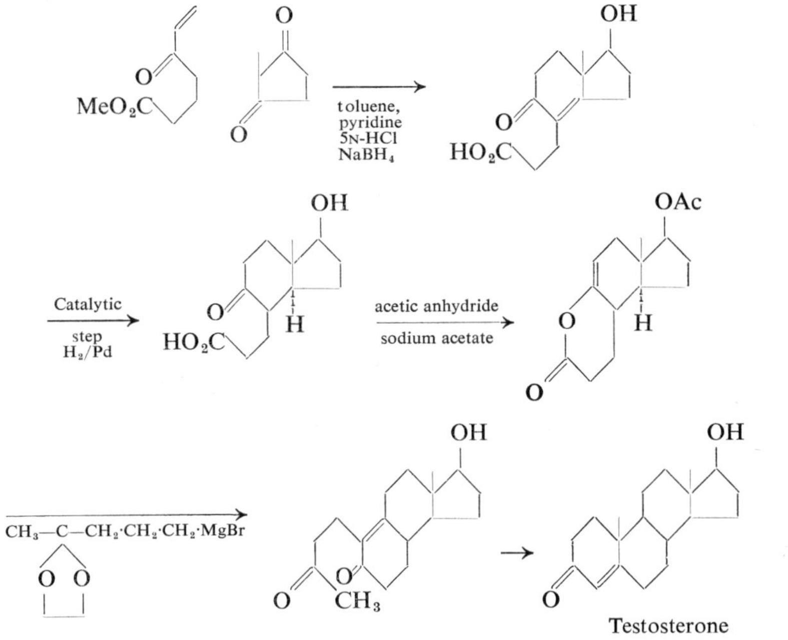

FIG. 14.3

Labelled preparations

Preparations of testosterone labelled with ^{14}C and ^3H are available. A method for the introduction of ^{14}C into ring A has already been mentioned on page 262.

A method for labelling at $C_{(19)}$ has been reported. In this, 19-nor-testosterone is treated with ozone to give the oxo-acid and with diazomethane to the methyl ester. It is alkylated with ^{14}C-labelled methyl iodide in t-butanol containing potassium t-butoxide. The product, 17β-acetoxy-4-oxoandrost-5-en-3-one-19-^{14}C is treated with CH_3MgI followed by hydrolysis and cyclization to [19-^{14}C]testosterone with an overall yield of 0·5 per cent (40, 129, 130).

Carrier-free [7-^3H]testosterone has been prepared from Δ^6-testosterone acetate (33), obtained by dehydrogenation of testosterone acetate with chloranil in t-butanol, or by conversion of 2,3-dichloro-5,6-dicyano-p-benzoquinone to the di-enone with HCl as catalyst. The latter method gives the better yield but the product is contaminated with 10 per cent of the 1,2 unsaturated isomer and the chromatographic separation of testosterone acetate and its Δ^1- and Δ^6-unsaturated derivatives is very difficult. Δ^6-testosterone acetate in dry methanol is now shaken with KOH in the presence of reduced 5 per cent palladium on charcoal as catalyst, in carrier-free tritium at 1 atmosphere pressure. After filtration, acidification and evaporation, testosterone acetate is separated in chloroform and crystallized from methanol. It is saponified in 0·2 N-alkali in aqueous methanol and the resulting testosterone separated by paper chromatography (iso-octane–toluene, 19:1 v/v/80 per cent methanol). The specific activity is reported to be 30·8 C/m. mole.

Properties

Testosterone recrystallizes from methylene chloride in colourless prisms. Its infra-red spectrum (KBr method) shows maxima at 3437, 3273, 2967, 2886, 1591, 1506 and 1299 cm^{-1}. It contains the Δ^4-3-one group and so absorbs maximally at 240 mμ and may be recognized by the soda fluorescence reaction. It forms a Girard T hydrazone which gives a polarographic wave at the characteristic half-wave potential of Δ^4-3-oxocompounds, i.e. $-1\cdot45$ V.

The thiosemicarbazone may be purified by chromatography on silica gel and crystallized from methylene dichloride as colourless prisms, m.p. 210–220°, decomp. (123, 131). This derivative may be acetylated to testosterone acetate thiosemicarbazone-2,4-diacetate which crystallizes from ether in pale yellow crystals, m.p. 176–179°, decomp.

Colour reactions

A relatively specific colour reaction was described by Koenig (93) and has been adapted for routine clinical use (117). Testosterone is heated with H_2SO_4 to which is added a saturated aqueous solution of thiocol with copper sulphate added to accelerate the reaction. A green oxidation product is formed which absorbs maximally at 635 mμ and quantitative measurements may be made down to about 0·2 μg testosterone per ml. The reaction is also given by androstenedione and compounds that hydrolyse to testosterone such

x

as the propionate, oxime or acetate (106). Epitestosterone also reacts but to a lesser degree than testosterone. An interesting method of detecting epitestosterone in the presence of testosterone was reported by Boscott (11) who found that it fluoresced if heated with 90 per cent formic acid.

A useful method for the detection of testosterone on thin layer chromatograms is to spray with ethanol–H_2SO_4 (1:1 v/v) and heat to 90° when a deep green stain appears.

Methods of estimation

In order to determine testosterone in urine or blood, methods of great sensitivity are required. At present there is available one interesting method making use of an enzymic conversion of testosterone to oestrone and oestradiol-17β and several others employing isotopes.

In the former method (56, 96) the enzyme is obtained from human placentae; it has been extracted and purified by Ryan (136). Methods for the determination of the resulting oestrogens are extremely sensitive, so that the method as a whole has both a high specificity and is sufficiently sensitive for determinations in reasonable amounts of plasma.

In the double-isotopic method of Riondel *et al.* (131), [1,2-³H]testosterone is used as an internal standard and [³⁵S] thiosemicarbazide for the preparation of a derivative. Thin layer chromatography on silica gel and paper chromatography in propylene glycol/toluene–acetone (200:1 v/v) are used to purify the product. The thiosemicarbazone is further purified by thin layer and paper chromatography after conversion to the 2,4-diacetyl derivative. The overall recovery is around 5 per cent but the final counting rates are sufficiently high for the estimation to be done on 10 ml plasma. The only steroid likely to interfere is 17-epitestosterone.

Another approach has been to use [³H]acetic anhydride for the preparation of the labelled acetate with [4-¹⁴C]testosterone as an internal standard (70). It is important to keep an excess of acetic anhydride present during the acetylation since the reaction is not as complete as for some other steroids. The acetyl derivative is partially purified by paper chromatography and then a second derivative, the thiosemicarbazone of the acetate, is prepared and purified on a further paper chromatogram. In recent modifications (19, 27) the labelled acetate is purified by thin layer chromatography on silica gel as well as by paper chromatography. The overall yields are reported to be around 13 per cent.

There are considerable problems attached to these radioactive methods, particularly in attempting to measure the small amounts present in the plasma of normal women. Specificity of labelling, for instance, in the method of Burger *et al.* (19) was checked by the behaviour of the derivative in no less than 7 chromatographic systems, by the constancy of the ³H/¹⁴C ratio and by the recovery of known amounts of testosterone. In spite of the number of chromatograms in the method, epitestosterone interferes to a certain extent.

The best yields from urine are obtained by extraction after hydrolysis with β-glucuronidase (25, 145). Extensive purification is required, by separation of the Girard hydrazones, by thin layer or by paper chromatography.

Recent work has demonstrated that epitestosterone is excreted with testosterone (13); it has previously been demonstrated in other biological fluids (99, 115, 147). These isomers are difficult to separate on thin layer chromatograms but are separated in the propylene glucol-ligroin paper chromatographic system or by gas liquid chromatography on QF-1 or SE-30.

The latter technique promises to be of great value in the future. The retention times for the trimethylsilyl ethers of testosterone and related steroids on SE-30 columns are: androstenedione 0·62, testosterone 0·66 and pregnenolone 0·69 (68). By the use of a flame detector it is possible to detect down to 0·01 μg testosterone by this technique (61, 62).

Metabolism

It has long been known that following the administration of testosterone to experimental animals and humans, increased amounts of androgens and 17-oxosteroids are excreted (for review see 45). The most important of these are androsterone, aetiocholanolone and epiandrosterone. Two diones have been reported, androstane-3,17-dione and aetiocholane-3,17-dione, and also the diol, aetiocholane-3α,17β-diol (170) and possibly androstane-3α,17α-diol.

The last two compounds have certainly been identified after intraperitoneal injection of testosterone to the rat (52, 53), the androstane derivative being the major initial metabolite. Other weakly polar C_{19} compounds were isolated, probably mono-oxygenated compounds such as have been isolated from human urine (15) and from *in vitro* experiments with testosterone (156, 157), namely androstenol, androst-16-en-3β-ol and androst-4,16-dien-3-one.

Androstenol was originally isolated from porcine testes and its structure established by partial synthesis (128). It is a member of an interesting group of steroids, the stenols. They have remarkable odours and androstenol is said to smell of musk. Its partial synthesis from androsterone by cyanohydrin dehydration, hydrolysis and decarboxylation was described by Brooksbank *et al.* (17).

It is excreted in urine as a glucosiduronate and may be extracted with ether following hydrolysis with β-glucuronidase. In the method Brooksbank and Haslewood (16) the extract from urine is purified on a column of alumina in a mixture of light petroleum and benzene (1:1 v/v). The estimation is by reaction with resorcylaldehyde in a mixture of H_2SO_4 and acetic acid which reacts with 17β-hydroxy or Δ^{16}-C_{19} steroids. The purple colour obtained shows maximal absorption at 580–585 mμ.

In working with androstenol it must be remembered that it is somewhat volatile.

Present evidence suggests that it is not a unique metabolite of testosterone since it may arise, for instance, from DHA (18). Its excretion in the urine of women with carcinoma of the breast correlates with the excretion of 11-deoxy-17-oxosteroids, and in normal human subjects it increases following treatment with corticotrophin (14). It may also be secreted by the normal or the polycystic ovary since on stimulation with follicle stimulating hormone and human chorionic gonadotrophin the amount in the urine increases considerably (23).

17-OXOSTEROIDS

Some of the commonest urinary 17-oxosteroids are shown in Table 14.1. Together these make up more than 90 per cent of the total 17-oxosteroids. 11β-hydroxyaetiocholanolone has only been found in the urine of patients with Cushing's Syndrome.

TABLE 14.1

Some 17-oxosteroids found in human urine

Trivial name	Derivatives with m.p.	
Androsterone	Acetate	160–162
	Benzoate	179–180
Aetiocholanolone	Acetate	92–93·5
	Benzoate	164–164·5
Dehydroepiandrosterone	Acetate	166–166·5
	Benzoate	256–257
Epiandrosterone	Benzoate	210–211
11-oxoandrosterone	Acetate	183·5–184·5
11β-hydroxyandrosterone	Acetate	240–242
11-oxoaetiocholanolone	Acetate	163–164

The main source of the urinary 11-deoxy-17-oxosteroids is the DHA secreted by the adrenal glands at a rate of approximately 20 mg for females and rather more for males per 24 hours (163). A secondary source is the testosterone secreted by the testis at 3 mg per 24 hours. The urinary 11-oxy-17-oxosteroids have their origin in the adrenal cortex, the major precursor being 11β-hydroxyandrost-4-ene-3,17-dione (43). They may also arise from cortisol and other C_{21} steroids (60) but only 5–7 per cent of radioactive cortisol given intravenously is recovered as 11-oxygenated-C_{19} steroid.

The 17-oxosteroids are excreted as glucosiduronates or sulphates. DHA and epiandrosterone are almost exclusively conjugated as sulphates, although traces of DHA glucosiduronate have been isolated from normal urine (150). Other types of conjugate such as phosphates, have been proposed from time to time (74, 118, 119, 121, 177). In human blood DHA (111) and androsterone (110) occur as the sulphates (32) and possibly as other conjugates (118). Some androsterone and aetiocholanolone glucosiduronate and small amounts of 11-oxoaetiocholanolone and 11β-hydroxyandrosterone (30, 85, 120, 161) have also been detected. DHA (or its sulphate) has also been isolated from adrenal cortex, ovary (103), testis (114) and from human sperm (39).

Androsterone is biologically active, being about one sixth as active as testosterone in the assay which depends on the growth of the capon's comb. DHA is only about one tenth as active as androsterone in the same assay.

Methods of extraction

Hydrolysis with hot mineral acid cleaves both the glucosiduronates and sulphates of the 17-oxosteroids. The free steroids are then extremely soluble in organic solvents such as ether, benzene and ethylene or methylene dichloride.

Hydrolysis with 10 per cent v/v HCl at 100° for 10 minutes is generally used in routine methods for 17-oxosteroids, but the use of 40 per cent H_2SO_4 instead leads to the production of fewer artifacts (9). These artifacts arise chiefly from DHA-sulphate which with hot HCl gives 3β-chloroandrost-5-en-17-one and androst-3,5-dien-17-one (10, 162). Dehydration may occur in other 17-oxosteroids, notably in androsterone giving Δ^2-androsten-17-one, in 11-hydroxyandrosterone giving 3α-hydroxyandrost-9-en-17-one and 11-hydroxyaetiocholanolone giving 3α-hydroxyaetiochol-9-en-17-one (38). To avoid this, other techniques have been tried. Simultaneous hydrolysis and extraction into benzene has some advantages but still leads to poor recoveries of 11-oxygenated 17-oxosteroids (166). Hydrolysis at room temperatures at pH 1 and solvolysis are mild techniques for the sulphates (20, 29, 37, 137, 146) and the recent modifications to the latter method with the use of perchloric acid as the acid catalyst extend this technique to the glucosiduronates (see p. 243).

A number of special methods have been described for the hydrolysis of DHAS. In urine, the conjugate may be broken down by boiling at neutral pH for 6 hours (59). For extraction from blood, the principle of transesterification has been used (47). DHAS is briefly heated with glacial acetic acid and so converted to the acetate, which in turn is extractable in ether. Since the reaction must be carried out in glacial acetic acid, it cannot be applied directly to blood. Extracts obtained by the salting-out procedure of Edwards *et al.* (50) cannot be used, due to the formation of interfering pigments. DHAS, however, and other sulphates form polar complexes with various basic dyes, and methyl green has been applied successfully in this procedure. The complex, after extraction, is best split by subsequent treatment with perchloric acid. Methylene blue also forms a complex which may be extracted in solvent and is split by treatment with Zeo Karb 225 in the Na^+ form (134).

The enzymic hydrolysis of the 17-oxosteroid conjugates with preparations of β-glucuronidase or with sulphatase requires at least 24 hours at 37° with an adequate excess of the enzyme present.

The conjugates themselves may be extracted by the salting-out procedures mentioned in Chapter 11 (pp. 243–244). For completeness of extraction, the urine should be acidified to below pH 5—some prefer pH 2—and partially saturated with ammonium sulphate (80 g per 100 ml). Extractions are made in ether-ethanol (3 : 1 v/v) (57, 73), ethyl acetate or tetrahydrofuran (37).

Methods of purification

Group separations are readily achieved by the use of Girard's Reagent T and digitonin.

The 17-oxosteroids form water-soluble Girard hydrazones and may be recovered by subsequent hydrolysis at pH 1 (126). The 3α- and 3β-hydroxy-17-oxosteroids may be separated since the 3β steroids form digitonides which precipitate from ether. They may be recovered as free 17-oxosteroids by treatment with pyridine (24).

CHROMATOGRAPHIC METHODS Adsorption chromatography has been much used in the past and some excellent results have been obtained. Thus crude extracts of ketonic steroids from urine have been fractionated into five groups by chromatography on magnesium silicate in carbon tetrachloride and mixtures of benzene and ether. Then further chromatography on several columns of alumina with benzene, benzene-ether and other solvents has produced, eventually, highly purified 17-oxosteroids (41).

Such methods served a useful purpose for the isolation and identification of urinary oxosteroids, but were obviously too cumbersome for routine clinical work. Dingemanse (38) devised a simpler procedure using alumina columns with stepwise elution, so that all the common 17-oxosteroids could be recognized. The elution patterns so obtained were often of clinical value and many modifications of the original method followed (79, 124, 127, 176), including very efficient gradient elution methods (87, 95, 166).

Good separations are obtained in modifications of the paper chromatographic methods of Bush and Zaffaroni (65, 72, 120, 138). Two-dimensional chromatography with a modified Bush A system in the first direction and benzene–light petroleum (15:85 v/v)/formic acid following esterification in the second, gives clear separations of androstane and pregnane derivatives of the 3α-, 5β-, 3α-5α-, and 3β-5-ene series and of 17α- and 17β-hydroxy-androstanes (49). Other suitable solvents are given in Table 11.3, p. 246. There are also several systems suitable for column partition chromatography (88, 150, 167).

Paper chromatographic separations of some Girard hydrazones is possible with development in water-saturated n-butanol, but isomeric steroids cannot be separated (173).

The method of glass-fibre chromatography has been used in a few centres. The sheets are impregnated with various salts including sodium tungstate, potassium silicate and ammonium chloride and they are developed with organic solvents such as cyclohexane and n-butanol. In runs lasting 50 minutes 11-deoxy and 11-oxygenated steroids are well separated. The individual steroids have much closer R_F values but by the use of derivatives, such as the

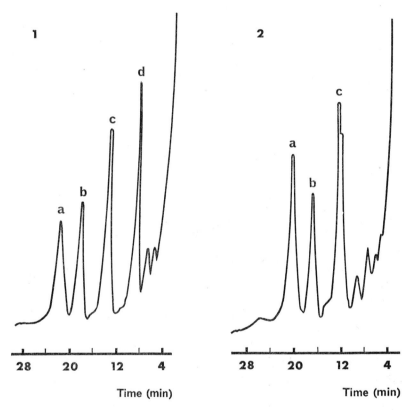

Fig. 14.4. Gas chromatography of 17-oxosteroids; (1) standards, (2) urinary extracts from a normal female

Chromatograms recorded on a Pye Panchromatograph with ^{90}Sr detector.
Column 1% HI-EFF 9B on Gas-Chrom P (mesh 100/120)   Flow rate 30 c.c./min.
Voltage 1000   Attenuation 10⁻⁸   Temperature 208°

Trimethyl silyl ethers of:

        (a) dehydroepiandrosterone
        (b) aetiocholanolone
        (c) androsterone
        (d) androstane-3,17-diol

dibromo compounds, adequate separations are obtained. Thus DHA and epiandrosterone with similar R_F values in most systems are well separated since after bromination 5,6-dibromo-epiandrosterone is formed from DHA and epiandrosterone is unchanged. In the system cyclohexane–n-butanol (100:0·05 v/v) the respective R_F values for the dibromo derivative and epiandrosterone are 1·0 and 0·45 (98).

Useful separations are obtained by thin layer chromatography on silica gel or alumina within 15–20 minutes. The method is being increasingly used in conjunction with gas liquid chromatography.

The trimethyl silyl ethers of the 17-oxosteroids are useful derivatives for gas chromatography (34, 90, 91, 164). Thus androsterone, aetiocholanolone, DHA and epiandrosterone separate on XE-60 with column temperature 187° and detector at 250° (64).

Columns of NPGA have also been used and the separation of the trimethyl silyl ethers for pure steroids and extracts from urine are shown in Figure 14.4.

Conjugated steroids

The glucosiduronates and sulphates are separable by chromatography on Florisil (6, 32) or alumina (4, 35). The sulphates are eluted first, from Florisil in acetone–methanol (98:2 v/v) or ethyl acetate–ethanol (1:9 v/v) and from alumina in aqueous ethanol, the concentration depending on the activity of the adsorbent. The glucosiduronates may be eluted in aqueous ethanol or acetate buffer at pH 5·0.

Further purification is achieved by partition chromatography on columns or on paper. With Celite as the support, ethylene dichloride–butanol–acetic acid–water (7·5:2·5:3:7 by vol.) separates the 17-oxosteroid conjugates from conjugated tetrahydrocortisol and related compounds. Rechromatography with the same solvents in the proportion 8·5:1·5:3:7 gives a partial separation of androsterone and aetiocholanolone glucosiduronates and a better resolution of the 11-oxygenated group. Further resolution of androsterone ($R_F = 0·16$) and aetiocholanolone ($R_F = 0·11$) is obtained in toluene–t-butanol–acetic acid–water (8:2:3:7 by vol.) and of the 11-oxygenated steroids in the same solvents in proportion 7·5:2·5:3:7. Satisfactory separations have also been obtained on columns of synthetic aluminium silicate with 50 per cent ethanol as the stationary phase and hexane mixed with increasing proportions of chloroform as the moving phase (100).

Several paper systems are available (5, 143). The R_F values of the conjugates in some of these are shown in Table 14.2.

Treatment with diazomethane affords another method of separating the glucosiduronates and sulphates, since the former form esters which are insoluble in water while the sulphates do not (86). Crystalline derivatives may be prepared in the form of triacetate methyl esters, the methylation being

TABLE 14.2

Solvents suitable for paper chromatography of conjugated 17-*oxosteroids*

References

Glucosiduronates:

Toluene–t-butanol (75 : 25 to 85 : 15 v/v)–acetic acid–water
(30 : 70 v/v)   (a)
Ethyl acetate–hexane–acetic acid–water (120 : 80 : 60 : 140 by vol.)   (143)
n-butyl ether–n-butanol–acetic acid–water (130 : 70 : 60 : 140 by vol.)   (143)

Sulphates:

2N-ammonium hydroxide–n-butanol (1 : 1 v/v)   (a)
Isopropyl ether–t-butanol–ammonium hydroxide–water
(120 : 80 : 20 : 180 by vol.)   (143)
Ethyl acetate–n-butanol–ammonium hydroxide–water
(180 : 20 : 20 : 180 by vol.)   (143)

Examples of separations

Glucosiduronates:

System: toluene–t-butanol–acetic acid–water (80 : 20 : 30 : 70 by vol.)   (57)

Steroid	R_F
11β-hydroxyaetiocholanolone	0·02
11β-hydroxyandrosterone	0·02
11-oxoaetiocholanolone	0·03
Aetiocholanolone	0·11
Androsterone	0·16

Glucosiduronates and sulphates:

System: isoamyl alcohol–ammonia–water (55 : 27 : 18 by vol.)   (6)

	R_F
Aetiocholanolone and androsterone glucosiduronates	0·30
11-oxoaetiocholanolone sulphate	0·48
Dehydroepiandrosterone and other 11-deoxy-17-oxosteroids	0·70

Sulphates:

System: isopropyl alcohol–ligroin–t-butanol–ammonia–water
(5 : 2 : 3 : 1 : 9 by vol.)   (6)

	Rate of flow (cm/36 hr)
11-oxoaetiocholanolone	3
Testosterone	7
Dehydroepiandrosterone	17
Epiandrosterone	22
Aetiocholanolone	24
Androsterone	29

Reference (a) BUSH, I. E. *Biochem. J.* **67,** 23P (1957).

carried out first, otherwise more than one product results, possibly because of the formation of a lactone ring (Fig. 14.5). The esters may be purified by chromatography on Celite in benzene–light petroleum–methanol–water (57) and they crystallize from light petroleum or benzene.

Syntheses of these compounds have been made possible by the preparation

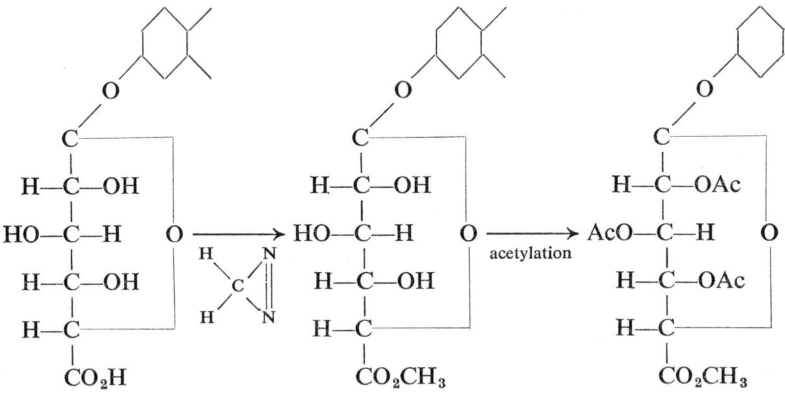

FIG. 14.5

of methyl 2,3,4-tri-O-acetyl-1-bromo-1-deoxy-D-glucuronate (64). The bromo ester in anhydrous ether is mixed with the steroid and dry Ag_2CO_3 is added and the reaction allowed to proceed for 5 hours. The extract is purified on Celite in light petroleum–methanol–water (10:8:2 by vol.). Refluxing in 3N-NaOH gives the glucosiduronate.

METHODS OF DETERMINATION OF 17-OXOSTEROIDS— Scores of methods have been described for the determination of the 17-oxosteroids in urine. In order that results in different laboratories are comparable some standardization is necessary and a recommended method has been published (108).

The extract of the hydrolysed steroids is usually washed with alkali to remove phenols and certain pigments. The use of pellets of NaOH has been recommended as being particularly efficient (46). Estimation is usually by reaction with alkaline m-dinitrobenzene (the Zimmermann reaction), which gives a purple colour with 17-oxosteroids. The 3- and 20-oxosteroids will also react, but they give colours of lower intensity and of slightly different absorption characteristics, and correction formulae have been introduced into the methods to account for them.

The formation of dyes with the reagent in alkali is a property of compounds with a carboxyl group adjacent to an active methylene group. High extinction at 520 mμ, however, is characteristic of the 17-oxosteroids. There are a few exceptions: similar properties have been noted with other compounds including cholestan-2-one and 2:3:6-trimethyl benzal acetone. On the other hand 3β-acetoxy-14-ξ-hydroxyandrost-5-en-17-one is reported to give no colour and when a carbonyl group is present at $C_{(16)}$, or there are two carbonyl groups at $C_{(16)}$ and $C_{(17)}$ with an active methylene group at $C_{(15)}$ no colour is produced (105).

These exceptions are of no importance in the determination of 17-oxosteroids in human urine. A limitation of the method, however, arises from the variation of colour intensity among the individual steroids. In general, the 11-hydroxy-17-oxosteroids give weaker, and the 11,17-dioxosteroids give stronger, colours than dehydroepiandrosterone (108).

The violet product is in a pH-dependent equilibrium with a colourless compound which for DHA has been isolated by paper chromatography (84). It has been crystallized from chloroform–di-iso-propyl ether in yellow prisms, m.p. 186–187. ((76) formula (a))

(a)   (b)

In ethanolic KOH the compound gives the characteristic violet colour of formula (b).

Many variations in the base used have been introduced, mainly to try to exclude as much non-specific colour as possible and to produce a more stable reagent. Quaternary ammonium hydroxides under certain conditions appear to give rise to very low reagent blanks.

The Zimmermann reaction has been modified for the detection of 17-oxosteroids on paper (54). It is prepared in 2·5 per cent aqueous hyamine 1622 and dimethyl benzyl ammonium chloride. This is mixed with KOH and the chromatograms are stained for 30 minutes. Excess reagent is washed away and the paper dried at 75°. The colour is then eluted quantitatively in dimethyl sulphoxide at 50° and the colours read at 540 mμ.

OTHER METHODS OF DETECTION AND DETERMINATION   The determination of DHA is often useful in the diagnosis of adrenal tumours, and a reliable method has been described by Fotherby (59). The colour reaction used in this method depends on the formation of a blue colour on heating with furfural in acetic acid (Pettenkofer reagent) in the presence of H_2SO_4 (112). The absorption maximum is 660 mμ. It also forms a blue colour (absorption max. 600 mμ) with H_2SO_4 and ethanol or ether (4:1 v/v) (78, 122).

Pincus (125) found that an intense blue colour (absorption max, 610 mμ) was developed by androsterone and its isomers on heating with $SbCl_3$ in a mixture of acetic acid and acetic anhydride. This reaction is not given by DHA and interference from 3- and 20-oxosteroids is negligible.

The 17-oxosteroids show some degree of fluorescence on heating with 90 per cent H_2SO_4 at 80° but it is much less than that of oestrogens (66). An early observation that testosterone, but not androstenedione or DHA, fluoresces with 38 per cent $SbCl_3$ in acetic anhydride-benzene does not appear to have been followed up (28).

Dinitrophenylhydrazine is a useful reagent for detection on paper or thin layer chromatograms. It reacts with ketone groups in descending order of sensitivity: Δ^4-3-oxo>3-oxo>20-oxo>17-oxo and 11-oxosteroids do not react (113). Isonicotinic acid hydrazide has also been used on thin layer chromatograms to differentiate between Δ^4 and $\Delta^{1,4}$-3-oxosteroids (153).

The $SbCl_3$ reagent has also been used on paper chromatograms and is suitable for Δ^5-3β-hydroxysteroids which give an orange to red colour. The fluorescence under ultraviolet light gives a useful differentiation, 3β-7-dihydroxy-Δ^5-steroids giving a blue colour.

The polarographic determination of 17-oxosteroids has been described and may be useful in some special circumstances. The Girard hydrazones of all the common 17-oxosteroids give cathodic waves at a half-wave potential of -1.45 V in buffer at pH 5·6. The height of the wave span is measured for the qualitative determination and is virtually identical for all the 17-oxosteroids.

DETERMINATION IN BLOOD Androsterone and DHA have been isolated and identified in plasma from peripheral blood and methods for their determination have been described (30, 71, 96, 120, 139). They occur as the sulphates and other conjugates; there is evidence also for the presence of other free and conjugated 17-oxosteroids including aetiocholanolone and 11β-hydroxyaetiocholanolone (120).

Special methods for the hydrolysis and extraction of conjugated DHA have been mentioned earlier (p. 309). Acid hydrolysis with continuous extraction (solvolysis) is more commonly used, followed by hot acid hydrolysis to release further oxosteroids. The hydrolysis is carried out after the preliminary removal of the plasma proteins by precipitation with methanol (71) or acetone-ethanol (120). Individual steroids are then separated by any of the chromatographic methods used for the urinary steroids, and are measured by the reactions already described.

HISTOCHEMICAL DETECTION Histochemical methods for the detection of oxosteroids lack specificity. Most depend on the condensation of the ketone group with reagents such as naphthoic acid hydrazide, but reaction is also given with non-reactive aldehydes. A method for differentiating ketones was proposed by Stoward and Adams-Smith (155). Ketones and aldehydes are converted to their methyl hydrazones by methyl hydrazine at pH 4–6. Immersion in sulpho-benzaldehyde regenerates the ketones within 2 hours, whereas aldehydes require 18 hours or more. Treatment with salicylyl hydrazide in 5 per cent acetic acid follows, and the excess reagent is removed with sodium pentacyanoaminine ferroate. When observed under a fluorescence microscope (excitation at 366 mμ) a greenish-yellow fluorescence is observed. Since this can be destroyed by alkali, it may be attributed to 3-oxosteroids (26).

REFERENCES

1 ACEVEDO, H. E., AXELROD, L. R., ISHIKAWA, E. and TAKAKI, F. *J. clin. Endocr.* **23,** 885 (1963).

2 AXELROD, L. R. and GOLDZIEHER, J. W. *J. clin. Endocr.* **22,** 431 (1962).

3 AXELROD, L. R. and GOLDZIEHER, J. W. *J. clin. Endocr.* **22,** 537 (1962).

4 BARLOW, J. J. and KELLIE, A. E. *Biochem. J.* **71,** 86 (1959).

5 BAULIEU, E.-E. *J. clin. Endocr.* **20,** 900 (1960).

6 BAULIEU, E.-E. *J. clin. Endocr.* **22,** 501 (1962).

7 BAULIEU, E.-E. and ROBEL, P. *Steroids* **2,** 111 (1963).

8 BAULIEU, E.-E., WALLACE, E. and LIEBERMAN, S. *J. biol. Chem.* **238,** 1316 (1963).

9 BIRKE, G. and PLANTIN, L.-O. *Acta med. scand.* **148,** Suppl. 291 (1954).

10 BORRELL, S. *J. clin. Endocr.* **21,** 955 (1961).

11 BOSCOTT, R. J. *Nature, Lond.* **164,** 140 (1949).

12 BOYCE, C. B. C. and WHITEHURST, J. S. *J. chem. Soc.* 4547 (1960).

13 BROOKS, R. V. and GIULIANI, G. *J. Endocr.* **29,** iv (1964).

14 BROOKSBANK, B. W. L. *J. Endocr.* **24,** 435 (1962).

15 BROOKSBANK, B. W. L. and HASLEWOOD, G. A. D. *Biochem. J.* **47,** 36 (1950).

16 BROOKSBANK, B. W. L. and HASLEWOOD, G. A. D. *Biochem. J.* **80,** 488 (1961).

17 BROOKSBANK, B. W. L., HASLEWOOD, G. A. D., POLLACK, J. A. and HEWETT, C. L. *Biochem. J.* **70,** 14P (1958).

18 BULBROOK, R. D., THOMAS, B. S. and BROOKSBANK, B. W. L. *J. Endocr.* **26,** 149 (1963).

19 BURGER, H. C., KENT, J. R. and KELLIE, A. E. *J. clin. Endocr.* **24,** 432 (1964).

20 BURSTEIN, S. and LIEBERMAN, S. *J. biol. Chem.* **233,** 331 (1958).

21 BUSH, I. E. *Pharmac. Rev.* **14,** 317 (1962).

22 BUTENANDT, A. and HANISCH, G. *Hoppe-Seyler's Z. physiol. Chem.* **237,** 89 (1935).

23 BUTT, W. R., CROOKE, A. C. and PALMER, R. Unpublished.

24 BUTT, W. R., HENLY, A. A. and MORRIS, C. J. O. R. *Biochem. J.* **42,** 447 (1948).

25 CAMACHO, A. M. and MIGEON, C. J. *J. clin. Endocr.* **23,** 301 (1963).

26 CAMBER, B. *Clin. Chim. Acta* **2,** 188 (1957).

27 CASEY, J. H. and KELLIE, A. E. *J. Endocr.* **29,** iv (1964).

28 CLARK, L. C. and THOMPSON, H. *Science* **107,** 429 (1948).

29 COHEN, S. L. and ONESON, I. B. *J. biol. Chem.* **204,** 245 (1953).
30 COHN, G. L., BONDY, P. K. and CASTIGLIONE, C. *J. clin. Invest.* **40,** 400 (1961).
31 COHN, G. L., MULROW, P. J. and DUNNE, V. C. *J. clin. Endocr.* **23,** 671 (1963).
32 CONRAD, S., MAHESH, V. B. and HERRMANN, W. L. *J. clin. Invest.* **40,** 947 (1961).
33 COOMBS, M. M. and RODERICK, H. R. *Nature, Lond.* **203,** 523 (1964).
34 COOPER, J. A. and CREECH, B. A. *Analyt. Biochem.* **2,** 502 (1961).
35 CRÉPY, O., JAYLE, M. F. and MESLIN, F. *Acta endocr. Copenh.* **24,** 233 (1957).
36 DAVID, K., DINGEMANSE, E., FREUD, J. and LAQUER, E. *Hoppe-Seyler's Z. physiol. Chem.* **233,** 281 (1935).
37 DE PAOLI, J. C., NISHIZAWA, E. and EIK-NES, K. B. *J. clin. Endocr.* **23,** 81 (1963).
38 DINGEMANSE, E., HUIS IN'T VELD, L. G. and HARTOGH-KATZ, S. L. *J. clin. Endocr.* **12,** 66 (1952).
39 DIRSCHERL, W. and BREUER, H. *Acta endocr. Copenh.* **44,** 403 (1963).
40 DJERASSI, C. and KIELCZEWSKI, M. A. *Steroids* **2,** 125 (1963).
41 DOBRINER, K., LIEBERMAN, S. and RHOADS, C. P. *J. biol. Chem.* **172,** 241 (1948).
42 DORFMAN, R. I. *A. Rev. Biochem.* **26,** 523 (1957).
43 DORFMAN, R. I. In *The Adrenal Cortex* (edited by A. R. Currie, T. Symington and J. K. Grant), p. 93 Livingstone, Edinburgh (1962).
44 DORFMAN, R. I., FORCHIELLI, E. and GUT, M. *Recent Prog. Horm. Res.* **19,** 251 (1963).
45 DORFMAN, R. I. and SHIPLEY, R. A. In *Androgens* p. 68, Chapman and Hall, London (1956).
46 DREKTER, I. J., HEISLER, A., SCISM, G. R., STERN, S., PEARSON, S. and McGAVACK, T. H. *J. clin. Endocr.* **12,** 55 (1952).
47 EBERLEIN, W. R. *J. clin. Endocr.* **22,** 963 (1962).
48 EDGAR, D. G. *J. Endocr.* **10,** 54 (1953).
49 EDWARDS, R. W. H. *J. Endocr.* **22,** xxvi (1960).
50 EDWARDS, R. W. H., KELLIE, A. E. and WADE, A. P. *Mem. Soc. Endocr.* **2,** 53 (1953).
51 EIK-NES, K. B. and KEKRE, M. *Biochim. biophys. Acta* **78,** 449 (1963).
52 EL ATTAR, T., DIRSCHERL, W. and MOSEBACH, K. O. *Acta endocr. Copenh.* **45,** 527 (1964).
53 EL ATTAR, T., MOSEBACH, K. O. and DIRSCHERL, W. *Acta endocr. Copenh.* **45,** 437 (1964).
54 EPSTEIN, E. and ZAK, B. *J. clin. Endocr.* **23,** 355 (1963).
55 EWALD, W., WERBIN, H. and CHAIKOFF, I. L. *Biochim. biophys. Acta* **81,** 199 (1964).

56 FINKELSTEIN, M., FORCHIELLI, E. and DORFMAN, R. I. *J. clin. Endocr.* **21,** 98 (1961).

57 FOGGITT, F. and KELLIE, A. E. *Biochem. J.* **91,** 209 (1964).

58 FORLEO, R. and COLLINS, W. P. *Acta endocr. Copenh.* **46,** 265 (1964).

59 FOTHERBY, K. *Biochem. J.* **73,** 339 (1959).

60 FUKUSHIMA, D. K., BRADLOW, H. L., HELLMAN, L., ZUMOFF, B. and GALLAGHER, T. F. *J. biol. Chem.* **235,** 2246 (1960).

61 FUTTERWEIT, W., MCNIVEN, N. L., NARCUS, L., LANTOS, C., DROSDOW-SKY, M. and DORFMAN, R. I. *Steroids* **1,** 628 (1963).

62 FUTTERWEIT, W., MCNIVEN, N. L., GUERRA-GARCIA, R., GIBREE, N., DROSDOWSKY, M., SIEGEL, G. L., SOFFER, L. J., ROSENTHAL, I. M. and DORFMAN, R. I. *Steroids* **4,** 137 (1964).

63 GIORGI, E. P. *J. Endocr.* **27,** 225 (1963).

64 GOEBEL, W. F. and BABERS, F. H. *J. biol. Chem.* **111,** 347 (1935).

65 GOLDZIEHER, J. W. and AXELROD, L. R. *J. clin. Endocr.* **22,** 1234 (1962).

66 GOLDZIEHER, J. W., BODENCHUK, J. M. and NOLAN, P. *Analyt. Chem.* **26,** 850 (1954).

67 GRIFFITHS, K., GRANT, J. K. and WHYTE, W. G. *J. clin. Endocr.* **23,** 1044 (1963).

68 GUERRA-GARCIA, R., CHATTORAJ, G. C., GABRILOVE, L. J. and WOTIZ, H. H. *Steroids* **2,** 605 (1963).

69 HUANG, W. Y. and PEARLMAN, W. H. *J. biol. Chem.* **238,** 1308 (1963).

70 HUDSON, B., COGHLAN, J., DULMANIS, A., WINTOUR, M. and EKKEL, I. *Aust. J. exp. Biol. med. Sci.* **41,** 235 (1963).

71 HUDSON, B. and OERTEL, G. W. *Analyt. Biochem.* **2,** 248 (1961).

72 JACADE, F. A., BAULIEU, E.-E. and JAYLE, M. F. *Acta endocr. Copenh.* **26,** 30 (1957).

73 JAMES, V. H. T. *J. Endocr.* **22,** 195 (1961).

74 JAMES, V. H. T. *Acta endocr. Copenh.* Suppl. **78,** 31 (1962).

75 JAMES, V. H. T. *Rep. Prog. Chem.* **59,** 426 (1962).

76 JAMES, V. H. T. and DE JONG, M. *J. clin. Path.* **14,** 425 (1961).

77 JAMES, V. H. T., LANDON, J. and WYNN, V. *J. Endocr.* **29,** ii (1964).

78 JENSEN, C. C. In *Androgens* (edited by R. I. Dorfman and R. A. Shipley), p. 562, Chapman and Hall, London (1956).

79 JOHNSEN, S. G. *Acta endocr. Copenh.* **21,** 127 (1956).

80 KAHNT, F. W., NEHER, R., SCHMID, K. and WETTSTEIN, A. *Experientia* **17,** 19 (1961).

81 KASE, N. and KOWAL, J. *J. clin. Endocr.* **22,** 925 (1962).

82 KASE, N., KOWAL, J., PERLOFF, W. and SOFFER, L. J. *Acta endocr. Copenh.* **44,** 15 (1963).

83 KASE, N., KOWAL, J. and SOFFER, L. J. *Acta endocr. Copenh.* **44,** 8 (1963).

84 KELLIE, A. E. and SMITH, E. R. *Nature, Lond.* **178,** 323 (1956).

85 KELLIE, A. E. and SMITH, E. R. *Biochem. J.* **66,** 490 (1957).

86 KELLIE, A. E. and WADE, A. P. *Biochem. J.* **62,** 1P (1956).

87 KELLIE, A. E. and WADE, A. P. *Biochem. J.* **66,** 196 (1957).

88 KELLY, W. G., BANDI, L., SHOOLERY, J. N. and LIEBERMAN, S. *Biochemistry* **1,** 172 (1962).

89 KINCL, F. A. and DORFMAN, R. I. *Acta endocr. Copenh.* **46,** 300 (1964).

90 KIRSCHNER, M. A. and LIPSETT, M. B. *J. clin. Endocr.* **23,** 255 (1963).

91 KIRSCHNER, M. A. and LIPSETT, M. B. *Steroids* **3,** 277 (1964).

92 KLEMPIEN, E. J., VOIGT, K. D. and TAMM, J. *Acta endocr. Copenh.* **36,** 498 (1961).

93 KOENIG, V. L., MELZER, F., SZEGO, C. M. and SAMUELS, L. T. *J. biol. Chem.* **141,** 487 (1941).

94 KRUSKEMPER, H. L., FORCHIELLI, E. and RINGOLD, H. J. *Steroids* **3,** 295 (1964).

95 LAKSHMANAN, T. K. and LIEBERMAN, S. *Archs. Biochem. Biophys.* **53,** 258 (1954).

96 LAMB, E. J., DIGNAM, W. J., PION, R. J. and SIMMER, H. H. *Acta endocr. Copenh.* **45,** 243 (1964).

97 LIEBERMAN, S., DOBRINER, K., HILL, B. R., FIESER, L. F. and RHOADS, C. P. *J. biol. Chem.* **172,** 263 (1948).

98 LIM, N. Y., FESLER, K. W. and DINGMAN, J. F. *J. clin. Endocr.* **24,** 68 (1964).

99 LINDNER, H. R. *Nature, Lond.* **183,** 1605 (1959).

100 LIPSETT, M. B. and WILSON, H. *J. Clin. Endocr.* **22,** 906 (1962).

101 MACDONALD, P. C., GONZALEZ, O., VAN DE WIELE, R. L. and LIEBERMAN, S. *J. clin. Endocr.* **23,** 665 (1963).

102 MAHESH, V. B. and GREENBLATT, R. B. *Acta endocr. Copenh.* **41,** 400 (1962).

103 MAHESH, V. B. and GREENBLATT, R. B. *J. clin. Endocr.* **22,** 441 (1962).

104 MAHESH, V. B. and GREENBLATT, R. B. *Recent Prog. Horm. Res.* **20,** 341 (1964).

105 MARLOW, H. W. *J. biol. Chem.* **183,** 167 (1950).

106 MARTIN, R. P. *Acta endocr. Copenh.* **40,** 263 (1962).

107 MATTHIJSSEN, C. and MANDEL, J. E. *Biochim. biophys. Acta* **82,** 138 (1964).

108 Medical Research Council Committee on Clinical Endocrinology, *Lancet* i. 1415 (1963).

109 MELI, A., HONRATH, W. L. and WOLFF, A. *Endocrinology* **74,** 79 (1964).

110 MIGEON, C. J. *J. biol. Chem.* **218,** 941 (1956).

111 MIGEON, C. J. and PLAGER, J. E. *J. biol. Chem.* **209,** 767 (1954).

112 MUNSON, P. L., JONES, M. E., McCALL, P. J. and GALLAGHER, T. F. *J. biol. Chem.* **176,** 73 (1948).

113 NEHER, R. In *Physical Properties of the Steroid Hormones* (edited by L. L. Engel), p. 37, Pergamon Press, Oxford (1963).

114 Neher, R. and Wettstein, A. *Acta endocr. Copenh.* **35,** 1 (1960).

115 Neher, R. and Wettstein, A. *Helv. chim. Acta* **43,** 1628 (1960).

116 O'Donnell, V. C. and McCaig, J. G. *Biochem. J.* **71,** 9P (1959).

117 Oertel, G. W. *Acta endocr. Copenh.* **37,** 237 (1961).

118 Oertel, G. W. *Clin. Chim. Acta* **8,** 154 (1963).

119 Oertel, G. W. and Eik-Nes, K. B. *Acta endocr. Copenh.* **30,** 93 (1959).

120 Oertel, G. W. and Kaiser, E. *Clin. Chim. Acta* **7,** 221 (1962).

121 Oertel, G. W., Kaiser, E. and Bruhl, P. *Biochem. Z.* **336,** 154 (1962).

122 Patterson, J. and Swale, J. *Mem. Soc. Endocr.* **2,** 41 (1953).

123 Pearlman, W. H. and Cerceo, E. *J. biol. Chem.* **203,** 127 (1953).

124 Pesonen, S. *Acta endocr. Copenh.* **40,** 387 (1962).

125 Pincus, G. *Endocrinology* **32,** 176 (1943).

126 Pincus, G. and Pearlman, W. H. *Endocrinology* **29,** 413 (1941).

127 Pond, M. H. *Lancet* ii, 906 (1951).

128 Prelog, V. and Ruzicka, L. *Helv. chim. Acta* **27,** 61 (1944).

129 Rakhit, S. and Gut, M. *J. Amer. chem. Soc.* **86,** 1432 (1964).

130 Rao, P. N. and Axelrod, L. R. *Chemy Ind.* 1838 (1963).

131 Riondel, A., Tait, J. F., Gut, M., Tait, S. A. S., Joachim, E. and Little, B. *J. clin. Endocr.* **23,** 620 (1963).

132 Rosner, J. M., Horita, S. and Forsham, P. H. *Endocrinology* **75,** 299 (1964).

133 Roversi, G. D., Polvani, F., Bompiani, A. and Neher, R. *Acta endocr. Copenh.* **44,** 1 (1963).

134 Roy, A. B. *Biochem. J.* **62,** 41 (1956).

135 Ruzicka, L. and Wettstein, A. *Helv. chim. Acta* **18,** 986 (1935).

136 Ryan, K. J. *J. biol. Chem.* **234,** 268 (1959).

137 Ryan, K. J. *Acta endocr. Copenh.* **46,** 170 (1964).

138 Sachs, L. *Acta endocr. Copenh.* **38,** 534 (1961).

139 Saier, E. L., Campbell, E., Strickler, H. S. and Grauer, R. C. *J. clin. Endocr.* **19,** 1162 (1959).

140 Saroff, J., Slaunwhite, W. R., Costa, G. and Sandberg, A. A. *J. clin. Endocr.* **23,** 629 (1963).

141 Savard, K., Dorfman, R. I., Baggett, B. and Engel, L. L. *J. clin. Endocr.* **16,** 1629 (1956).

142 Savard, K., Gut, M., Dorfman, R. I., Gabrilove, J. L. and Soffer, L. J. *J. clin. Endocr.* **21,** 165 (1961).

143 Schneider, J. J. and Lewbart, M. L. *Recent Prog. Horm. Res.* **15,** 201 (1959).

144 Schubert, K. *Acta endocr. Copenh.* Suppl. 51, 1019 (1960).

145 Schubert, K. and Wehrberger, K. *Naturwissenschaften* **47,** 281 (1960).

146 Segal, L., Segal, B. and Nes, W. R. *J. biol. Chem.* **235,** 3108 (1960).

147 SHORT, R. V. *J. Endocr.* **20**, 147 (1960).

148 SHORT, R. V. *J. Endocr.* **23**, 401 (1962).

149 SHORT, R. V. *J. Endocr.* **24**, 359 (1962).

150 SIITERI, P. K., VAN DE WIELE, R. L. and LIEBERMAN, S. *J. clin. Endocr.* **23**, 588 (1963).

151 SLAUNWHITE, W. R. and SAMUELS, L. T. *J. biol. Chem.* **220**, 341 (1956).

152 SMITH, H., HUGHES, G. A. and McLOUGHLIN, B. J. *Experientia* **19**, 177 (1963).

153 SMITH, L. L. and FOELL, T. *Analyt. Chem.* **31**, 102 (1959).

154 SOLOMON, S., VANDE WIELE, R. L. and LIEBERMAN, S. *J. Amer. chem. Soc.* **78**, 5453 (1956).

155 STOWARD, P. J. and ADAMS-SMITH, W. N. *J. Endocr.* **30**, 273 (1964).

156 STYLIANOU, M., FORCHIELLI, E. and DORFMAN, R. I. *J. biol. Chem.* **236**, 1318 (1961).

157 STYLIANOU, M., FORCHIELLI, E., TUMONILLO, M. and DORFMAN, R. I. *J. biol. Chem.* **236**, 692 (1961).

158 SUCHOWSKY, G. K. and BALDRATTI, G. *J. Endocr.* **30**, 159 (1964).

159 SWEAT, M. L., BERLINER, D. L., BRYSON, M. J., NABORS, C., HASKEL, J. and HOLMSTROM, E. G. *Biochim. biophys. Acta* **40**, 289 (1960).

160 TALALAY, P. and WANG, V. S. *Biochim. biophys. Acta* **18**, 300 (1955).

161 TAMM, J., BECKMANN, I. and VOIGT, K. D. *Acta endocr. Copenh.* **27**, 403 (1958).

162 TEICH, S., ROGERS, J., LIEBERMAN, S., ENGEL, L. L. and DAVIS, J. W. *J. Amer. chem. Soc.* **75**, 2523 (1953).

163 VANDE WIELE, R. L., MACDONALD, P. C., GURPIDE, E. and LIEBERMAN, S. *Recent Prog. Horm. Res.* **19**, 275 (1963).

164 VANDEN HEUVEL, W. J. A., CREECH, B. G. and HORNING, E. C. *Analyt. Biochem.* **4**, 191 (1962).

165 VELLUZ, L., NOMINÉ, G., AMIARD, G., TORELLI, V. and CÉRÈDE, J. *C.R. Acad. Sci. Paris* **257**, 3086 (1963).

166 VESTERGAARD, P. and CLAUSEN, B. *Acta endocr. Copenh.* Suppl. **64**, 35 (1962).

167 WALLACE, E. and LIEBERMAN, S. *J. clin. Endocr.* **23**, 90 (1963).

168 WARD, P. J. and GRANT, J. K. *J. Endocr.* **26**, 139 (1963).

169 WARREN, J. C. and SALHANICK, H. A. *J. clin. Endocr.* **21**, 1218 (1961).

170 WEST, C. D., REICH, H. and SAMUELS, L. T. *J. biol. Chem.* **193**, 219 (1951).

171 WETTSTEIN, A. *Experientia* **17**, 329 (1961).

172 WIELAND, P., ULBERWASSER, H., ARMER, G. and MIESCHER, K. *Helv. chim. Acta* **36**, 376, 646 and 1231 (1953).

173 ZAFFARONI, A., BURTON, R. B. and KEUTMANN, E. H. *J. biol. Chem.* **177**, 109 (1949).

174 ZANDER, J. *J. biol. Chem.* **232**, 117 (1953).

175 ZARROW, M. X., NEHER, G. M., LAZO-WASEM, E. A. and SALHANICK, H. A. *J. clin. Endocr.* **17,** 658 (1957).

176 ZYGMUNTOWICZ, A. S., WOOD, M., CHRISTO, E. and TALBOT, N. B. *J. clin. Endocr.* **11,** 578 (1951).

177 ZUMOFF, B. and BRADLOW, H. L. *J. clin. Endocr.* **23,** 799 (1963).

15

CORTICOSTEROIDS

The steroids of the adrenal cortex have three main biological activities which are concerned with (1) electrolyte balance, (2) carbohydrate metabolism and (3) gonadal function. The steroids affecting gonadal function consist of the androgens and oestrogens and have been described in Chapters 13 and 14. Those steroids which maintain the electrolyte balance are called the *mineralocorticosteroids*, whilst those concerned with carbohydrate metabolism are the *glucocorticosteroids*. However, this division can sometimes be confusing, since many corticosteroids contribute to both activities.

Biological activity

1. *Mineralocorticosteroids* control the balance of salt and water, their action being to retain sodium and to prevent the retention of too much potassium. Sensitive methods of bioassay have been developed, which make use of these properties (247). Aldosterone is the most potent adrenal steroid of this type, being 20–30 times as active as deoxycorticosterone.
2. *Glucocorticosteroids* promote the deposition of glycogen in the liver, produce glucose from amino acids and retard the oxidation of glucose; they are thus diabetogenic and act as insulin antagonists. They are relatively, but not completely, inactive with respect to electrolyte metabolism.

The glucocorticosteroids are essential for the maintenance of life, and they play an important part in resistance to shock and infection. The principal steroid of this group is cortisol; it is likely that cortisone when administered systemically is rapidly and completely reduced by the liver to cortisol.

There has been an exceptional amount of interest in the chemistry and biological properties of these steroids because of the discovery of the anti-inflammatory activity of cortisone and its therapeutic usefulness in the treatment of rheumatoid arthritis and of other diseases where the symptoms can be attributed to inflammatory reactions.

Structure and activity

The structures and activities of some of the common natural and synthetic steroids are given in Fig. 15.1. The mechanism of action of these steroids at

	Mineralo-corticoid activity	Glucocorticoid activity	Anti-inflammatory activity	Anti-haemolytic activity
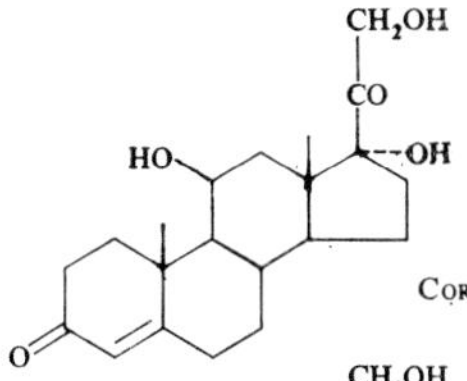 CORTISOL	1	1	1	1
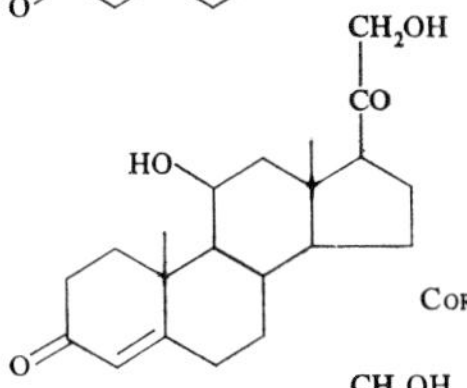 CORTICOSTERONE	5	0·5	0·3	10
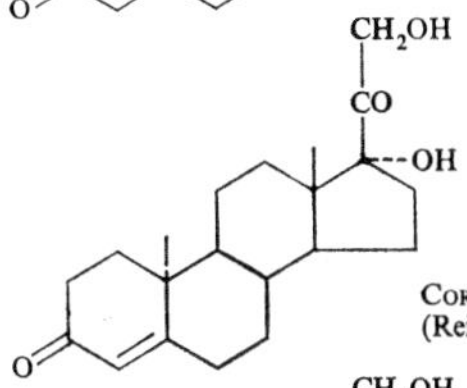 CORTEXOLONE (Reichstein's S)	0	0	—	10
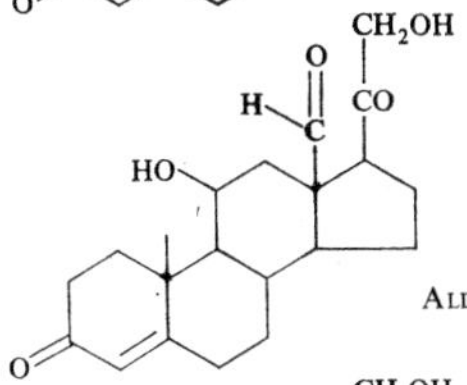 ALDOSTERONE	800	0·2	—	0
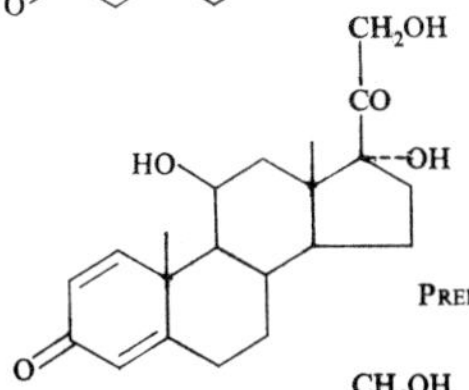 PREDNISOLONE	0·6	4	3	1-2
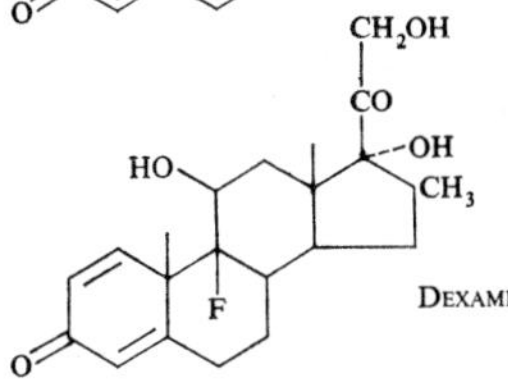 DEXAMETHASONE	0	30	190	5-10

FIG. 15.1. Structure and relative activities of some corticosteroids

the cellular level is largely unknown. The natural steroids possess a Δ^4-3-one group and an α-ketol side chain from $C_{(17)}$. Only aldosterone possesses an aldehyde function at $C_{(18)}$. An oxygen substituent at $C_{(11)}$ is a characteristic of the glucocorticosteroids, and cortisol appears to owe its physiological activity largely to the presence of a hydroxyl group in this position.

The reduction of an 11-oxo group to an 11-hydroxyl group seems essential for glucocorticosteroid activity and is dependent on the stereochemistry of the A and B rings (39, 44). Little if any reduction of the 11-oxo group occurs in 5β steroids, i.e. those with a *cis* A/B ring junction (Fig. 15.2). The 11-oxo group of the 5α epimers with *trans* A/B junctions is extensively reduced however. The reaction must presumably occur by association of the α side of the steroid with the enzyme responsible for this reaction, and steroids with the *cis* A/B junction are not likely to combine firmly with such enzymes.

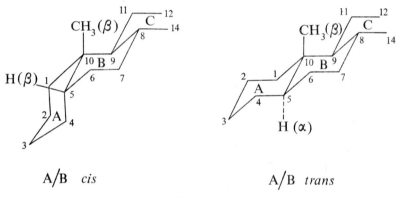

A/B *cis*   A/B *trans*

FIG. 15.2

In the synthetic steroid, prednisone, the angulation of the A/B ring junction is intermediate between the flat *trans* and fully bent *cis* of the saturated 3-hydroxysteroids. On administration of prednisone only 50 per cent is reduced at $C_{(11)}$ as compared with 90 per cent of cortisone (43). This correlates with the significantly reduced activity of prednisone compared with prednisolone.

It is also suggested that the oxidation-reduction at $C_{(11)}$ may act as an essential cofactor in a redox system (267). Steroid dehydrogenases use both NAD and NADP as co-enzymes and steroid hormones in general may exert their action by catalysed transhydrogenation of $NADH_2$ to NADP.

Certain corticosteroids can inhibit *in vitro* the lysis of erythrocytes caused by mechanical stress (295) or by the action of certain chemicals, e.g. sulphydryl inhibitors (2). As seen by examination of Fig. 15.1, the anti-haemolytic activity seems to depend largely on the configuration around $C_{(18)}$ and $C_{(20)}$, the non-polar 18-methyl group and the oxy configuration at

$C_{(20)}$ being important. Different esters at $C_{(21)}$, e.g. phosphate or hemisuccinate, do not alter the effect appreciably (2).

An interesting synthetic compound, 9α-fluoro-11β-hydroxyprogesterone, seems to act like a 'skeleton key' to many of the receptors for steroid hormones. Thus it possesses considerable glucocorticoid, sodium-retaining and progestational activities (100).

Biosynthesis

The main pathway for the biosynthesis of cortisol has been established as cholesterol →pregnenolone →progesterone →17-hydroxyprogesterone →cortisol. The evidence for this is extensive, and only some of the more recent work will be described here. In an extensive review of the subject Wettstein (287) has reported over 70 steroids of adrenal origin isolated from the gland or from urine.

Cholesterol is an obligatory precursor of cortisol; in studies with labelled acetate it is found that the labelling of individual carbon atoms of cortisol formed from the acetate is identical with that found in cholesterol derived from labelled acetate (52).

Corticotrophin plays an important part in the partial degradation of the side chain of cholesterol (121). Firstly, hydroxylating enzymes convert cholesterol to 20β-hydroxycholesterol and 20β, 22-dihydroxycholesterol, and then with 20,22-desmolase and $NADPH_2$ as co-factor, corticotrophin stimulates the production of pregnenolone. This steroid has been isolated from the adrenals of the pig (187).

Adrenocortical tissue retains much of its activity *in vitro* so that incubation studies have yielded valuable information regarding the biosynthetic pathways. Thus the biosynthesis of corticosteroids from labelled cholesterol has been demonstrated in the presence of adrenal tissue from the rat (206), dog (157) and human (115).

There have been numerous studies using labelled progesterone with tissue from human adrenal adenoma (281), hyperplastic adrenal tissue (15, 228, 283, 285), foetal (280) and pig (297) adrenals. The addition of $NADPH_2$ to the incubation medium results in an enhanced conversion of progesterone to the more polar corticosteroids.

Although substantial amounts of deoxycorticosterone are not found in the normal human adrenal this steroid is a major product of *in vitro* experiments (281). In addition, adrenal tissue taken from a patient with Cushing's syndrome who excreted excess amounts of 17-hydroxycorticosteroids, when incubated with [4-^{14}C]progesterone produced no labelled cortisol but instead, 11-deoxycorticosterone and corticosterone (283). This may indicate that progesterone is not the only natural precursor of cortisol or that the 17-hydroxylating mechanism is less efficient *in vitro*. It has in fact been observed in experiments with normal, hyperplastic or neoplastic adrenals that 17α-hydroxypregnenolone may be at least as good a precursor of cortisol as 17α-hydroxyprogesterone (166, 183, 284, 297). This alternative pathway would, therefore, be cholesterol →pregnenolone →17α-hydroxypregnenolone →17α-hydroxyprogesterone. The normal adrenal probably secretes 17α-hydroxypregnenolone since the metabolite, pregn-5-ene-3β, 17α, 20α-triol, occurs in urine (95, 290).

Catabolism

The liver is the main organ responsible for the formation of water-soluble conjugates of the corticosteroids (260). Cortisol is reduced in ring A to a 3α-ol-5β structure giving tetrahydrocortisol and oxidized at $C_{(11)}$ to give tetrahydrocortisone. Almost all the [^{14}C]cortisol administered to human subjects is excreted as these two compounds, conjugated as the glucosiduronates, with the hexahydro metabolites, cortol and cortolone (107). A minor route involves the removal of the side chain to yield 17-oxosteroids (Fig. 15.3).

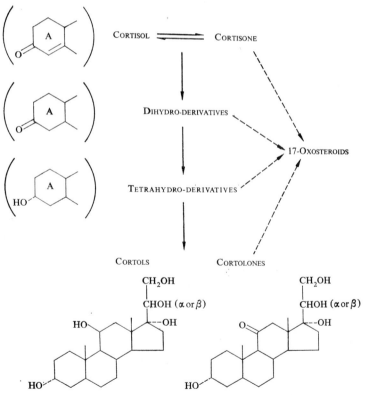

FIG. 15.3. Some excretory products of cortisol

Tetrahydroderivatives may be prepared by incubating corticosteroids with rat liver 3α-hydroxysteroid dehydrogenase and co-factors (267). Such methods have been used for the preparation of tritium-labelled metabolites of cortisol from cortisol of high specific activity (243).

It has been shown by *in vitro* experiments that the adrenal is capable of conjugating corticosteroids as sulphates (159). Corticosterone and deoxycorticosterone are most readily conjugated in this way. They are also conjugated as sulphates by liver homogenates, but cortisol and cortisone are not (238).

Occurrence and extraction

(a) IN BLOOD

The corticosteroids circulate as 'free' steroids, as loosely bound complexes with protein and as conjugates. The free steroids may be separated from those bound to protein by dialysis (59, 67, 68, 175, 184, 213) or by gel filtration (28, 72, 76, 213), after which the steroid-protein binding is easily broken down by extraction with organic solvents such as ethyl acetate or chloroform. The conjugated steroids are not extracted by these solvents and must first be hydrolysed or be extracted by special methods described later.

PROTEIN BINDING Cortisol circulates largely as a complex formed with an α-globulin (cortisol-binding globulin, CBG, or transcortin) and partly with albumin. CBG has been purified by using stepwise elution in phosphate buffers from DEAE-cellulose (241) or by gel filtration through Sephadex G-25 (242). Contaminating proteins are then removed by adsorption on hydroxyl apatite and after several such treatments CBG is eluted as a single symmetrical peak. When prepared in this way CBG is homogeneous in the ultracentrifuge with a sedimentation constant, $S_{20,w}$ of 3·0, it migrates as an $α_1$-globulin during electrophoresis and in immunoelectrophoresis gives a single precipitin line against antiserum to whole human serum. It contains 5·4 per cent hexose, 4·7 per cent hexosamine, 3·2 per cent sialic acid and 0·8 per cent fucose. If one binding site is present per molecule of glycoprotein, the calculated molecular weight is 45,000 which is consistent with the sedimentation constant. CBG constitutes about 0·1 per cent of the total serum proteins and 1·2 per cent of the total $α_1$-globulin.

The binding sites are virtually saturated when the concentration of cortisol in plasma is between 20 and 30 μg/100 ml, and only at higher concentrations is significant binding to albumin or other plasma proteins observed. Increased binding occurs during pregnancy and in the plasma of patients receiving oestrogens (69, 233).

FACTORS AFFECTING BINDING CAPACITY The binding capacity of CBG for many other steroids has been studied. Binding occurs not only with cortisol but also with corticosterone, deoxycorticosterone, a few synthetic steroids and to a much lesser degree with cortisone. It has been found that for maximal displacement of cortisol or corticosterone from their binding sites the presence of at least two hydroxyl groups at the 11β-, 17α- or 21-positions and a Δ^4-3-one structure is required (67). Competition for binding sites is greatly decreased by the presence of 6α-CH_3, 11-oxo, 11α-OH, 16α-OH, 16α-CH_3, 18-al or 9α-F groups on a corticosterone molecule (67, 92, 184). Dehydrogenation at the $C_{(1)}$ and $C_{(2)}$ positions partly reverses this. Thus 17-hydroxyprogesterone displaces almost 50 per cent of previously bound cortisol, whereas tetrahydroderivatives have much less affinity for CBG than their respective parent steroids (71, 233). Certain synthetic steroids do not react uniformly; prednisone (11-oxo group) displaces much less cortisol than prednisolone ($11\beta,17\alpha,21$-trihydroxypregn-1,4-diene-3,20-dione) but triamcinolone (9α-F-$11\beta,16\alpha,17\alpha,21$-tetrahydroxypregna-1,4-diene-3,20-dione) and betamethasone (9α-F-16β-methyl-$11\beta,17\alpha,21$-trihydroxypregna-1,4-diene-3,20-dione) hardly compete at all. Presumably the 9α-F group has a powerful influence here.

The effect of temperature on binding affinity of CBG has been widely studied (59, 72, 185, 213, 236, 242, 249). The binding affinity of the purified α-globulin decreases with rise of temperature (242) and is greatly increased at 4° (69). The increased binding capacity which is induced by oestrogen, however, is not greater at 4°. This suggests that the binding sites induced by oestrogens are qualitatively different from those on normal CBG. Binding capacity is destroyed by heating at 60° for 20 minutes (68) or by boiling for 5 minutes (184) but under these conditions cortisol still binds albumin.

Cortisol which is bound to CBG is biologically inert and is unavailable for metabolism (232). This has been demonstrated by *in vitro* experiments with the enzyme systems of human or rat liver microsomes which are responsible for the metabolism of cortisol. In the presence of CBG the metabolism is reduced. The binding protein may therefore act as a kind of buffer mechanism against rapid changes in available cortisol. After a rapid increase in secretion of cortisol, most of it will become bound to protein and so will not be immediately available. Conversely, if the secretion decreases, the protein-bound fraction provides a reserve (178).

The nature of the linkage between cortisol and CBG is unknown. Extraction of plasma with solvents at low temperatures—conditions under which denaturation should be slight—is sufficient to reduce the binding capacity to about half the original value (76). This suggests a possible lipid linkage but no positive evidence for this is yet available. The binding between cortisol and albumin is certainly weak and dissociation occurs even during gel filtration (68). It is reported, however, that dissociation from CBG may also occur on Sephadex (213).

There is some evidence that erythrocytes contain a substance which can bind cortisol, but which has a lower capacity than CBG (72). Later work, however, does not support the concept of a specific cortisol-binding agent in erythrocytes (74). Even so, there appears to be an uptake of around 80 per cent of cortisol by erythrocytes, most of which may be easily washed off in buffer (2, 279). It has been suggested that the corticosteroids may pack themselves into the phospholipid layer of cell membranes so that the lipophilic structure intermixes with the aliphatic chains of the phospholipids, while the hydrophilic side chain remains outside (288).

Aldosterone is bound primarily to albumin but at 4° it is about equally bound to albumin and CBG (69). There may well be other proteins involved (70, 175).

(b) IN URINE

Free steroids may be extracted from urine by solvents such as chloroform or ethyl acetate. A useful table of partition coefficients between water and various solvents for several corticosteroids has been published (29). These free steroids are of interest clinically (78, 83, 227) but constitute only a minor proportion of the total urinary corticosteroids in the human. They are excreted largely as the tetrahydroderivatives conjugated with glucuronic or sulphuric acids and possibly others. In the cat, however, corticosteroids are not excreted as glucosiduronates (26, 220) and the bulk of the corticosteroids in the guinea-pig are excreted unconjugated (207).

Hot-acid hydrolysis cannot be used to split these conjugates if the steroids are to be recovered intact since degradation of the $C_{(17)}$ side chain occurs (108). Instead the enzymic or solvolytic methods must be used (see p. 243).

The conjugates themselves may be extracted with n-butanol (214), a mixture of n-butanol and chloroform (153) or with n-propanol (190). The method of Edwards et al. (81) and several modifications of this (12, 42, 154, 155) are convenient since they employ more volatile solvents. This is a great advantage since the corticosteroids are easily destroyed during evaporation of the solvent at elevated temperatures; such evaporations should be carried out under reduced pressure at temperatures of not more than about 40°.

The conjugates are adsorbed on to the weakly basic exchange resin 'Decolorite' (Permutit Co. Ltd.) from urine at pH 3·0, and are eluted in methanol and ammonium hydroxide (42). The resin requires careful treatment before use (44, 45), and it is possible that the conjugates are not retained by a true ion-exchange reaction but rather by non-ionic adsorption; it is probable that the technique of gel filtration will be preferred in future (13).

Methods of Separation and Purification

(a) FREE (UNCONJUGATED) STEROIDS

Preliminary purification of extracts from biological fluids usually consists of washing with alkali and water. To prevent losses, the alkaline washing is done in the cold with weak NaOH or even milder alkali such as sodium or

potassium carbonate (46, 117). It must be remembered that some corticosteroids are very polar and β-cortolone for instance is extracted by NaOH
(111, 223).

Lipids may be removed by partitioning between organic solvents and
aqueous alcohols. Satisfactory results are obtained with 50 per cent aqueous
methanol and carbon tetrachloride (181), 70 per cent methanol and pentane
or toluene-hexane (143), or 70 per cent ethanol and hexane-pentane (263).
Further purification of crude extracts is conveniently achieved on columns of
silica gel (46).

Chromatographic methods

PAPER   Methods based on the original techniques of Zaffaroni (37) and
Bush (38) have been adequately reviewed (41). There are some reports on
the use of similar solvent systems on glass fibre sheets, very rapid separations
then being possible (227, 255). Thus cortisol is easily separated from cortisone
and the tetrahydroderivatives in the system benzene–N,N-dimethyl formamide (100:1·3 v/v) or benzene–formamide (100:10 v/v) with a running time
of about 20 minutes.

THIN LAYER CHROMATOGRAPHY   In a remarkable paper Lisboa (167) has
demonstrated the separation of over 30 steroids by means of one- and two-
dimensional chromatography, and of repeated chromatography in the same
direction with different solvents. Suitable mixtures for steroid separation on
thin layers of silica gel are benzene or chloroform with ethanol or methanol.
Good separations of some of the principal corticosteroids are also obtained
in the solvents used in the Zaffaroni systems with thin layers of Kieselguhr
(114). Cortisol and prednisolone separate on Kieselguhr in chloroform-
formamide, whereas it is difficult to separate steroids differing by one double
bond in ring A by thin layer chromatography on silica gel (259).

ADSORPTION CHROMATOGRAPHY   Column chromatography with mixtures
of magnesium silicate and Celite was used in much of the early work on the
separation of the corticosteroids and a special form of magnesium silicate,
Florisil, was introduced into the widely used routine method for cortisol of
Nelson and Samuels (189).

Alumina is not suitable as it has been shown to alter the molecular structure
of many of these steroids (160). Even silica gel has been reported to have a
similar effect (170, 251, 269) although for most purposes it is perfectly satisfactory (262).

Adsorption chromatography is very suitable for the separation of a limited
number of pure steroids and the columns have a relatively high capacity.
For finer separations, however, the partition methods are preferable.

PARTITION COLUMN CHROMATOGRAPHY   Morris and Williams (181) first
used partition columns for the separation of corticosteroids, and the technique has been widely used since with a variety of solvent systems. In the

original method, the separation of individual steroids is achieved on two columns. The first, toluene with 25 per cent aqueous ethanol on Celite, separates the less polar steroids from cortisol and cortisone. The former group is resolved on a second column of light petroleum: toluene (20:80 v/v) with ethylene glycol as the stationary phase. A later development has been the introduction of gradient elution to this form of column so that only one column is required (280). The system, hexane with a gradient of dichloroethane and 90 per cent aqueous methanol as stationary phase gives good separation of deoxycorticosterone, 11-dehydrocorticosterone, corticosterone and cortisol.

COUNTERCURRENT DISTRIBUTIONS Some systems suitable for the corticosteroids are given in Table 15.1.

TABLE 15.1

Partition coefficients for some corticosteroids (concentration in upper phase/concentration in lower phase)

	(1)	(2)	(3)	(4)	(5)
Cortisol	<0·02	0·14	0·24	1·4	2·85
Cortisone	<0·02	0·26	0·32	1·55	2·93
11-dehydrocorticosterone	0·21	2·6	0·51	1·91	—
11-deoxycorticosterone	—	16	—	17·8	—
Corticosterone	—	1·57	0·96	3·73	7
Cortexolone	—	1·22	2·85	—	—
Aldosterone	—	—	—	—	1·44
Tetrahydrocortisone	—	—	—	—	3·6
Tetrahydrocortisol	—	—	—	—	5·3

(1) Petroleum ether–34·5% aqueous ethanol.
(2) Benzene–50% aqueous methanol.
(3) 75% n-hexane–25% s-butanol–water
(4) 2,2,4-trimethyl pentane–s-butanol–water (3 : 2 : 4 by vol)
(5) 50% n-hexane–s-butanol–water

(1) DICZFALUSY, E. *Acta endocr. Copenh.* **10**, 373 (1952).
(2) CARSTENSEN, H. *Acta chem. scand.* **9**, 1026 (1955).
(3) and (5) CARSTENSEN, H. *Methods in Biochemical Analysis* **9**, 127 (1962).
(4) TALBOT, N. B., ULICK, S., KOUPREIANOW, A. and ZYGMUNTOWICZ, A. *J. clin. Endocr.* **15**, 301 (1955).

GAS LIQUID CHROMATOGRAPHY The application of this technique to the corticosteroids is restricted because of their lability under the conditions usually required. The 17α,21-dihydroxy-20-ones are easily degraded to 17-oxosteroids (275) while 21-deoxy-17α-hydroxy-corticosteroids may undergo D-homo-annulation (225).

It has been found that some corticosteroids are transformed while others are stable on columns of 1 per cent SE-30 at 225° (31). The 21-acetoxy derivatives of 17α,21-dihydroxy-20-oxosteroids give several peaks resulting from rearrangements but the 17α,21-diacetoxy derivatives are stable. Steroids with 21-hydroxy-20-oxo groups give a main peak of the unchanged compound. In general, fully acetylated derivatives may be subjected to this form of chromatography without substantial alteration of structure.

The trimethyl silyl ethers promise to be useful derivatives, although several products may be formed according to the solvent employed (pyridine or chloroform) during the reaction. Satisfactory chromatography is reported on silicone columns at 280°. Cortisone may be protected by forming the bis-methylenedioxy derivative by reaction with formaldehyde in acid solution

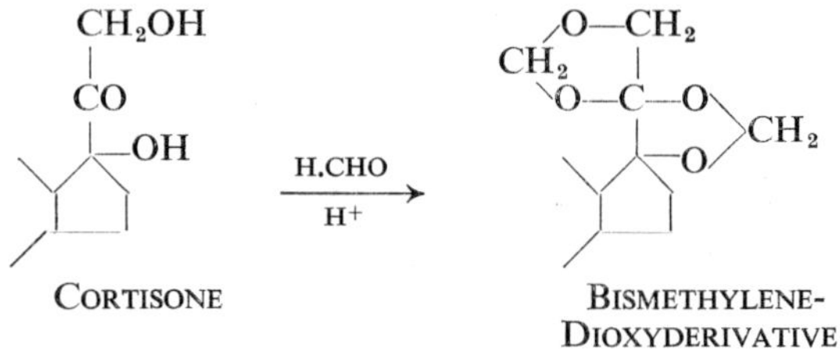

$$CORTISONE \xrightarrow[H^+]{H.CHO} BISMETHYLENE-DIOXYDERIVATIVE$$

FIG. 15.4

(Fig. 15.4). Other hydroxylated analogues give more complex chromatograms however (149).

Another approach is to convert the 17-hydroxycorticosteroids to 17-oxosteroids since the latter compounds may readily be applied to gas liquid chromatography (9, 150). If periodate is used for the oxidation, steroids with a 21-hydroxyl-20-oxo side chain give 17-carboxylic acids which may be esterified with diazomethane (172). These substances are satisfactorily separated on SE-30 columns.

Aldosterone presents some difficulties but tetrahydroaldosterone as the triacetate is readily separated from other compounds on SE-30 columns (296).

(b) CONJUGATED STEROIDS

The glucosiduronates and sulphates are separated easily by paper chromatography (239). Bush (40) used a number of alkaline and acidic systems and reported that the conjugates were only a little more difficult to separate than the free steroids. The systems octanol–pyridine–water (5:3:2 by vol.) and amyl alcohol–pyridine–acetic acid–octanol–water (3:1:1:3:4 by vol.) are useful for the separation of conjugates of both the natural and synthetic corticosteroids (264).

The sulphates are eluted by 50 per cent ethanol from columns of alumina, and the glucosiduronates may then be removed by 0·5 M-acetate at pH 5·0. Separation of the individual steroids is possible by partition chromatography in the system ethylene dichloride–t-butanol–acetic acid–water (7·5:2·5:3·7) (93); or by countercurrent distribution on 0·2 per cent NH_4OH–n-butanol–ethyl acetate (100:50:50 by vol.).

Crystalline derivatives of the glucosiduronates in the form of triacetate methyl ethers may be obtained (93). After methylation with diazomethane acetylation is carried out in pyridine and acetic anhydride. Purification is achieved on Celite columns in benzene–light petroleum–aqueous methanol. The methylation must be performed first; otherwise more than one product is obtained, possibly because of lactone ring formation.

Chemical reactions useful for identification

The early methods for the determination of corticosteroids were based on the reducing properties of the α-ketolic side chain ($—CO—CH_2OH$) and made use of reagents such as copper sulphate or phosphomolybdic acid. Since they are neither specific, nor very sensitive, they will not be discussed further here.

(1) Reduction of tetrazolium salts

Water-soluble tetrazolium salts may be reduced by many substances in alkaline solution with opening of the ring and production of a red formazan compound (Fig. 15.5).

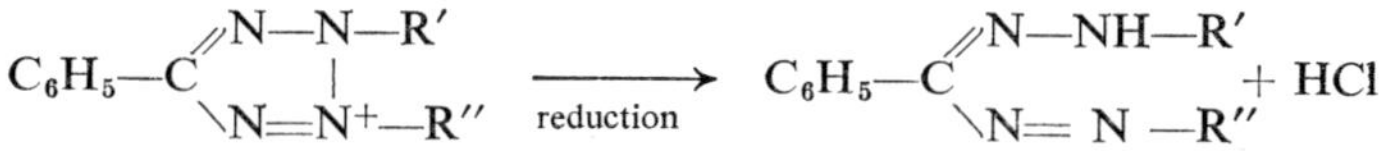

$$C_6H_5-C\begin{matrix} \diagup N-N-R' \\ | \\ \diagdown N=N^+-R'' \end{matrix} \xrightarrow[\text{reduction}]{} C_6H_5-C\begin{matrix} \diagup N-NH-R' \\ \\ \diagdown N= N -R'' \end{matrix} + HCl$$

Tetrazolium Salt   Formazan
(colourless) I   (coloured) II

FIG. 15.5

Triphenyl-tetrazolium chloride (Formula I $R',R''=C_6H_5$) is reduced to a red formazan, insoluble in water but soluble in many organic solvents. The reagent, however, is rather easily reduced on exposure to light, and derivatives are usually used which are less photosensitive. One such derivation is 2-(p-iodophenyl)-3-(p-nitrophenyl)-5-phenyl tetrazolium chloride, (Formula I $R' = C_6H_4NO_2$, $R'' = C_6H_4I$) (124), another is 2:5-diphenyl-3-(4-styryl phenyl)-tetrazolium chloride (32), but the most commonly used is blue tetrazolium (3,3'-dianisole-bis-4,4'-3,5-diphenyl tetrazolium chloride) (58, 168, 191).

Certain non-ketolic substances react with the reagent, and variations in the base used and the time and temperature of the reaction have been investigated in order to determine the conditions which minimize interference from such substances (135, 174). Non-ketolic steroids possessing a Δ^4-3-oxo group reduce the reagent, but they produce less colour and react more slowly. The presence of an 11-oxo or 17-oxo group enhances the reaction but a 6-oxo or 6β-hydroxy group decreases the reaction.

Alkaline blue tetrazolium is a useful reagent for the detection of corticosteroids on paper. After the development of the red formazan Δ^4-3-oxosteroids may be observed on heating by the soda-fluorescence reaction (38). The styryl derivative mentioned above is useful for detection on thin layer chromatograms; it reacts with 21-acetates better on alumina than silica gel.

(2) *Oxidation*

(a) PERIODATE   In acid or neutral media the oxidation potential is high and the rate of oxidation is rapid. C_{21} steroids with α-ketol or α-glycol side chains give formaldehyde and are converted to etianic acids or products with a $C_{(17)}$ formyl group respectively (Fig. 15.6). Aldosterone gives a hemiacetal

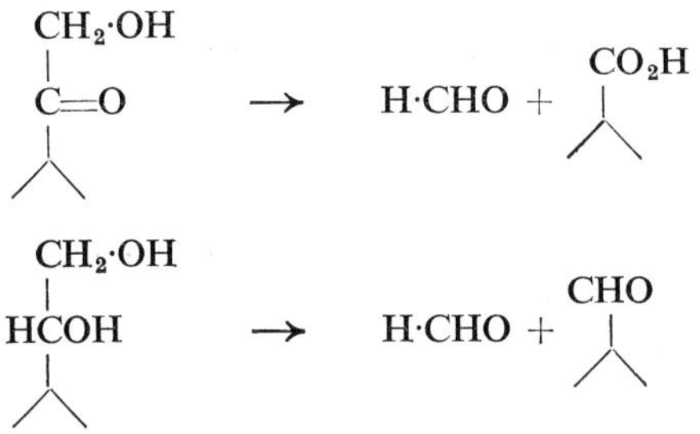

FIG. 15.6. Oxidation of 17-deoxycorticosteroids by periodate or bismuthate

lactone of 11β-hydroxy-18-aldo-3-oxo-androst-4-ene-17β-carboxylic acid.

17-,20-,21-trihydroxy steroids or 17-,20-dihydroxy steroids give 17-oxosteroids, the second group yielding acetaldehyde (63) (Fig. 15.7).

In alkaline media the oxidation potential is lower, and the oxidation rate for glycols is reduced; only those 17-hydroxysteroids with a glycerol side chain yield 17-oxosteroids, i.e. 17-,20-,21-trihydroxysteroids (221). This reaction has been developed for the detection of such compounds on paper chromatograms (289). Only weakly positive reactions are given with 20α-,21- and 20β-,21-dihydroxysteroids.

Reactions with periodate are much used in clinical studies (64, 89, 137, 173, 177, 231) particularly for cortisol and its major metabolites which are oxidized to 17-oxosteroids and may then be measured by the Zimmermann reaction. The products may be separated into 11-oxygenated and 11-deoxy fractions by chromatography on silica gel (182), on paper (82) or by partition chromatography using Celite columns (88).

Periodate also degrades the glucosiduronic group in conjugated steroids giving the free steroids or formate esters (134). It does not affect the 11β-hydroxy groups as may sodium bismuthate (44). This is of importance when

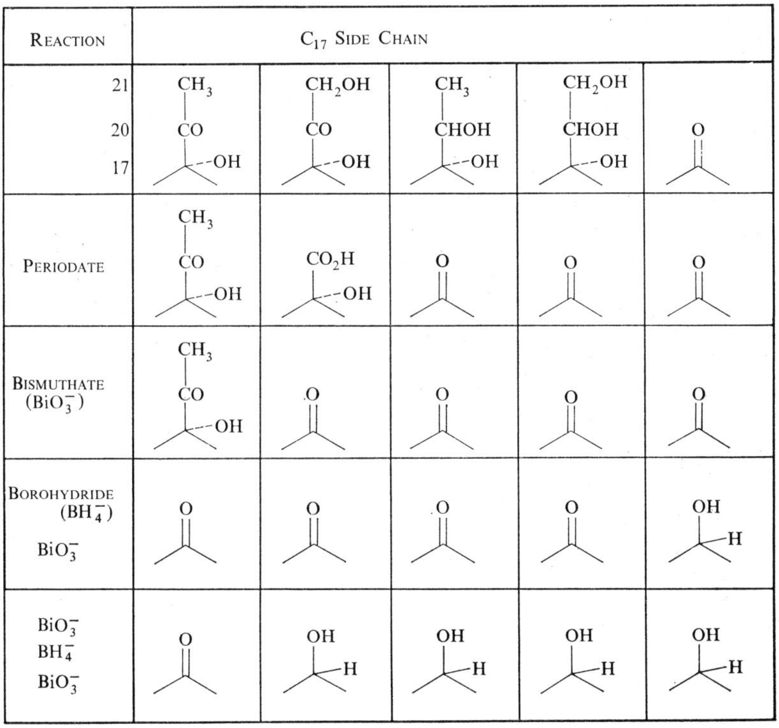

REACTION	C₁₇ SIDE CHAIN				
21 20 17	CH₃ CO �--OH	CH₂OH CO ⎢--OH	CH₃ CHOH ⎢--OH	CH₂OH CHOH ⎢--OH	O (ketone)
PERIODATE	CH₃ CO ⎢--OH	CO₂H ⎢--OH	O	O	O
BISMUTHATE (BiO₃⁻)	CH₃ CO ⎢--OH	O	O	O	O
BOROHYDRIDE (BH₄⁻) BiO₃⁻	O	O	O	O	OH—H
BiO₃⁻ BH₄⁻ BiO₃⁻	O	OH—H	OH—H	OH—H	OH—H

FIG. 15.7

the Zimmermann reaction is used for the final estimation since 11β-hydroxy and 11-oxo-17-oxosteroids may have different colour equivalents.

(b) SODIUM BISMUTHATE 17-deoxycorticosteroids with an α-ketol or α-glycol side chain are oxidized by sodium bismuthate, as shown above in Fig. 15.6. The α-ketols give formaldehyde and an etianic acid while the α-glycols give formaldehyde and a 20-aldo compound.

The reactions of this reagent with 17-hydroxysteroids are shown in Fig. 15.7. Cortisol and its metabolites give mainly 11-oxoaetiocholanolone, the 11β-hydroxyl group being oxidized to the 11-ketone by most batches of the reagent. It will be noticed that 21-deoxyketols are resistant to oxidation.

In routine clinical methods sodium borohydride is often used first to reduce any 17-oxosteroids to compounds containing the structure $\overset{\text{OH}}{\underset{}{\bigwedge}}$—H at C$_{(17)}$ (4). Subsequent oxidation with bismuthate does not affect this product, but the 21-deoxyketols which are reduced by borohydride to 17,20-glycols and the other 17-hydroxysteroids give 17-oxosteroids on subsequent oxidation (Fig. 15.7).

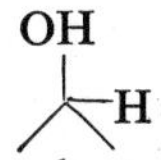

The 21-deoxyketols may be measured separately by including three steps,

z

bismuthate, borohydride and bismuthate (4, 298). Then only these steroids give 17-oxosteroids as the final product.

During oxidation with sodium bismuthate, as with periodate, the steroid glucosiduronates are oxidized to the free steroids or the formate esters. It has also been observed that sodium borohydride reduces 11-oxo groups but the reaction is slower than with 20-oxo groups.

(c) OTHER OXIDANTS　Chromium trioxide (1 per cent w/v CrO_3 in 50 per cent acetic acid) oxidizes the $C_{(17)}$ side chains of corticosteroids to 17-oxo-steroids (164). Under these rather mild conditions, however, the oxidation proceeds slowly and is complete only after 8–16 hours at 20–22° (41). The 11β- and 11α-hydroxyl groups in corticosteroids, however, are completely oxidized in 10–20 minutes.

Aldosterone diacetate is oxidized to the 18→11-lactone-21-acetate (170) under these conditions. It is reported that 16α- and 16β-hydroxyl groups in certain C_{21} steroids are not oxidized (186).

Manganese dioxide is a specific oxidant for equatorial allylic alcohols (235, 252) dissolved in chloroform. The oxidation is complete in 24 hours. More vigorous conditions are required for the oxidation of axial groups. This reagent has been used as an aid to the identification of 6β-hydroxyandros-tenedione in urine (235).

(3) Phenylhydrazine

In acid solution this reagent forms hydrazones with steroids containing a dihydroxyacetone side chain ($\overset{\diagdown}{\underset{\diagup}{C}}H \cdot OH \cdot CO \cdot CH_2 \cdot OH$) which have maximum absorption at 410 mμ (212). 3-hydrazones are formed with Δ^4-3-ones and these absorb maximally at 340–360 mμ.

This reagent is widely used for clinical investigations of cortisol in plasma and urine (Porter-Silber reaction). Various colour corrections have been suggested to improve the specificity of the reaction (27, 125), but since the reagent contains strong sulphuric acid it is not suitable for direct application to crude extracts. It is also not completely specific for the dihydroxyacetone side chain since it reacts with the 21-aldehydes of deoxycorticosterone, corticosterone, 18-hydroxydeoxycorticosterone (204, 246) and a number of non-steroidal compounds.

The hydrazones formed with 2,4-dinitrophenylhydrazine are coloured compounds that separate well on paper or alumina (216). The reaction may be used for quantitative estimations, but although it is quite sensitive, it is less specific than the Porter-Silber reaction (117). Δ^4-3-oxo compounds react within 5 minutes at 20° and give hydrazones with maximum absorption at 450 mμ. After 90 minutes at 59°, 20-oxosteroids react as well, giving maximum absorption at 460 mμ (116). Aldosterone gives greater colour intensity than deoxycorticosterone, so that the 18-aldo group probably also reacts (180).

Iso-nicotinic acid hydrazide is another useful reagent; it reacts at different rates with different ketones. In 1 per cent ethanolic acetic acid it reacts with Δ^4-3-ones at 37° giving 3-hydrazones with maximum absorption at 380 mμ(273). These derivatives are well separated by thin layer chromatography on silica gel in benzene–methanol (75:25 v/v (167)).

(4) Fluorescence

(a) SODA FLUORESCENCE This reaction is a most useful and sensitive method for detection on paper chromatograms (see p. 251). It is particularly sensitive for 11β-hydroxy compounds. The reaction has been developed for quantitative determinations on paper (e.g. 6) or in solution when 0·1–0·3N-potassium t-butoxide is used instead of NaOH (1, 255). In the latter method the wavelength of the incident light is 365 mμ and the fluorescence is measured at 560–580 mμ. Under these conditions the reaction is sensitive to 0·01 μg steroid.

(b) IN ACID Cortisol and corticosterone exhibit a fairly specific fluorescence after heating in 75–80 per cent H_2SO_4, and this reaction has been widely used in clinical work (30, 55, 73, 75, 77, 83, 94, 140, 169, 229, 245, 261). A micro-method has been described in which the sensitivity is such that 0·5 ng may be measured, the quantity present in a drop or two of blood or in less than 1 per cent of a rat adrenal (113).

For the quantitative determination of cortisol or corticosterone in plasma, an activating wavelength of 470 mμ is used and the fluorescence is measured at 550 mμ. Corticosterone gives more than 2·5 times the fluorescence of cortisol; these steroids are easily separated by partitioning between solvents, and may be measured independently (209, 230, 276). In extracts of plasma, fluorescence may arise from substances other than corticosteroids, and several methods of eliminating this interference have been suggested (30, 66, 179). These are not wholly satisfactory, but none the less, fluorimetric methods are extremely useful and give results sufficiently accurate for most clinical investigations.

Phosphoric acid may be used instead for H_2SO_4 for the fluorimetric detection of some adrenal steroids. Thus 3α,17α,20α-trihydroxypregnan-11-one may be detected on paper chromatograms by a blue fluorescence under u.v. light after treatment with 70 per cent H_3PO_4 at 85–87° for 10 minutes (90). A variety of colours is given with other steroids which may be observed in daylight or in u.v. light (89, 140).

(5) Polarographic methods

Morris and Williams (181), using a modification of the Girard procedure, heated the steroid at 100° for 2 minutes with Girard T reagent in t-butanol and acetic acid. After evaporation of the solvents the residue is dissolved in KCl–KOH solution adjusted to pH 5·6 with acetic acid. After washing with toluene the solution is ready for polarography. Under these conditions, cathodic waves are given with Δ^4-3-ones at $E_{\frac{1}{2}}$ about $-1·10$ V and with the 20-ketone in 11-dehydrocorticosterone, corticosterone and deoxycorticosterone at $-1·36$ V.

(6) *Other reactions*

(a) It will be remembered (p. 337) that the 17-deoxy steroids containing a 20:21 diol group are oxidized by bismuthate to 20-aldo compounds. The latter may be detected by the Angeli-Rimini reaction; they are treated with benzene sulpho-hydroxamic acid in weakly alkaline solution to give hydroxamic acids. These are detected by conversion to their purple ferric complexes (84, Fig. 15.8).

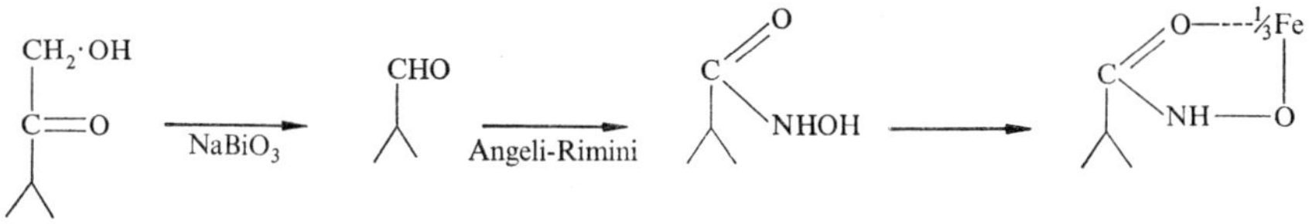

FIG. 15.8

(b) A limited number of corticosteroids react with *p*-hydroxybenzaldehyde in H_2SO_4 (Komanowsky's reagent) even when they are substituted at $C_{(20)}$. Thus the 20-semicarbazone of 4:5α-dihydrocortisone acetate reacts with this reagent but not with tetrazolium.

(c) Methanolic zinc chloride reacts with all C_{21} steroids which contain a 3-hydroxy or 3-oxo group, provided this is activated in some way. Thus all 11-hydroxy derivatives react but 11-oxo derivatives will not, except when a conjugated diene system exists in ring A. 4,5α-dihydrocortisone acetate for instance will not react, whereas prednisone acetate will.

The reagent probably has the same specificity as antimony trichloride but it is relatively non-toxic. It is useful as a reagent for thin layer chromatograms, and produces a variety of colours in visible and u.v. light (259).

Some corticosteroids occurring in biological fluids

(a) THE GLUCOCORTICOSTEROIDS

The remarkable clinical effects of cortisone and related steroids, particularly in rheumatoid arthritis, which were first recognized about fifteen years ago, stimulated interest in the synthesis of these steroids from other more plentiful naturally occurring substances. The chief difficulty was in the introduction of the 11-oxygen atom into ring C, since most naturally occurring steroids in plants, for instance, contained a saturated ring C and at the time there were no known methods of introducing this substituent. The construction of the dihydroxy acetone side chain was another difficulty.

These problems were soon overcome and satisfactory syntheses were described from several laboratories (e.g. 11, 51, 211). Extensive reviews of these methods have appeared (17, 62, 226). Here it may be mentioned that the introduction of the oxygen function at $C_{(11)}$ may be achieved by transferring an oxygen at $C_{(12)}$, as in deoxycholic acid, to $C_{(11)}$ by forming the 11:12-disubstituted intermediate. Alternatively 7:9(11)-dienes(I) (see Fig. 15.9) may be prepared from naturally occurring substances such as ergosterol and stigmasterol. Epoxidation leads to the formation of the 7-ene-9α,11α-epoxide (II) which when treated with boron trifluoride-ether complex or ferric chloride in benzene gives the 8-en-11-one structure (III). This is then reduced to the required structure by lithium in liquid ammonia (IV).

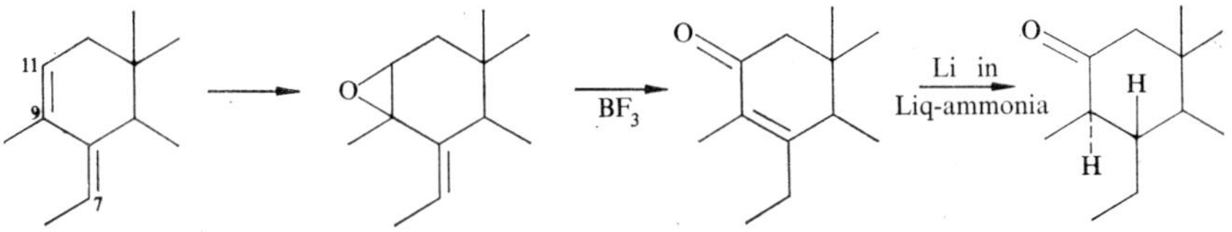

FIG. 15.9

New methods of synthesis are still appearing: one starting with 2-methyl-cyclopentane-1,3-dione (277) has already been mentioned, since it is suitable also for oestrone and testosterone (p. 304).

The synthesis of the glucosiduronates is possible by the methods given on p. 314 for the 17-oxosteroid conjugates, namely by the use of methyl-2,3,4-tri-O-acetyl-1-bromo-1-deoxy-D-glucuronate (93).

METABOLIC PRODUCTS   At least 50 per cent of injected ^{14}C-labelled cortisol is excreted as tetrahydroderivatives of cortisol and cortisone (see Fig. 15.3). Tetrahydrocortisone and tetrahydrocortisol are well known urinary metabolites and methods for their determination have been described (41, 156). The amount of allotetrahydrocortisone, however, is believed to be quite small, but allotetrahydrocortisol occurs in adrenal glands (291) and has been shown to be a metabolite of cortisol in perfusion experiments with rat livers (53, 54). It has also been recognized in urine (47); it runs slightly ahead of tetrahydrocortisol in benzene–methanol–water (2:1:1 by vol.), but after acetylation the order is reversed in the system light petroleum–benzene–methanol–water (66:33:80:20 by vol.). The isomers are more easily separated after oxidation by sodium bismuthate to the 17-oxosteroids.

Experiments in which ^{14}C-labelled tetrahydrocortisol was injected into humans showed that the 5β-H structure was quite stable since no labelled allotetrahydrocortisol was excreted. This suggests that the allo form in urine must arise directly from cortisol on reduction of ring A. Furthermore, only a small amount of the cortisone derivative was recovered, so small that it is possible that the 11-oxo derivatives in urine derive directly from cortisol rather than through tetrahydrocortisol.

There is evidence that a certain amount of cortisol is excreted in the form of sulphate conjugates (155, 198, 199). After administration of cortisol to human subjects, the 21-sulphate conjugate of cortisol has been identified; suitable systems for its separation by chromatography are butyl acetate–toluene–n-butanol–water–acetic acid (50:10:40:9:10 by vol.) and butyl acetate–toluene–n-butanol–4N-NH₄OH–methanol (60:30:10:50:50 by vol.). Methods for the preparation of the sulphate conjugates have been known for a long time (250). The steroid in pyridine is mixed with pyridine-SO₃ and the sulphation is allowed to proceed for 60 hours at room temperature. The sulphate conjugates may be recognized by use of the methylene blue reagent (see p. 310).

Most of the remaining cortisol can be accounted for in other reduced products such as the cortols and cortolones in which the 20-oxo group, in addition to the ring A, has been reduced (Fig. 15.3).

Both 20α- and 20β-cortolones have been recognized in urine (111, 222, 223) and there is some evidence that they occur as sulphates (8). They may be separated by paper chromatography in the benzene–formamide system, the R_F value of the β form being slightly greater than that for the α. The cortols are more polar in this system and are therefore nearer the origin; they may be recognized by their glycerol side chain (223) and by periodate oxidation to 17-oxosteroids.

The 20β-hydroxy compound derived from cortisol, 11β,17α,20β,21-tetrahydroxypregn-4-en-3-one, was the major compound isolated from a group of five steroids more polar than cortisol in the urine of hypertensive dogs (16).

Corticosterone is also excreted as a tetrahydroderivative. In the benzene–formamide or petroleum ether–benzene–methanol–water (30:70:50:50 by vol.) systems it may be separated from other metabolites including the 3β-allo derivative (3β,11β,21-trihydroxy-5α-pregnane-20-one).

The 21-sulphate conjugates of both corticosterone and tetrahydrocorticosterone have been detected in urine (200) and both 3α,5β and 3β,5α derivatives of the tetrahydro compound have been isolated from experiments with slices of rat liver (198).

(b) THE MINERALOCORTICOSTEROIDS

Deoxycorticosterone was known to influence electrolyte balance in mammals long before the discovery of the most active naturally occurring steroid in this group, aldosterone. The effects are generally believed to be by the action on the cationic transport processes in the membranes of the renal tubules. The action is not confined to the kidney, however, and effects have been noted in *in vitro* systems with yeasts (61). Deoxycorticosterone inhibits the excretion of sodium ions from a sodium yeast suspended in a medium containing potassium ions. Conway interprets this effect in terms of a 'redox pump'.

Deoxycorticosterone also effects the growth of the mould *Neurospora crassa* (161). Potassium or rubidium is required for growth and deoxycorticosterone inhibits the uptake of both. This is an extremely sensitive reaction, concentrations as low as 10^{-5}M being employed. Closely related steroids such as corticosterone or 17-hydroxydeoxycorticosterone have no effect.

Traces of deoxycorticosterone may be recognized in adrenal extracts and in *in vitro* perfusion experiments, but the amount secreted is so small that it is doubtful if it exerts a significant metabolic effect. It is more likely that it occurs as an intermediate in the biosynthesis of other corticosteroids.

The release of aldosterone from the adrenal cortex, unlike that of the other major corticosteroids, is not completely controlled by corticotrophin (e.g. 20); moreover, aldosterone does not markedly influence the release of corticotrophin by the pituitary. Two other substances have been suggested as stimulators of aldosterone; these are glomerulotrophin which has been isolated from the region of the pineal gland (21, 85, 86), and angiotensin (158).

A fair amount of information is available about the angiotensins which are among the most potent hypertensive compounds known. They arise from a constituent of the plasma, angiotensinogen. Renin, a proteolytic enzyme present in the kidney, cleaves a leucyl-leucyl bond in angiotensinogen to liberate angiotensin I, a decapeptide:

Asp-Arg-Val-Tyr-Ile-His-Pro-Phe-His-Leu

This peptide is inactive *in vitro* but is transformed *in vivo* by a 'converting enzyme', a peptidase, to the active angiotensin II which is an octapeptide:

Asp-Arg-Val-Tyr-Ile-His-Pro-Phe

Synthesis of this compound and of several analogues has been reported (219, 240). It seems that the secondary structure of angiotensin II is necessary for activity (218, 292, 293). This is destroyed by treatment with urea (194). Angiotensin has been labelled with tritium and ^{131}I, but some chemical alteration in the molecule results as judged by the changes in chromatographic mobilities (10).

The first synthesis of aldosterone was described in 1957 (237) and among the later methods are the 17-stage synthesis from 3β-acetoxy-11-oxo-5α-conessine (147) and the total synthesis described by Johnson *et al.* (139).

Labelled preparations of aldosterone are conveniently obtained by biosynthetic methods from labelled progesterone. Thus [7-^{3}H] and [16-^{3}H]aldosterone have been prepared by the incubation of the corresponding progesterone derivatives with capsule strippings of bovine adrenal glands. This tissue contains mainly *zona glomerulosa* and produces much more aldosterone per gramme of tissue than does whole adrenal tissue (7, 91).

In vitro experiments have shown that [4-^{14}C]aldosterone is converted by human liver slices to tetrahydroaldosterone glucosiduronate (234) and other products. The principal metabolites in urine include a 3-oxo conjugate, the tetrahydro derivative (271) excreted as the glucosiduronate and an 11,18,20-cyclic diacetal (146) and 3β- and 5α-compounds (145) which are observed after the administration of large quantities of aldosterone. The 3-oxo conjugate is acid labile, and yields aldosterone but is not readily hydrolysed by β-glucuronidase although there is evidence that it is a glucosiduronate (274). This could be accounted for by its position at $C_{(3)}$ or by some features of its linkage, e.g. it may be of the α configuration.

Methods for the estimation of aldosterone in urine involve continuous extraction in chloroform or methylene dichloride at pH 1 for the major fraction, followed by treatment with β-glucuronidase. The extracts may then be purified by the usual methods of chromatography. On paper in the chloroform-formamide system, aldosterone runs close to cortisone and in the Bush B5 system it runs midway between cortisol and cortisone. These two systems together give a useful purification of the aldosterone, which may then be modified by treatment with acetic anhydride to give the diacetate. After further chromatography the soda fluorescence may be used directly on the paper as in the method of Ayres *et al.* (6). This reaction is sensitive down to about 0·05 μg; the more lengthy method of elution and measurement of fluorescence in potassium t-butoxide is even more sensitive (255).

However, the method of choice is probably the double-isotope derivative method of Kliman and Peterson (151) in which tritium-labelled acetic anhydride is used for the preparation of the derivative and ^{14}C-labelled aldosterone diacetate is added as internal standard. This method will routinely determine 0·01 μg of aldosterone.

The same labelled derivatives are employed for the estimation of aldosterone in plasma (294). After extensive purification by paper chromatography the diacetate is oxidized by $KClO_4$ and the resulting $^{14}CO_2$ and ^3H_2O are separated and measured as ^{14}C and ^3H after reduction in the presence of Zn.

18-HYDROXYSTEROIDS

18-hydroxysteroids are intermediates in the biosynthesis of aldosterone (188, 270). 18-hydroxydeoxycorticosterone and 18-hydroxycorticosterone have been isolated after incubating cholesterol, pregnenolone or progesterone with rat adrenal tissue (19, 203, 205). There are reports also of the occurrence of these steroids in the adrenals of rats and other animals (171, 215, 282).

They may be purified in the Bush system of paper chromatography, or on

Celite partition columns (202, 205). 18-hydroxydeoxycorticosterone, how-ever, appears to be somewhat unstable, and decomposition has been noted on re-chromatography. Oxidation with chromic acid or lead tetra-acetate leads to the production of 18,20 lactones (196). An 18,20 lactone isolated from pig adrenals is probably formed from the 18-hydroxycorticosterone originally present (188).

An interesting property of 18-hydroxydeoxycorticosterone is that it reacts with the Porter-Silber phenylhydrazine reagent although it is not a 17-hydroxysteroid (18, 202, 204). 18-hydroxycorticosterone, however, does not react.

PREGNANETRIOL

This steroid is found in high concentration in the urine of patients with congenital adrenal hyperplasia. The disease arises from an inability to syn-thesize certain enzymes and is inherited as an autosomal recessive. In the commonest form there is a partial or complete lack of the enzyme catalysing steroid hydroxylation at $C_{(21)}$ (Fig. 15.10) so that 17-hydroxyprogesterone is

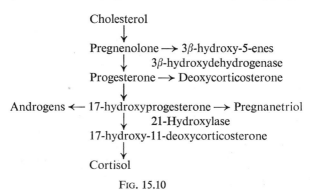

FIG. 15.10

not converted to cortisol. Corticotrophin secretion from the pituitary there-fore increases, and this leads to excessive production of 17α-hydroxy pro-gesterone and thus of androgens and pregnanetriol in the urine. In other forms of the disease, a defect of 11β-hydroxylation leads to excessive produc-tion of deoxycorticosterone and 17α-hydroxy-deoxycorticosterone. These are sodium-retaining steroids and cause hypertension; tetrahydro-11-deoxy-corticosterone appears in the urine. Lastly a deficiency of 3β-hydroxysteroid dehydrogenase gives rise to an excess of 3β-hydroxy-Δ^5-steroids in the urine (24).

Pregnanetriol was originally detected in urine by Marrian (48) and several methods for its estimation have been described (25, 65, 192). It is excreted as a glucosiduronate, so that the β-glucuronidase method of hydrolysis is usually employed, either directly in the urine or on an extract of the conjugated steroid as in the method of Stern (257). It is then easily separated from the less polar steroids by chromatography on alumina, and determined spectrophotometrically by reaction with concentrated H_2SO_4. The yellow chromogen absorbs maximally at 435 mμ.

Purification of urinary extracts is also possible on glass fibre paper (256). The solvent mixture, cyclohexane–acetone (100:12 v/v), is suitable with paper impregnated with potassium silicate.

Pregnanetriol is a 17-oxogenic steroid and gives aetiocholanolone on oxidation with sodium bismuthate. A simple method for its estimation by means of this reaction has been described by Morris (182) and developed by Hill (128) for clinical use. The 17-oxosteroids initially present in the urine are reduced by sodium borohydride, and after oxidation with sodium bismuthate the aetiocholanolone produced from pregnanetriol is separated from the 11-oxygenated-17-oxosteroids which arise from cortisol metabolites by chromatography on silica gel. They are measured by the Zimmermann reaction, their ratio giving a useful clinical index. This ratio

$$\frac{\text{aetiocholanolone}}{\text{11-oxygenated-17-oxosteroids}}$$

is high in the adreno-genital syndrome and low normally. It is not subject to diurnal variation so may be measured on isolated samples of urine.

Edwards *et al.* (82) have described a modified procedure in which periodate oxidation and paper chromatography are employed.

Pregnanetriol arises from the ovary as well as the adrenal cortex and a cyclical fluctuation has been noted during the menstrual cycle (96, 210). Its production is increased by stimulation with gonadotrophins (34, 50).

Pregnanetriolone is also found in the urine of patients with congenital adrenal hyperplasia. Moreover, in such conditions as Cushing's syndrome, the Stein-Leventhal syndrome (244) and pseudohermaphroditism (109), it has been found in association with other hydroxylated compounds including 5β-pregnane-3α,11β,17α,20α-tetrol. It is excreted as the glucosiduronate and is best extracted by chloroform after enzymic hydrolysis. Zaffaroni-type chromatograms have been used for purification, and it may be detected by its fluorescence in H_3PO_4. It may be determined fluorimetrically (299), or as an acetaldehydogenic steroid (64).

Neither cortisol nor cortisone is converted biosynthetically to this steroid (106, 110) and its most probable precursor is deoxycorticosterone or 21-deoxycortisol (136).

Elevated quantities of another steroid, pregn-5-ene-3β,17α,20α-triol, occur in the urine of patients with the specific deficiency of 3β-hydroxysteroid dehydrogenase, with adrenocortical tumours and in some patients with the Stein-Leventhal syndrome. This steroid appears as the 3-sulphate and may be extracted in solvents after hydrolysis at 100° and neutral pH. Extracts are purified by gradient elution chromatography on alumina with mixtures of benzene and ethanol (258). The steroid gives a transient yellow colour with a mixture of sulphuric acid and 90 per cent v/v ethanol (77·5:22·5 v/v) which turns a pink-purple colour with absorption maximum at 525 mμ. The 20β isomer also gives this reaction but other 3β-hydroxy-Δ^5-steroids do not.

6β-HYDROXYCORTISOL

The *in vivo* 6β-hydroxylation of steroids was indicated by the reports of the isolation of 6β-hydroxypregnanediols in urine by Lieberman *et al.* (163). There followed reports of 6-hydroxylase systems in several tissues including hog adrenals (119), corpora lutea of bovine ovaries (120), rat liver (5), human placentae (14, 118) and neoplastic tissue (79). 6β-hydroxycortisol itself was then isolated from human urine (35) and from guinea-pig urine (36) and 6β-hydroxycortisone was isolated from the urine of a patient with Cushing's syndrome (197).

A review of much of the early work on 6-hydroxylated steroids has appeared (80). Since the excretion of 6β-hydroxycortisol is increased by administration of corticotrophin, it would seem that the origin of this steroid is the adrenal. It also increases in the last trimester of pregnancy (98) but this does not appear to be related to any general rise in total 17-hydroxysteroids. It is probable that there is an increased conversion from endogenous cortisol rather than an increased endogenous production. It may also be related to the fact that 6-hydroxylation is known to be increased by oestrogens (144).

Ulstrom *et al.* (272) found that 6-hydroxylation was an important pathway for the metabolism of cortisol in the newborn, and it may be that this observation provides further evidence of the effect of the high levels of maternal oestrogens circulating. 6β-hydroxycortisol is much more polar than cortisol, and presumably, in the metabolic disposal of cortisol, conversion by 6-hydroxylation is an alternative to ring A reduction and conjugation to glucuronic acid.

Work with labelled steroids has shown that [4-^{14}C]cortisol is converted *in vivo* by human cirrhotic liver to [4-^{14}C]6β-hydroxycortisol (60) and *in vitro* by liver, adrenal, kidney, placenta and skeletal muscle (165). In the *in vitro* experiments the liver was by far the most efficient tissue. Evidence is collecting that the measurement of 6β-hydroxycortisol in urine may give an even better indication of the level of free cortisol circulating in the body than the measurement of the urinary excretion of cortisol itself (87, 268).

Extraction and purification

Since it is so soluble in water, 6β-hydroxycortisol is extracted from urine with difficulty. Solvents such as ethyl acetate, or ethyl acetate mixed with chloroform are the most efficient, especially when used with the addition of salt to the urine (99). No hydrolysis appears to be necessary although Touchstone and Blakemore (268) preferred to use β-glucuronidase.

After the extract has been washed with dilute alkali and water, the 6β-hydroxycortisol may be separated from less polar steroids in the propylene glycol or aqueous methanol systems of paper chromatography. The systems ethyl acetate–chloroform–methanol–water (25:75:50:50 by vol.) and benzene –t-butanol–water (70:43:86 by vol.) separate the 6α-hydroxy isomer from 6β-hydroxycortisol. It is seen in Table 15.2 that the R_F values of the isomers are reversed in the two systems (99). The diacetates tend to separate less

TABLE 15.2

R_F values of 6-hydroxylated steroids compared with tetrahydrocorticosteroids in system A: ethyl acetate–chloroform–methanol–water (25 : 75 : 50 : 50 by vol) and system B: benzene–t-butanol–water (70 : 43 : 86 by vol). [From Reference 99]

	A	B
6α-hydroxycortisol	0·39	0·53
6β-hydroxycortisol	0·43	0·49
6β-hydroxycortisone	0·69	0·75
Tetrahydrocortisol	0·83	0·82
Tetrahydrocortisone	0·88	0·85

easily chromatographically, but the 17-oxosteroids produced by oxidation with bismuthate are easily separated in the Bush B5 system. Frantz et al. (99) have produced some evidence for the occurrence of the 6α isomer in urine.

Properties

6β-hydroxycortisol gives many of the reactions of cortisol. It reacts with the blue tetrazolium and the Porter-Silber reagents and gives maximum absorption in ethanol at 240 mμ. It may be detected on paper chromatograms by the soda fluorescence reaction.

It gives a transient red colour with H_2SO_4 and fluoresces (460–510 mμ). Oxidation with sodium bismuthate gives a 17-oxosteroid and with chromic acid both the 6α and 6β isomers give a 6,17-dioxosteroid.

Treatment with acetic anhydride in pyridine gives the acetate which may be crystallized as colourless needles, m.p. 119–123° (60), from ethyl acetate or 95 per cent ethanol. The H_2SO_4 chromogen gives peaks at 238, 280, 340, 390 and 475 mμ.

OTHER 6-HYDROXYLATED STEROIDS

Many other 6-hydroxylated compounds have been prepared by microbiological methods (105). Derivatives of 17-hydroxydeoxycorticosterone, 17α-

hydroxyprogesterone and deoxycorticosterone have been obtained by using the organism, *Rhizopus arrhigus*.

It has been calculated that up to 10 per cent of administered progesterone is excreted as 6-oxygenated metabolites (97). Progesterone incubated with human placental tissue yields 6-hydroxy- and 6-oxo-progesterone; three isomeric 3,6-diols of the 5α- and 5β-pregnane series have been isolated from pregnancy urine (152). 5α-pregnane-3α,6α,20α-triol has been isolated from the urine of rabbits injected with progesterone (152).

Synthetic steroids with corticosteroid activity

Because of the great clinical value of cortisone there has been a continued search for new and better analogues. Interest in synthetics has been stimulated by the fact that the dose levels of cortisone necessary to suppress the symptoms of rheumatoid arthritis may give rise to objectionable side effects. These include excessive retention of sodium, negative nitrogen balance, osteoporosis and mooning of the face as in Cushing's syndrome.

Nearly every position in the molecule has been modified in the course of this work. The main modifications have been the substitution of halogen, hydroxy or alkyl groups for H, and the introduction of double bonds. In order to control this work it has been necessary to develop assay procedures, usually using rodents, to give information about the activities of the new compounds. Unfortunately such information often gives only a crude estimate of their potencies in man. The assays giving the most reliable information have been those depending on the deposition of liver glycogen in the rat (193) or mouse (278), the effect on thymus involution (112) and the anti-inflammatory activity in the rat (248). Even so they compare unfavourably with the results obtained from human clinical assays in which the eosinopenic and hypoglycaemic potencies are measured (286). In a study of 31 synthetic steroids the clinical assays showed excellent agreement with the anti-rheumatic activity in man in contrast to the bioassays which contained several anomalous results (217).

MODIFICATIONS OF THE STRUCTURE AND ACTIVITY OF CORTICOSTEROIDS

A summary of some of the main modifications and the effects on activity are presented in Table 15.3.

Fluorination in the 9α position of cortisol enhances the gluco- and particularly the mineralo-corticosteroid activities. The other halogens generally have less effect on activity with the exception of the chloro compounds of cortisol and cortisone which are more active in sodium retention than the corresponding fluoro compounds.

Dehydrogenation to give a Δ^1 compound increases the gluco- but not the

TABLE 15.3

Modifications to corticosteroids and the subsequent effects on biological activity (+increase, − decrease)

Modification	Mineralocorticoid activity	Glucocorticoid activity
9α-F	+++	++
1-ene	−	++
1-ene + 9α-F	+	+++
2α-CH$_3$	+	+
2α-CH$_3$ + 9α-F	++	+
6α-CH$_3$	−	+
16α-OH	− −	+
16α-CH$_3$	− −	+++

mineralo-corticosteroid activity. Dehydrogenation of the 9α-fluoro compounds increases both types of activity, but chiefly the glucocorticosteroid activity.

2α-methylation increases the glycogenic activity in the rat but the most striking change is in mineral metabolism. When this group is introduced into 9α-fluorocortisol, the resulting steroid is three times as active as aldosterone.

The 6α-methyl compounds are useful in that they show enhanced glycogenic activity with no increase in mineral activity. Thus there is a striking change in mineralocorticosteroid activity in shifting the methyl group from 2α to 6α. The change is even greater in the 16α-hydroxy and 16α-methyl compounds where the mineral activity is even lower than in the 6α-methyl steroids, and the glycogenic activity is very much higher, e.g. in 9α-fluoro-16α-methyl-prednisolone.

The effects of some modifications in structure on the anti-rheumatic activities in man are indicated in Table 15.4 (23, 122, 217).

Methods of synthesis

9α-*halogenated steroids.* Certain micro-organisms (e.g. *Rhizopus nigricans* and *Aspergillus nidulans*) may be used to introduce an 11α-hydroxyl group in corticosteroids unsubstituted in ring c (104, 208) and so give rise to 11α inactive derivatives of cortisone (II, Fig. 15.11). After protection of the 21-group by acetylation the 11α-tosylate (III) is prepared and on heating with sodium acetate in acetic acid gives the 9(11)-dehydro derivative (IV). Reaction with N-bromoacetamide and perchloric acid gives a 9α-bromo compound (V) which is converted to the 9β,11β-epoxide (VI) by means of potassium acetate in alcohol and then to the halogen compound (VII) by the appropriate halogen acid (103, 130). In place of halogen the groups —OH,

TABLE 15.4

The effect of certain modifications to corticosteroids on their anti-rheumatic activity in man

Steroid	Modification	Relative anti-rheumatic activity in man
Corticosterone	natural	<0·1
Cortisol	natural	1
Prednisone	1-ene	4
Prednisolone	1-ene	4
9α-fluorocortisol acetate	9α-F	10
9α-fluoro prednisolone	9α-F + 1-ene	15–17
6α-methyl prednisolone	6α-CH$_3$	3–5
9α-fluoro-16α-hydroxy prednisolone	9α-F + 1-ene + 16α-OH	3–5
9α-fluoro-16α-methyl prednisolone	9α-F + 1-ene + 16α-CH$_3$	29

—OCH$_3$ or —OC$_2$H$_5$ etc. may be introduced by treatment with water or the requisite alcohol in the presence of perchloric acid. The 9α-fluoro derivative of cortisol was one of the first synthetic steroids shown to be effective in the treatment of rheumatoid arthritis. As seen in Table 15.4, it is active in much lower doses than the natural hormone.

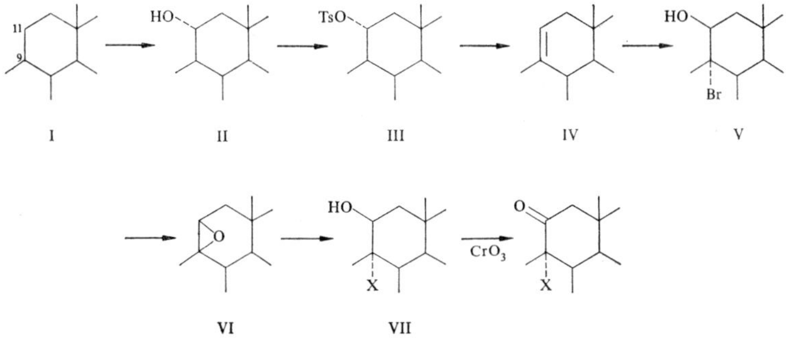

X = F, Cl, Br or I

FIG. 15.11

1-dehydrosteroids. Microbiological methods are again useful in the preparation of Δ^1-steroids. An extensive list of these is given in the review by Fried and Borman (101). *Corynebacterium simplex, Didymella lycopersici* and *Bacillus sphaericus* have each been applied to a wide range of corticosteroids.

There are several chemical methods available. Thus 2,4-dibromides of 5α- and 5β-dihydrocortisone may be dehydrobrominated by refluxing with collidine to the Δ¹ structure (127); the 11α-hydroxy derivative of progesterone obtained by a microbiological method is converted by several steps through a dienolate (Fig. 15.12, I), a bromo-compound (II), and by subsequent dehydrohalogenation with collidine to the Δ¹ structure (133); or

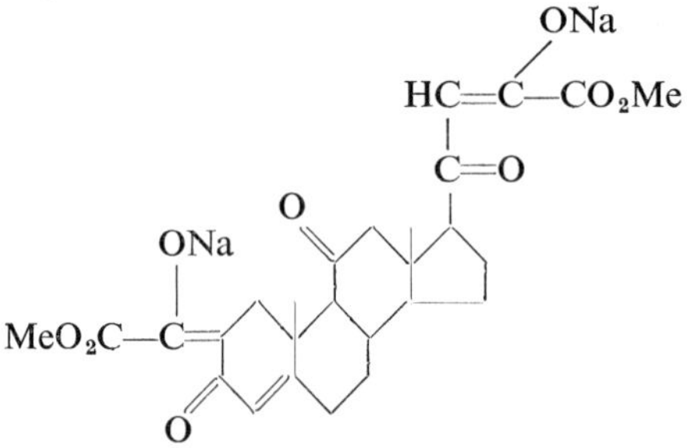

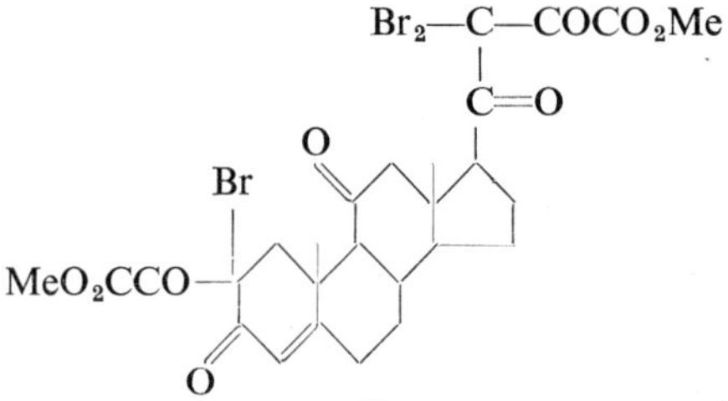

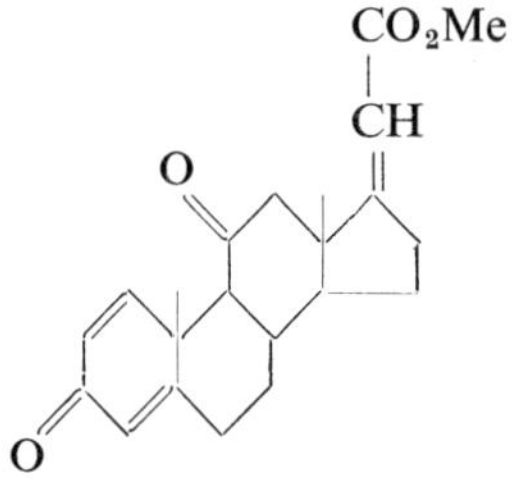

FIG. 15.12

again good yields of these compounds are obtained by dehydrogenation with SeO_2 (176).

The effectiveness of prednisone and prednisolone in the treatment of rheumatoid arthritis was first reported by Bunim et al. (33) and by Herzog et al. (126). They are most useful in that they are four to five times as active as cortisone and cortisol, and at the doses required do not cause retention of sodium or water.

The Δ^1-dihydro derivatives of 9α-halogenated steroids are also of great clinical value. They may be obtained microbiologically with *Corynebacterium simplex* in good yield (101) or chemically by such methods as those of Hirschmann *et al.* (129) or Fried *et al.* (102).

ALKYLATED STEROIDS *2α-methyl* derivatives of cortisol are synthesized from 11-oxoprogesterone with the intermediate formation of a 2-enolate (Fig. 15.12, I). Treatment with methyl iodide in acetone in the presence of potassium carbonate gives the 2α-methyl compound (132).

The 2α-methyl steroids are noted for their powerful salt-retaining properties; they also appear to be metabolized rather differently from the natural steroids and remain in the circulation longer.

6α-methyl steroids with greatly reduced salt-retaining activity may be obtained microbiologically, e.g. with *Septomixa affinis* (254). For chemical synthesis 11α-hydroxyprogesterone is converted into the 3,20-bisethylene-ketal-11-acetate and then epoxidized with perchloric acid to a mixture of 5α-,6α- and 5β,6β-epoxides. The α-epoxide is opened with CH_3MgBr to give the 6β-methyl-5α-ol structure. The 6β isomer is readily isomerized by base to the more stable α isomer (131, 253, 254).

The important *16α-methyl compounds* may be obtained from Δ^{16}-20-oxo-steroids by reaction with bromoform and t-butoxide and subsequent hydrogenation of the 16α-tribromo-methyl-20-oxosteroid (142). In another method a 16α,17α-epoxy-16β-methyl-20-oxo compound (Fig. 15.13, I) is treated with HBr to give a 16-methylene-17α-hydroxy-20-one (Fig. 15.13, II). Hydrogenation with Pd gives a mixture of 16α- and 16β-methyl isomers (Fig. 15.13, III) with the former predominating (148, 265).

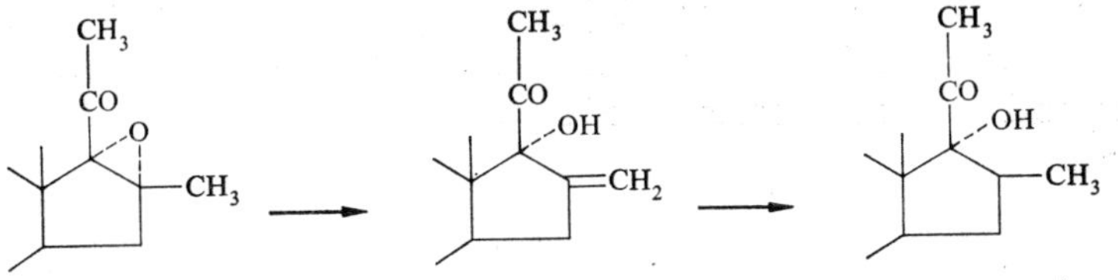

FIG. 15.13

The clinical effects of these highly active compounds were originally reported in 1958 (22) and numerous studies on the uses of these compounds have been made ever since.

16α-hydroxylated steroids are conveniently prepared by microbiological methods, from progesterone by using an *actinomycete* culture (201), or from deoxycorticosterone with *Streptomyces roseochromogenus* (105).

In the synthesis of the important compound 9α-fluoro-16α-hydroxypredni-solone (triamcinolone) the micro-organisms *Corynebacterium simplex* or

AA

Mycobacterium rhodochrons have been used to convert 16α-hydroxy-9α-fluoro-cortisol to the required compound (266).

Several other types of steroid have been synthesized including 4,6 or 21-halogenated, and 19-nor compounds. The methods used have been reviewed by Fried (101).

Methods of separation of synthetic corticosteroids

Much useful information on the urinary metabolites of some of the synthetic corticosteroids, and of paper chromatographic methods for separating them has appeared in a paper by Bush and Mahesh (45). The fluorinated steroids are metabolized in much the same way as the natural steroids as far as reduction of ring A, and reduction of the side-chain are concerned. However, 11-oxo compounds seem to be absent from the urine, and this seems to hold for the metabolism of the Δ^1-derivatives as well.

In the aqueous methanol systems, prednisolone runs with allotetrahydrocortisol and is only separated by inconveniently long runs. After acetylation, however, the monoacetate of prednisone is completely separated from the diacetates of allotetrahydrocortisol and related steroids in the Bush B5 system. Alternatively the 3:17-dioxosteroid obtained by oxidation with bismuthate is more easily separated from the oxosteroids derived from cortisol metabolites than the original steroids.

The metabolites of 9α-fluorocortisol are also difficult to separate from the metabolites of cortisol. The problem may be solved in the same way, by careful chromatography after acetylation (4, p. 345).

Methods are also described for the separation of synthetic corticosteroids by thin layer chromatography (236) and by gas-liquid chromatography (9). In the latter method the steroids are oxidized with bismuthate to give the corresponding 17-oxosteroids. Good separations are then obtained on NPGA columns.

Non-steroidal compounds which affect adrenocortical secretions

A number of compounds related to Amphenone B, 3,3-bis-(*p*-amino-phenyl)-2-butanone (Fig. 15.14), have been shown to affect the secretion rate of corticosteroids by the adrenal cortex. Amphenone B itself seems to cause a generalized inhibition of steroid production by interfering with a number of different enzymes (138, 224). It is one of a number of substituted deoxy-benzoins synthesized by Allen and Corwen (3). A more specific action is exhibited by 2-methyl-1,2-bis(3-pyridyl)-1-propanone (SU-4885, Metapyrone etc., 56) which inhibits 11β-hydroxylase and therefore the synthesis of cortisol. The compensatory increase in release of corticotrophin gives rise to increased production of 11-deoxycortisol by the adrenal.

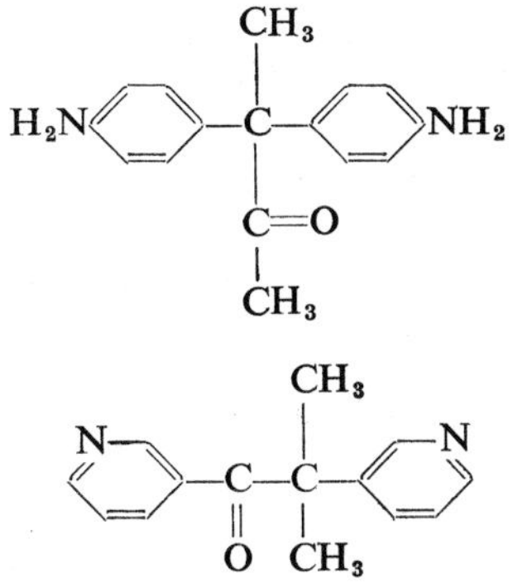

Amphenone

Metapyrone

Fig. 15.14

The compound is therefore useful in investigations of pituitary function (162). The increase in endogenous corticotrophin which occurs after administration of the compound may be observed by measuring the changes in secretion of 11-deoxycortisol. Urinary metabolites of this steroid may be selectively extracted from urine in CCl_4 (123) although it has been reported that recoveries are only of the order of 30 per cent by results based on the use of a tritium-labelled internal standard (141).

Alternatively the 11-deoxycorticosteroids may be separated from the 11-oxycorticosteroids by chromatography on silica gel of the 17-oxosteroids produced on oxidation with bismuthate (49).

Of the many other compounds affecting the secretion of corticosteroids, special mention may be made of Triporanol, 1-(4-diethylaminoethoxyphenyl)-1-(p-tolyl)-2-(p-chlorophenyl)-ethanol which inhibits the biosynthesis of cholesterol (195). It has been shown to decrease the excretion of corticosteroids, probably by modifying the extra-adrenal metabolism of cortisol. Compounds inhibiting 17α-hydroxylation have also been reported (57). The tetralone, SU-9055—3-(1,2,3,4,-tetrahydro-1-oxo-2-naphthyl)-pyridine,

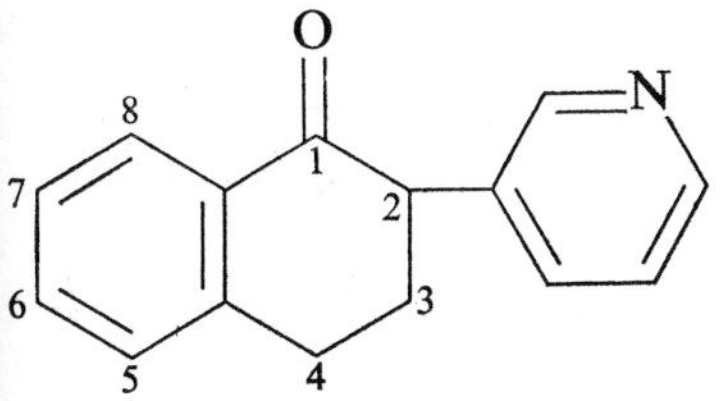

SU - 9055 and
analogues (6, 7, 8, Cl:
6, OCH_3 etc.)

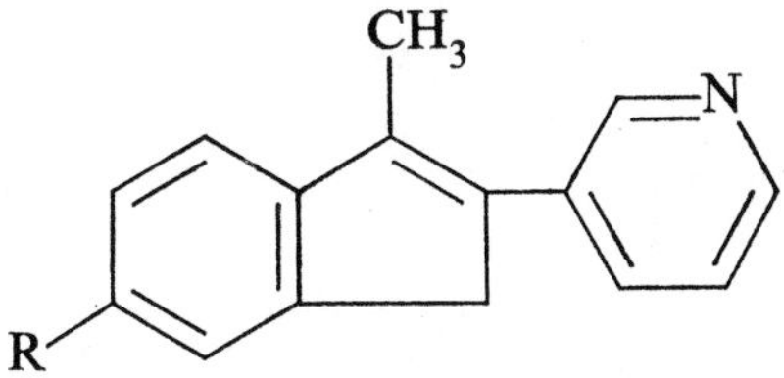

SU - 8000
(R = Cl) and
analogues (R=H, NO_2, NH_2)

Fig. 15.15

and the indene, SU-8000—3-(6-chloro-3-methyl-2-indenyl)-pyridine (Fig. 15.15) decrease the excretion of cortisol and 11-deoxycortisol and increase deoxycortisone and corticosterone, but lack the 17-hydroxyl group. *In vitro* studies have shown that the production of 17-hydroxycorticosteroids from progesterone is inhibited by these compounds.

The 3-pyridyl residue is common to several of these inhibitors but the activity is not wholly dependent on this structure since modifications in other parts of the molecules alter the type of activity.

REFERENCES

1 ABELSON, D. and BONDY, P. K. *Archs Biochem. Biophys.* **57,** 208 (1955).

2 AGARWAL, K. N. and GARBY, L. *Acta endocr. Copenh.* Suppl. 93, 3 (1964).

3 ALLEN, M. J. and CORWIN, A. H. *J. Amer. chem. Soc.* **72,** 117 (1950).

4 APPLEBY, J. I., GIBSON, G., NORYMBERSKI, J. K. and STUBBS, R. D. *Biochem. J.* **60,** 453 and 460 (1955).

5 AXELROD, L. R. and MILLER, L. L. *Archs. Biochem. Biophys.* **49,** 248 (1954).

6 AYRES, P. J., GARROD, O., SIMPSON, S. A. and TAIT, J. F. *Biochem. J.* **65,** 639 (1957).

7 AYRES, P. J., PEARLMAN, W. H., TAIT, J. F. and TAIT, S. A. *Biochem. J.* **70,** 230 (1958).

8 BAGNALL, A. V., GUPTA, D. and TANNER, J. M. *J. Endocr.* **22,** xxv (1961).

9 BAILEY, E. *J. Endocr.* **28,** 131 (1964).

10 BARBOUR, B. H. and BARTTER, F. C. *J. clin. Endocr.* **23,** 313 (1963).

11 BARKLEY, L. B., FARRAR, M. W., KNOWLES, W. S. and RAFFELSON, M. *J. Amer. chem. Soc.* **76,** 5017 (1954).

12 BARLOW, J. J. and KELLIE, A. E. *Biochem. J.* **71,** 86 (1959).

13 BELING, C. G. *Acta endocr. Copenh.* Suppl. 79 (1963).

14 BERLINER, D. L. and SALHANICK, H. A. *J. clin. Endocr.* **16,** 903 (1956).

15 BERLINER, M. L., BERLINER, D. L. and DOUGHERTY, T. F. *J. clin. Endocr.* **18,** 109 (1958).

16 BESCH, P. K., BROWNELL, K. A., HARTMAN, F. A. and WATSON, D. J. *Acta endocr. Copenh.* **39,** 355 (1963).

17 BIRCH, A. J. *Rep. Prog. Chem.* **48,** 184 (1951).

18 BIRMINGHAM, M. K. *Nature, Lond.* **184,** BA 67 (1959).

19 BIRMINGHAM, M. K. and KURLENTS, E. *Can. J. Biochem. Physiol.* **37,** 510 (1959).

20 BLAIR-WEST, J. R., COGHLAN, J. P., DENTON, D. A., GODING, J. R., WINTOUR, M. and WRIGHT, R. D. *Endocrinology* **77,** 501 (1965).

21 BLAIR-WEST, J. R., COGHLAN, J. P., DENTON, D. A., GODING, J. R., WINTOUR, M. and WRIGHT, R. D. *Recent Prog. Horm. Res.* **19,** 311 (1963).

22 BOLAND, E. W. *Calif. Med.* **88,** 417 (1958).

23 BOLAND, E. W. and LIDDLE, G. W. *Ann. rheum. Dis.* **16,** 297 (1959).

24 BONGIOVANNI, A. M. *J. clin. Invest.* **41,** 2086 (1962).

25 BONGIOVANNI, A. M. and CLAYTON, G. W. *Johns Hopk. Hosp. Bull.* **94,** 180 (1954).

26 BORRELL, S. *Biochem. J.* **70,** 727 (1958).

27 BORTH, R. *Acta endocr. Copenh.* **22,** 125 (1956).

28 BOULOUARD, R. and FONTAINE, Y.-A. *C.R. Acad. Sci. Paris* **257,** 1379 (1963).

29 BRAUNSBERG, H. and JAMES, V. H. T. *J. clin. Endocr.* **21,** 1146 (1961).

30 BRAUNSBERG, H. and JAMES, V. H. T. *J. Endocr.* **25,** 309 (1962).

31 BROOKS, C. J. W. *Biochem. J.* **92,** 8P (1964).

32 BROOKS, S. G., EVANS, R. M., GREEN, G. F. H., HUNT, J. S., LONG, A. G., MOONEY, B. and WYMAN, L. J. *J. chem. Soc.* 4614 (1958).

33 BUNIM, J. J., PECHET, M. M. and BOLLET, A. J. *J. Amer. med. Ass.* **157,** 311 (1955).

34 BURGER, H. G. and SOMMERVILLE, I. F. *Acta endocr. Copenh.* **43,** 95 (1963).

35 BURSTEIN, S., DORFMAN, R. I. and NADEL, E. M. *Archs. Biochem. Biophys.* **53,** 307 (1954).

36 BURSTEIN, S. and KIMBALL, H. L. *Analyt. Biochem.* **4,** 132 (1962).

37 BURTON, R. B., ZAFFARONI, A. and KEUTMANN, E. H. *J. biol. Chem.* **188,** 763 (1951).

38 BUSH, I. E. *Biochem. J.* **50,** 370 (1952).

39 BUSH, I. E. *Experientia* **12,** 325 (1956).

40 BUSH, I. E. *Biochem. J.* **67,** 23P (1957).

41 BUSH, I. E. In *The Chromatography of Steroids,* Pergamon Press, Oxford (1961).

42 BUSH, I. E. and GALE, M. *Biochem. J.* **67,** 29P (1957).

43 BUSH, I. E. and MAHESH, V. B. *Biochem. J.* **69,** 21P (1958).

44 BUSH, I. E. and MAHESH, V. B. *Biochem. J.* **71,** 705 (1959).

45 BUSH, I. E. and MAHESH, V. B. *Biochem. J.* **71,** 718 (1959).

46 BUSH, I. E. and SANDBERG, A. A. *J. biol. Chem.* **205,** 783 (1953).

47 BUSH, I. E. and WILLOUGHBY, M. *Biochem. J.* **67,** 689 (1957).

48 BUTLER, G. C. and MARRIAN, G. F. *J. biol. Chem.* **119,** 565 (1937).

49 BUTT, W. R., CROOKE, A. C., HILL, E. E. and MORRIS, R. *J. Endocr.* **20,** xvi (1960).

50 BUTT, W. R., CROOKE, A. C. and PALMER, R. Unpublished.

51 CARDWELL, H. M. E., CORNFORTH, J. W., DUFF, S. R., HOLTERMANN, H. and ROBINSON, R. *J. chem. Soc.* 361 (1953).

52 CASPI, E., DORFMAN, R. I., KHAN, B. T., ROSENFELD, G. and SCHMID, W. *J. biol. Chem.* **237,** 2085 (1962).

53 CASPI, E. and HECHTER, O. *Archs. Biochem. Biophys.* **53,** 478 (1954).

54 CASPI, E., LEVY, H. and HECHTER, O. *Archs. Biochem. Biophys.* **45,** 169 (1953).

55 CHANCE, B., SCHOENER, B. and FERGUSON, J. J. *Nature, Lond.* **195,** 776 (1962).

56 CHART, J. J., SHEPPARD, H., ALLEN, M. J., BENCZE, W. L. and GAUNT, R. *Experientia* **14,** 151 (1958).

57 CHART, J. J., SHEPPARD, H., MOWLES, T. and HOWIE, N. *Endocrinology* **71,** 479 (1962).

58 CHEN, C., WHEELER, J. and TEWELL, H. *J. Lab. clin. Med.* **42,** 749 (1953).

59 CHEN, P. S., MILLS, I. H. and BARTTER, F. C. *J. Endocr.* **23,** 129 (1961).

60 COHN, G. L., UPTON, V. and BONDY, P. K. *J. clin. Endocr.* **21,** 1328 (1961).

61 CONWAY, E. J. and HINGERTY, D. *Biochem. J.* **55,** 455 (1953).

62 CORNFORTH, J. W. *Rep. Prog. Chem.* **49,** 190 (1952).

63 COX, R. I. *Biochem. J.* **52,** 339 (1952).

64 COX, R. I. *J. biol. Chem.* **234,** 1693 (1959).

65 COX, R. I. *Acta endocr. Copenh.* **33,** 477 (1960).

66 DALY, J. R. and SPENCER-PEET, J. *J. Endocr.* **30,** 255 (1964).

67 DAUGHADAY, W. H. *J. clin. Invest.* **37,** 511 and 519 (1958).

68 DAUGHADAY, W. H., ADLER, R. E., MARIZ, I. K. and RAMINSKI, D. C. *J. clin. Endocr.* **22,** 704 (1962).

69 DAUGHADAY, W. H., HOLLOSZY, J. and MARIZ, I. K. *J. clin. Endocr.* **21,** 53 (1961).

70 DAVIDSON, E. T., DE VENUTO, F. and WESTPHAL, U. *Endocrinology* **71,** 893 (1962).

71 DE MOOR, P., DECKX, R. and STEENO, O. *J. Endocr.* **27,** 355 (1963).

72 DE MOOR, P., HEIRWEGH, K., HEREMANS, S. F. and DECLERCK-RASKIN, M. *J. clin. Invest.* **41,** 816 (1962).

73 DE MOOR, P., OSINKI, P., DECKX, R. and STEENO, O. *Clin. Chim. Acta* **7,** 475 (1962).

74 DE MOOR, P. and STEENO, O. *J. Endocr.* **26,** 301 (1963).

75 DE MOOR, P. and STEENO, O. *J. Endocr.* **28,** 59 (1963).

76 DE MOOR, P., STEENO, O. and DECKX, R. *Acta endocr. Copenh.* **44,** 107 (1963).

77 DE MOOR, P., STEENO, O., RASKIN, M. and HENDRIKX, A. *Acta endocr. Copenh.* **33,** 297 (1960).

78 DOE, R. P., ZINNEMAN, H. H., FLINK, E. B. and ULSTROM, R. A. *J. clin. Endocr.* **20,** 1484 (1960).

79 DOMINGUEZ, O. V. *J. clin. Endocr.* **21,** 663 (1961).

80 DORFMAN, R. I. *A. Rev. Biochem.* **26,** 523 (1957).

81 EDWARDS, R. W. H., KELLIE, A. E. and WADE, A. P. *Mem. Soc. Endocr.* **2,** 53 (1953).

82 EDWARDS, R. W. H., MAKIN, H. L. J. and BARRATT, T. M. *J. Endocr.* **30,** 181 (1964).

83 ESPINER, E. A. *J. Endocr.* **33,** 233 (1965).

84 EXLEY, D., INGALL, S. C., NORYMBERSKI, J. K. and WOODS, G. F. *Biochem. J.* **81,** 428 (1961).

85 FARRELL, G. *Recent Prog. Horm. Res.* **15,** 275 (1959).

86 FARRELL, G. and MCISAAC, W. M. *Archs. Biochem. Biophys.* **94,** 543 (1961).

87 FERGUSON, H. C., BARTRAM, A. C. G., FOWLIE, H. C., CATHRO, D. M., BIRCHALL, K. and MITCHELL, F. L. *Acta endocr. Copenh.* **47,** 58 (1964).

88 FEW, J. D. *J. Endocr.* **22,** 31 (1961).

89 FINKELSTEIN, M. In *Methods in Hormone Research* (edited by R. I. Dorfman) Vol. 1, p. 169, Academic Press, New York (1962).

90 FINKELSTEIN, M. and GOLDBERG, S. *J. clin. Endocr.* **17,** 1063 (1957).

91 FLOOD, C., LAYNE, D. S., RAMCHARAN, S., ROSSIPAL, E., TAIT, J. F. and TAIT, S. A. S. *Acta endocr. Copenh.* **36,** 237 (1961).

92 FLORINI, J. R. and BUYSKE, D. A. *J. biol. Chem.* **236,** 247 (1961).

93 FOGGITT, F. and KELLIE, A. E. *Biochem. J.* **91,** 209 (1964).

94 FORTIER, C. *Can. J. Biochem. Physiol.* **37,** 571 (1959).

95 FOTHERBY, K. *Biochem. J.* **69,** 596 (1958).

96 FOTHERBY, K. *J. Endocr.* **25,** 19 (1962).

97 FOTHERBY, K., JAMES, F., KAMYAB, S., KLOPPER, A. and WILSON, G. R. *J. Endocr.* **31,** xxv (1965).

98 FRANTZ, A. G., KATZ, F. H. and JAILER, J. W. *Proc. Soc. exp. Biol. Med.* **105,** 41 (1960).

99 FRANTZ, A. G., KATZ, F. H. and JAILER, J. W. *J. clin. Endocr.* **21,** 1290 (1961).

100 FRIED, J. *Cancer* **10,** 752 (1957).

101 FRIED, J. and BORMAN, A. *Vitams Horm.* **16,** 303 (1958).

102 FRIED, J., FLOREY, K., SABO, E. F., HERZ, J. E., RESTIVO, A. R., BORMAN, A. and SINGER, F. M. *J. Amer. chem. Soc.* **77,** 4181 (1955).

103 FRIED, J. and SABO, E. F. *J. Amer. chem. Soc.* **79,** 1130 (1957).

104 FRIED, J., THOMA, R. W., GERKE, J. R., HERZ, J. E., DONIN, M. N. and PERLMAN, D. *J. Amer. chem. Soc.* **74,** 3962 (1952).

105 FRIED, J., THOMA, R. W., PERLMAN, D., HERZ, J. E. and BORMAN, A. *Recent Prog. Horm. Res.* **11,** 149 (1955).

106 FUKUSHIMA, D. K., BRADLOW, H. L., HELLMAN, L. and GALLAGHER, T. F. *J. clin. Endocr.* **19,** 393 (1959).

107 FUKUSHIMA, D. K., BRADLOW, H. L., HELLMAN, L., ZUMOFF, B. and GALLAGHER, T. F. *J. biol. Chem.* **235,** 2246 (1960).

108 FUKUSHIMA, D. K. and GALLAGHER, T. F. *J. biol. Chem.* **226,** 725 (1957).

109 FUKUSHIMA, D. K. and GALLAGHER, T. F. *J. biol. Chem.* **229,** 85 (1957).

110 FUKUSHIMA, D. K. and GALLAGHER, T. F. *J. clin. Endocr.* **18,** 694 (1958).

111 FUKUSHIMA, D. K., LEEDS, N. S., BRADLOW, H. L., KRITCHEVSKY, T. H., STOKEM, M. B. and GALLAGHER, T. F. *J. biol. Chem.* **212,** 449 (1955).

112 GAUNT, R., LEATHEM, J. H., HOWELL, C. and ANTONCHAK, N. *Endocrinology* **50,** 521 (1952).

113 GLICK, D., VON REDICH, D. and LEVINE, S. *Endocrinology* **74,** 653 (1964).

114 GOLDEL, L., ZIMMERMANN, W. and LOMMER, D. *Hoppe Seyler's Z. physiol. Chem.* **333,** 35 (1953).

115 GOLDSTEIN, M., GUT, M., DORFMAN, R. I., SOFFER, L. J. and GABRILOVE, J. L. *Acta endocr. Copenh.* **42,** 187 (1963).

116 GORNALL, A. G. and GWILLIAM, C. *Can. J. Biochem. Physiol.* **35,** 71 (1957).

117 GORNALL, A. G. and MCDONALD, M. P. *J. biol. Chem.* **201,** 279 (1953).

118 HAGOPIAN, M., PINCUS, G., CARLO, J. and ROMANOFF, E. B. *Endocrinology* **58,** 387 (1956).

119 HAINES, W. J. *Recent Prog. Horm. Res.* **7,** 255 (1952).

120 HAYANO, M., WIENER, M. and LINDBERG, M. C. *Fedn Proc.* **12,** 216 (1953).

121 HECHTER, O. In *Cholesterol* p. 337, Academic Press, New York (1958).

122 HELLMAN, L. D., ZUMOFF, B., SCHWARTZ, M. K., GALLAGHER, T. F., BERNTSEN, C. A. and FREYBERG, R. A. *Ann. rheum. Dis.* **16,** 141 (1957).

123 HENKE, W. J., DOE, R. P. and JACOBSON, M. E. *J. clin. Endocr.* **20,** 1527 (1960).

124 HENLY, A. A. *Nature, Lond.* **169,** 877 (1952).

125 HERTOGHE, J., CRABBÉ, J., DUCKERT-MAULBETSCH, A. and MULLER, A. F. *Acta endocr. Copenh.* **20,** 139 (1955).

126 HERZOG, H. L., NOBILE, A., TOLKSDORF, S., CHARNEY, W., HERSHBERG, E. B. and PERLMAN, P. L. *Science* **121,** 176 (1955).

127 HERZOG, H. L., PAYNE, C. C., JERNICK, M. A., GOULD, D., SHAPIRO, E. L., OLIVETO, E. P. and HERSCHBERG, E. B. *J. Amer. chem. Soc.* **77,** 4781 (1955).

128 HILL, E. E. *Acta endocr. Copenh.* **33,** 230 (1960).

129 HIRSCHMANN, R. F., MILLER, R., BEYLER, R. E., SARETT, L. H. and TISHLER, M. *J. Amer. chem. Soc.* **77,** 3166 (1955).

130 HIRSCHMANN, R. F., MILLER, R., WOOD, J. and JONES, R. E. *J. Amer. chem. Soc.* **78,** 4956 (1956).

131 HOGG, J. A., BEAL, P. F., NATHAN, A. H., LINCOLN, F. H., SCHNEIDER, W. P., MAGERLEIN, B. J., HANZE, A. R. and JACKSON, R. W. *J. Amer. chem. Soc.* **77,** 4436 (1955).

132 HOGG, J. A., LINCOLN, F. H., JACKSON, R. W. and SCHNEIDER, W. P. *J. Amer. chem. Soc.* **77,** 6401 (1955).

133 HOGG, J. A., LINCOLN, F. H., NATHAN, A. H., HANZE, A. R., SCHNEIDER, W. P., BEAL, P. F., KORMAN, J. and MAGERLEIN, B. J. *J. Amer. chem. Soc.* **77,** 4438 (1955).

134 HUEBNER, C. F., LOHMAR, R., DIMLER, R. J., MOORE, S. and LINK, K. P. *J. biol. Chem.* **159,** 503 (1945).

135 IZZO, A. T., KEUTMANN, E. H. and BURTON, R. B. *J. clin. Endocr.* **17,** 889 (1957).

136 JAILER, J. W., GOLD, J. J., VANDE WIELE, R. and LIEBERMAN, S. *J. clin. Invest.* **34,** 1639 (1955).

137 JAMES, V. H. T. and CAIE, E. *J. clin. Endocr.* **24,** 180 (1964).

138 JENKINS, J. S., MEAKIN, J. W. and NELSON, D. H. *Endocrinology* **64,** 572 (1959).

139 JOHNSON, W. S., COLLINS, J. C., PAPPO, R., RUBIN, M. B., KROPP, P. J., JOHNS, W. F., PIKE, J. E. and BARTMANN, W. *J. Amer. chem. Soc.* **85,** 1409 (1963).

140 KALANT, H. *Biochem. J.* **69,** 79 and 93 (1958).

141 KAPLAN, N. M. *J. clin. Endocr.* **23,** 945 (1963).

142 KASPAR, E. and WIECHERT, R. *Ber. dt. chem. Ges.* **91,** 2664 (1958).

143 KASSENAAR, A., MOOLENAAR, A. and NIJLAND, J. *Acta endocr. Copenh.* **18,** 60 (1955).

144 KATZ, F. H., LIPMAN, M. M., FRANTZ, A. G. and JAILER, J. W. *J. clin. Endocr.* **22,** 71 (1962).

145 KELLY, W. G., BANDI, L. and LIEBERMAN, S. *Biochemistry* **1,** 792 (1962).

146 KELLY, W. G., BANDI, L., SHOOLERY, J. N. and LIEBERMAN, S. *Biochemistry* **1,** 172 (1962).

147 KERWIN, J. P., WOLFF, M. E., OWINGS, F. F., LEWIS, B. B., BLANK, B., MAGNANI, A., KARASH, C. and GEORGIAN, V. *J. org. Chem.* **27,** 3628 (1962).

148 KIRK, D. N., PETROW, V., STANSFIELD, M. and WILLIAMSON, D. M. *J. chem. Soc.* 2385 (1960).

149 KIRSCHNER, M. A. and FALES, H. M. *Analyt. Chem.* **34,** 1548 (1962).

150 KITTINGER, G. W. *Steroids* **3,** 21 (1964).

151 KLIMAN, B. and PETERSON, R. E. *J. biol. Chem.* **235,** 1639 (1960).

152 KNIGHTS, B. A., ROGERS, A. W. and THOMAS, G. H. *Biochem. biophys. Res. Commun.* **8,** 253 (1962).

153 KORNEL, L. *Metabolism* **8,** 432 (1959).

154 KORNEL, L. *J. clin. Endocr.* **22,** 1079 (1962).

155 KORNEL, L. *J. clin. Endocr.* **23,** 1192 (1963).

156 KORNEL, L. and HILL, S. R. *Metabolism* **10,** 18 (1961).

157 KRUM, A. A., MORRIS, M. D. and BENNETT, L. L. *Endocrinology* **74,** 543 (1964).

158 LARAGH, J. H., ANGERS, M., KELLY, W. G. and LIEBERMAN, S. *J. Amer. med. Ass.* **174,** 234 (1960).

159 LEBEAU, M. C. and BAULIEU, E.-E. *Endocrinology* **73,** 832 (1963).

160 LEDERER, E. and LEDERER, M. *Chromatography* 2nd edn p. 62, Elsevier, Amsterdam (1957).

161 LESTER, G., STONE, D. and HECHTER, O. *Archs. Biochem. Biophys.* **75,** 196 (1958).

162 LIDDLE, G. W., ISLAND, D., LANCE, E. M. and HARRIS, A. P. *J. clin. Endocr.* **18,** 906 (1958).

163 LIEBERMAN, S., FUKUSHIMA, D. K. and DOBRINER, K. *J. biol. Chem.* **182,** 299 (1950).

164 LIEBERMAN, S., KATZENELLENBOZEN, E. R., SCHNEIDER, R., STUDER, P. E. and DOBRINER, K. *J. biol. Chem.* **205,** 87 (1953).

165 LIPMAN, M. M., KATZ, F. H. and JAILER, J. W. *J. clin. Endocr.* **22,** 268 (1962).

166 LIPSETT, M. B. and HOCKFELT, B. *Experientia* **17,** 449 (1961).

167 LISBOA, B. P. *Acta endocr. Copenh.* **43,** 47 (1963).

168 MADER, W. J. and BUCK, R. R. *Analyt. Chem.* **24,** 666 (1952).

169 MATTINGLY, D. *J. clin. Path.* **15,** 374 (1962).

170 MATTOX, V. R. and MASON, H. L. *J. biol. Chem.* **223,** 215 (1956).

171 MCKERNS, K. W., COULOMB, B., KALUTA, E. and DE RENZO, E. C. *Endocrinology* **63,** 709 (1958).

172 MERITS, I. *Lipid Res.* **3,** 126 (1962).

173 METCALF, M. G. *J. Endocr.* **26,** 415 (1963).

174 MEYER, A. S. and LINDBERG, M. C. *Analyt. Chem.* **27,** 813 (1955).

175 MEYER, C. J., LAYNE, D. S. TAIT, J. F. and PINCUS, G. *J. clin. Invest.* **40,** 1663 (1961).

176 MEYSTRE, C., FREY, H., VOSER, W. and WETTSTEIN, A. *Helv. chim. Acta* **39,** 734 (1956).

177 MICHELAKIS, A. M. *J. clin. Endocr.* **22,** 1071 (1962).

178 MILLS, I. H. *Mem. Soc. Endocr.* **11,** 81 (1961).

179 MONCLOA, F., PÉRON, F. G. and DORFMAN, R. I. *Endocrinology* **65,** 717 (1959).

180 MOOLENAAR, A. J. *Acta endocr. Copenh.* **25,** 161 (1957).

181 MORRIS, C. J. O. R. and WILLIAMS, D. C. *Biochem. J.* **54,** 470 (1953).

182 MORRIS, R. *Acta endocr. Copenh.* **32,** 596 (1959).

183 MULROW, P. J., COHN, G. L. and KULJIAN, A. *J. clin. Invest.* **41,** 1584 (1962).

184 MURPHY, B. P., ENGELBERG, W. and PATTEE, C. J. *J. clin. Endocr.* **23,** 293 (1963).

185 MURPHY, B. P. and PATTEE, C. J. *J. clin. Endocr.* **23,** 459 (1963).

186 NEHER, R., DESAULLES, P., VISCHER, E., WIELAND, P. and WETTSTEIN, A. *Helv. chim. Acta* **41,** 1667 (1958).

187 NEHER, R. and WETTSTEIN, A. *Acta endocr. Copenh.* **35,** 1 (1960).

188 NEHER, R. and WETTSTEIN, A. *Helv. chim. Acta* **43,** 623 (1960).

189 NELSON, D. H. and SAMUELS, L. T. *J. clin. Endocr.* **12,** 519 (1952).
190 NIELSEN, J. *Acta endocr. Copenh.* Suppl. 90, 173 (1964).
191 NOWACZYNSKI, W., GOLDNER, M. and GENEST, J. *J. Lab. clin. Med.* **45,** 818 (1955).
192 NOWACZYNSKI, W., KOIW, E. and GENEST, J. *J. clin. Endocr.* **20,** 1503 (1960).
193 PABST, M. L., SHEPPARD, R. and KUIZENGA, M. H. *Endocrinology* **41,** 55 (1947).
194 PAGE, I. H. and BUMPUS, F. M. *Recent Prog. Horm. Res.* **18,** 167 (1962).
195 PALOPOLI, F. B. *Prog. cardiovasc. Dis.* **2,** 489 (1960).
196 PAPPO, R. *J. Amer. chem. Soc.* **81,** 1010 (1959).
197 PASQUALINI, J. R., DE GENNES, J. L. and JAYLE, M. F. *J. clin. Endocr.* **23,** 651 (1963).
198 PASQUALINI, J. R. and FAGGETT, J. *J. Endocr.* **31,** 85 (1964).
199 PASQUALINI, J. R. and JAYLE, M. F. *Biochem. J.* **81,** 147 (1961).
200 PASQUALINI, J. R. and JAYLE, M. F. *C.R. Soc. Biol. Paris,* **157,** 96 (1963).
201 PERLMAN, D., TITUS, E. D. and FRIED, J. *J. Amer. chem. Soc.* **79,** 4818 (1957).
202 PÉRON, F. G. *Endocrinology* **66,** 458 (1960).
203 PÉRON, F. G. *J. biol. Chem.* **236,** 1764 (1961).
204 PÉRON, F. G. *Endocrinology* **69,** 39 (1961).
205 PÉRON, F. G. *Endocrinology* **70,** 386 (1962).
206 PÉRON, F. G. *Biochim. biophys. Acta* **82,** 125 (1964).
207 PÉRON, F. G. and DORFMAN, R. I. *Endocrinology* **62,** 1 (1958).
208 PETERSON, D. H., MURRAY, H. C., EPPSTEIN, S. H., REINECKE, L. M., WEINTRAUB, A., MEISTER, P. D. and LEIGH, H. M. *J. Amer. chem. Soc.* **74,** 5933 (1952).
209 PETERSON, R. E. *J. biol. Chem.* **225,** 25 (1957).
210 PICKETT, M. T., KYRIAKIDES, E. C., STERN, M. I. and SOMMERVILLE, I. F. *Lancet* ii, 829 (1959).
211 POOS, G. I., LUKES, R. M., ARTH, G. E. and SARETT, L. H. *J. Amer. chem. Soc.* **76,** 5031 (1954).
212 PORTER, C. C. and SILBER, R. H. *J. biol. Chem.* **185,** 201 (1950).
213 QUINCEY, R. V. and GRAY, C. H. *J. Endocr.* **26,** 509 (1963).
214 REDDY, W. J. *Metabolism* **3,** 489 (1954).
215 REIF, A. E. and LONGWELL, B. B. *Endocrinology* **62,** 573 (1958).
216 RIECH, H., SANFILIPPO, S. J. and CRANE, K. F. *J. biol. Chem.* **198,** 713 (1952).
217 RINGLER, I., WEST, K., DULIN, W. E. and BOLAND, E. W. *Metabolism* **13,** 37 (1964).
218 RINIKER, B. *Metabolism* **13,** 1247 (1964).
219 RITTEL, W, ISELIN, B., KAPPELER, H., RINIKER, B. and SCHWYZER, R. *Helv. chim. Acta* **40,** 614 (1957).

220 ROBINSON, D. and WILLIAMS, R. T. *Biochem. J.* **68,** 23P (1958).

221 ROMANOFF, E. B. and HUNT, C. A. *Endocrinology* **57,** 499 (1955).

222 ROMANOFF, L. P., MORRIS, C. W., WELCH, P., RODRIGUEZ, R. M. and PINCUS, G. *J. clin. Endocr.* **21,** 1413 (1961).

223 ROMANOFF, L. P., PARENT, C., RODRIGUEZ, R. M. and PINCUS, G. *J. clin. Endocr.* **19,** 819 (1959).

224 ROSENFELD, G. and BASCOM, W. D. *J. biol. Chem.* **222,** 565 (1956).

225 ROSENFELD, R. S., LEBEAU, M. C., JANDORCK, R. D. and SALUMAA, T. *J. Chromat.* **8,** 355 (1962).

226 ROSENKRANZ, G., SONDHEIMER, F., MANCERA, O., PATAKI, J., RINGOLD, H. F. and ROMO, J. *Recent Prog. Horm. Res.* **8,** 1 (1953).

227 ROSNER, J. M., COS, J. J., BIGLIERI, E. G., HANE, S. and FORSHAM, P. H. *J. clin. Endocr.* **23,** 820 (1963).

228 ROVERSI, G. D., POLVANI, F., BOMPIANI, A. and NEHER, R. *Acta endocr. Copenh.* **44,** 1 (1963).

229 RUDD, B. T., COWPER, J. M. and CRAWFORD, N. *Clin. Chim. Acta* **6,** 686 (1961).

230 RUDD, B. T., SAMPSON, P. and BROOKES, B. N. *J. Endocr.* **27,** 317 (1963).

231 RUTHERFORD, E. R. and NELSON, D. H. *J. clin. Endocr.* **23,** 533 (1963).

232 SANDBERG, A. A. and SLAUNWHITE, W. R. *J. clin. Invest.* **42,** 51 (1963).

233 SANDBERG, A. A., SLAUNWHITE, W. R. and CARTER, A. C. *J. clin. Invest.* **39,** 1914 (1960).

234 SANDOR, T. and LANTHIER, A. *Acta endocr. Copenh.* **39,** 87 (1962).

235 SAROFF, J., SLAUNWHITE, W. R., COSTA, G. and SANDBERG, A. A. *J. clin. Endocr.* **23,** 629 (1963).

236 SCHEIFFARTH, F., ZICHA, L., FUNCK, F. W. and ENGELHARDT, M. *Acta endocr. Copenh.* **43,** 227 (1963).

237 SCHMIDLIN, J., ANNER, G., BILLETER, J. R., HEUSLER, K., UEBERWASSER, H., WIELAND, P. and WETTSTEIN, A. *Helv. chim. Acta* **40,** 1034 and 2291 (1957).

238 SCHNEIDER, J. J. and LEWBART, M. L. *J. biol. Chem.* **222,** 787 (1956).

239 SCHNEIDER, J. J. and LEWBART, M. L. *Recent Prog. Horm. Res.* **15,** 201 (1959).

240 SCHWARZ, H., BUMPUS, F. M. and PAGE, I. H. *J. Amer. chem. Soc.* **79,** 5697 (1957).

241 SEAL, U. S. and DOE, R. P. *J. biol. Chem.* **237,** 3136 (1962).

242 SEAL, U. S. and DOE, R. P. *Endocrinology* **73,** 371 (1964).

243 SHAW, D. A. and QUINCEY, R. V. *J. Endocr.* **26,** 577 (1963).

244 SHEARMAN, R. P., COX, R. I. and GANNON, A. *Lancet* i, 260 (1961).

245 SILBER, R. H., BUSCH, R. D. and OSLAPAS, R. *Clin. Chem.* **4,** 278 (1958).

246 SILBER, R. H. and PORTER, C. C. *Meth. biochem. Analysis* **4,** 139 (1957).

247 SIMPSON, S. A. and TAIT, J. F. *Endocrinology* **50,** 150 (1952).

248 SINGER, F. M. and BORMAN, A. *Proc. Soc. exp. Biol. Med.* **92,** 23 (1956).

249 SLAUNWHITE, W. R. and SANDBERG, A. A. *J. clin. Invest.* **38,** 384 (1959).
250 SOBEL, A. E. and SPOERRI, P. E. *J. Amer. chem. Soc.* **63,** 1259 (1941).
251 SOLOWAY, A. H., CONSIDINE, W. J., FUKUSHIMA, D. K. and GALLAGHER, T. F. *J. Amer. chem. Soc.* **76,** 2941 (1954).
252 SONDHEIMER, E., AMENDOLLA, C. and ROSENKRANZ, G. *J. Amer. chem. Soc.* **75,** 5930 (1953).
253 SPERO, G. B., THOMPSON, J. L., LINCOLN, F. H., SCHNEIDER, W. P. and HOGG, J. A. *J. Amer. chem. Soc.* **79,** 1515 (1957).
254 SPERO, G. B., THOMPSON, J. L., MAGERLEIN, B. J., HANZE, A. R., MURRAY, H. C., SEBEK, O. K., and HOGG, J. A. *J. Amer. chem. Soc.* **78,** 6213 (1956).
255 STAUB, M. C. and DINGMAN, J. F. *J. clin. Endocr.* **21,** 148 (1961).
256 STAUB, M. C., GAITAN, E. and DINGMAN, J. F. *J. clin. Endocr.* **22,** 87 (1962).
257 STERN, M. I. *J. Endocr.* **16,** 180 (1957).
258 STERN, M. I. and BARWELL, J. O. H. *J. Endocr.* **27,** 87 (1963).
259 STEVENS, P. J. *Proc. Ass. clin. Biochem.* **2,** 156 (1963).
260 STEVENS, W., BERLINER, D. L. and DOUGHERTY, T. F. *Endocrinology* **68,** 875 (1961).
261 SWEAT, M. L. *Analyt. Chem.* **26,** 773 (1954).
262 SWEAT, M. L. *Analyt. Chem.* **26,** 1964 (1954).
263 TAMM, J., BECKMANN, I. and VOIGT, K. D. *Acta endocr. Copenh.* **27,** 292 (1958).
264 TAMM, J., VOIGT, K. D. and VOLKWEIN, U. *Steroids,* **2,** 271 (1963).
265 TAUB, D., HOFFSOMMER, R. D., SLATES, H. L., KUO, C. H. and WENDLER, N. L. *J. Amer. Chem. Soc.* **82,** 4012 (1962).
266 THOMA, R. W., FRIED, J., BONANNO, S. and GRABOWICH, P. *J. Amer. chem. Soc.* **79,** 4818 (1957).
267 TOMPKINS, G. and ISSELBACHER, K. *J. J. Amer. chem. Soc.* **76,** 3100 (1954).
268 TOUCHSTONE, J. C. and BLAKEMORE, W. S. *J. clin. Endocr.* **21,** 263 (1961).
269 TRAPPE, W. *Biochem. Z.* **306,** 316 (1940).
270 ULICK, S. and KUSCH, K. *J. Amer. chem. Soc.* **82,** 6421 (1960).
271 ULICK, S., KUSCH, K. and AUGUST, J. T. *J. Amer. chem. Soc.* **83,** 4482 (1961).
272 ULSTROM, R. A., COLLE, E., BURLEY, J. and GUNVILLE, R. *J. clin. Endocr.* **20,** 1080 (1960).
273 UMBERGER, E. J. *Analyt. Chem.* **27,** 768 (1955).
274 UNDERWOOD, R. H. and TAIT, J. F. *J. Clin. Endocr.* **24,** 1110 (1964).
275 VANDEN HEUVEL, W. J. A. and HORNING, E. C. *Biochem. biophys. Res. Commun.* **3,** 356 (1960).
276 VAN DER VIES, J. *Acta endocr. Copenh.* **38,** 399 (1961).
277 VELLUZ, L., NOMINÉ, G., AMIARD, G., TORELLI, V. and CÉRÈDE, J. *C.R. Acad. Sci. Paris,* **257,** 3086 (1963).

278 VENNING, E. H. and KAZMIN, V. *Endocrinology* **39,** 131 (1946).
279 VERMEULEN, A. *Acta endocr. Copenh.* **37,** 348 (1961).
280 VILLEE, D. B., ENGEL, L. L., LORING, J. M. and VILLEE, C. A. *Endocrinology* **69,** 354 (1961).
281 VILLEE, D. B., VILLEE, C. A., ENGEL, L. L. and TALBOT, N. B. *J. clin. Endocr.* **22,** 481 (1962).
282 WARD, P. J. and BIRMINGHAM, M. K. *Biochem. J.* **76,** 269 (1960).
283 WARD, P. J. and GRANT, J. K. *J. Endocr.* **26,** 139 (1963).
284 WELIKY, I. and ENGEL, L. L. *J. biol. Chem.* **237,** 2089 (1962).
285 WELIKY, I. and ENGEL, L. L. *J. biol. Chem.* **238,** 1302 (1964).
286 WEST, K. M. *Metabolism* **7,** 441 (1958).
287 WETTSTEIN, A. *Experientia* **17,** 329 (1961).
288 WILLMER, E. N. *Biol. Rev.* **36,** 368 (1961).
289 WILSON, H. and LIPSETT, M. B. *Analyt. Biochem.* **5,** 217 (1963).
290 WILSON, H., LIPSETT, M. B. and RYAN, D. W. *J. clin. Endocr.* **21,** 1304 (1961).
291 WINTERSTEINER, O. and PFIFFNER, J. J. *J. biol. Chem.* **111,** 599 (1935).
292 WOLF, R. L., MENDLOWITZ, M., PICK, J., GITLOW, S. E. and NAFTCHI, N. *J. Lab. clin. Med.* **60,** 150 (1962).
293 WOLF, R. L., MENDLOWITZ, M., PICK, J., GITLOW, S. E. and NAFTCHI, N. *Proc. Soc. exp. Biol. Med.* **109,** 308 (1962).
294 WOLFF, H. P. and TORBICA, M. *Lancet* i, 1346 (1963).
295 WOSEGIEN, F., DOSE, K. and FISCHER, H. *Klin. Wschr.* **40,** 589 (1962).
296 WOTIZ, H. H. *Recent Prog. Horm. Res.* (discussion) **19,** 98 (1963).
297 YUDAEV, N. A. and PANKOV, Y. A. *Vop. med. Khim.* **9,** 507 (1963).
298 ZANDER, J., SCHRÖDER, G., WALTER, B. and BORTH, R. *Acta endocr. Copenh.* **42,** 321 (1963).
299 ZONDEK, B. and FINKELSTEIN, M. *Acta endocr. Copenh.* **11,** 297 (1952).

EXAMPLE OF A QUANTITATIVE BIOASSAY

Calculations of relative potencies of two preparations of human pituitary follicle stimulating hormone (U^1 and U^2) in terms of a common standard (S) by the ovarian augmentation method.

Preparation U^1 was tested at three dose levels, U_1^1, U_2^1 and U_3^1, U^2 at two levels, U_1^2 and U_2^2 and S at three levels, S_1, S_2 and S_3. The log dose interval, I, was 0·301 throughout.

Measured effects (ovarian weight) in mg

U_1^1	U_2^1	U_3^1	U_1^2	U_2^2	S_1	S_2	S_3
7·2	7·2	9·0	2·0	13·8	7·2	17·6	8·0
9·2	8·4	10·6	7·4	6·5	7·1	9·0	20·2
5·9	14·5	14·6	5·5	10·4	7·8	10·8	10·4
7·0	13·7	16·7	6·8	6·0	12·3	9·8	8·9
8·1	11·8	20·6	8·5	13·6	6·4	11·1	23·9
3·7	7·3	14·2	10·2		6·8	9·5	23·9
	8·9	12·7					
	11·6						
Sum 41·1	83·4	98·4	40·4	50·3	47·6	67·8	95·3
Mean 6·9	10·4	14·1	6·8	10·1	7·9	11·3	15·9

Total degrees of freedom = $S(n-1)$ where n is the number of animals at each dose level = 42.

(1) Calculation of slope

The combined slope $b_c = E_c/I$ where E_c is a contrast for the difference of effect corresponding to the log dose interval I.

367

It equals $S(C)/S(D)$ where $C = \frac{1}{2}(\bar{U}_2 - \bar{U}_1)$ and $D = 0.5$ when the number of dose levels $(k) = 2$, and $C = \bar{U}_3 - \bar{U}_1$ and $D = 2$ when $k = 3$. (For other values of k see Ref. 1.)

Here
$$S(C) = 7.2 + 1.65 + 8.0 = 16.85$$
$$S(D) = 2 + 0.5 + 2 = 4.5$$
$$E_c = \frac{16.85}{4.5} = 3.74$$

and
$$b_c = \frac{3.74}{0.301} = 12.4$$

(2) Calculation of variances

The mean standard deviation, s_c, is:

$$\frac{S\left(\dfrac{\text{Range}}{dn}\right)}{S(k)}$$

where the range is the difference between the highest and lowest effects at each dose level and dn varies according to n as follows:

n	2	3	4	5	6	7	8	9	10
dn	1·13	1·69	2·06	2·33	2·53	2·70	2·85	2·97	3·08

Here
$$S\left(\frac{\text{Range}}{dn}\right) = \frac{5.5}{2.53} + \frac{7.3}{2.85} + \ldots + \frac{15.9}{2.53} = 27.64$$

$$S(k) = 8$$

and
$$s_c = \frac{27.64}{8} = 3.46$$

The index of precision, λ, or

$$\frac{s_c}{b_c} = \frac{3.46}{12.4} = 0.28.$$

The mean variance $(V) = s_c^2/\bar{n}$ where $\bar{n}$ is the mean number of observations per dose level $= \dfrac{50}{8} = 6.25$

$$\therefore V = \frac{3.46^2}{6.25} = 1.92$$

(3) Validity tests

(a) REGRESSION

Variance of the combined slope, $V(b_c)$, is:

$$\frac{V}{I^2 \times S(D)} = \frac{1 \cdot 92}{0 \cdot 301^2 \times 4 \cdot 5}$$

$$= 4 \cdot 71$$

Index of significance of $b_c = g_c = V(b_c)t^2/b_c^2$ where t is obtained from statistical tables and depends on the arbitrary choice of probability, P (usually $P = 0 \cdot 05$) and on the total degrees of freedom.

$$\therefore g_c = \frac{4 \cdot 71 \times 2 \cdot 02^2}{12 \cdot 4^2} = 0 \cdot 125$$

(b) CURVATURE

The contrast, H, is calculated for each dose response line with $k = 3$ or more. When $k = 3$, $H = U_1 + U_3 - 2U_2$

and when $k = 4$, $H = U_1 + U_4 - U_2 - U_3$.

Then $t = H/\{V(H)\}^{\frac{1}{2}}$ where $V(H) = 6V$ for $k = 3$ and $4V$ for $k = 4$

Now
$$H_1 = 0 \cdot 2 \qquad V(H) = 11 \cdot 52$$

$$\therefore t = \frac{0 \cdot 2}{3 \cdot 4} = 0 \cdot 06$$

and
$$H_2 = 1 \cdot 2 \qquad V(H) = 11 \cdot 52$$

$$\therefore t = \frac{1 \cdot 2}{3 \cdot 4} = 0 \cdot 35$$

Since neither of these t values reaches significance at the $P = 0 \cdot 05$ level for 42 degrees of freedom, any curvature in the dose-response lines may be ignored.

The combined curvature, H_c, of the lines is also checked by using the equation $H_c^2 = S(H_k^2)/S(k - 2)$ to calculate H_c^2 and then estimating its significance by reference to standard analysis of variance tables from the calculated value of $F_c = H_c^2/V$, the degrees of freedom being $n_1 = S(k - 2)$ and $n_2 =$ total degrees of freedom. Here $H_k^2 = H^2/6$ (see Ref. 1) and

$$\therefore H_c^2 = \frac{0 \cdot 2^2 + 1 \cdot 2^2}{6(1 + 1)} = 0 \cdot 12$$

and
$$F_V = \frac{0 \cdot 12}{1 \cdot 92} = 0 \cdot 06 \; (n_1 = 2, \, n_2 = 42)$$

This variance ratio is insignificant and therefore the combined curvature may be ignored.

BB

(c) Variation in slope

G is a measure of the difference between the slopes of the dose response lines and the combined difference is calculated from the equation

$$G_c^2 = \frac{S(C^2/D) - E_cS(C)}{p' - 1}$$

where p' = number of preparations used at two or more dose levels and then $F_v = G_c^2/V$. The significance of F_v is again obtained by reference to standard tables, the degrees of freedom being $n_1 = p' - 1$ and n = total degrees of freedom.

$$G_c^2 = \frac{\left(\dfrac{7\cdot2^2}{2} + \dfrac{1\cdot65^2}{0\cdot5} + \dfrac{8\cdot0^2}{2}\right) - 3\cdot74 \times 16\cdot85}{3 - 1}$$

$$= 0\cdot173$$

$F_v = 0\cdot173/1\cdot92 = 0\cdot09$ ($n_1 = 2$, $n_2 = 42$). P is greater than $0\cdot2$ and any difference in slope may therefore be ignored.

These tests have demonstrated the validity of the assays and the relative potencies and fiducial limits may now be calculated.

(4) Calculation of relative potencies

The potency ratios are calculated from the contrast, F, which is the difference between the mean effects of each unknown preparation and the standard, i.e. $F = \bar{U} - \bar{S}$.

Then the log potency ratio $M = F/b_c$

$$\text{Preparation } U^1. \quad F = \frac{31\cdot4}{3} - \frac{35\cdot1}{3} = -1\cdot233$$

$$M = -0\cdot0994 \text{ or } \bar{1}\cdot9006$$

$$\text{Potency ratio} = \text{antilog } M = 0\cdot795$$

$$\text{Preparation } U^2. \quad F = \frac{16\cdot9}{2} - \frac{35\cdot1}{3} = -3\cdot25$$

$$M = -0\cdot2621 \text{ or } \bar{1}\cdot7379$$

$$\text{Potency ratio} = \text{antilog } M = 0\cdot547$$

The fiducial limits are calculated from the expression

$$\frac{M}{1 - g_c} \pm \frac{t}{b_c(1 - g_c)} \left\{A(1 - g_c) + M^2V(b_c)\right\}^{\frac{1}{2}}$$

A, the variance of F, depends on the number of dose levels of the two preparations, being $2V/3$ when there are 3 levels of each and $5V/6$ when there

are 3 levels of one and 2 levels of the other preparation. The value of t is obtained from the tables for $P = 0.05$ and degrees of freedom $= 42$.
The limits for U^1 are:

$$-\frac{0.0994}{0.875} \pm \frac{2.02}{12.4 \times 0.875} (1.28 \times 0.875 + 0.0994^2 \times 4.71)^{\frac{1}{2}}$$

$$= -0.1136 \pm 0.1973 \quad \text{or} \quad \bar{1}.6891 \text{ and } 0.0837$$

Conservation of these logarithms gives the limits as 0.489 and 1.575
The limits for U^2 are:

$$-\frac{0.2621}{0.875} \pm \frac{2.02}{12.4 \times 0.875} (1.6 \times 0.875 + 0.2621^2 \times 4.71)^{\frac{1}{2}}$$

$$= -0.2995 \pm 0.2439 \quad \text{or} \quad \bar{1}.4566 \text{ and } \bar{1}.9444$$

The limits are therefore 0.286 and 0.880.

These results show that the potency of the mean dose of U^1 is 79.5 per cent with limits of 48.9 and 157.5 per cent of the mean dose of the standard. The corresponding results for U^2 are 54.7 (28.6 — 88.0) per cent. Such conclusions are likely to be correct in 95 per cent of cases.

REFERENCE

1 BORTH, R. *Acta endocr. Copenh.* **35**, 454 (1960).

TRIVIAL AND SYSTEMATIC NAMES OF STEROIDS

Trivial name	Systematic name
Progesterone	Pregn-4-ene-3,20-dione
Pregnanediol	5β-Pregnane-3α,20α-diol
Allopregnanediol	5α-Pregnane-3α,20α-diol
Pregnenolone	3β-Hydroxypregn-5-en-20-one
Pregnanetriol	5β-Pregnane-3α,17α,20α-triol
Pregnanetriolone	3α,17α,20α-Trihydroxypregnane-11-one
Testosterone	17β-Hydroxyandrost-4-en-3-one
Epitestosterone	17α-Hydroxyandrost-4-en-3-one
Androsterone	3α-Hydroxy-5α-androstan-17-one
Epi-androsterone	3β-Hydroxy-5α-androstan-17-one
Dehydroepiandrosterone	3β-Hydroxyandrost-5-en-17-one
Aetiocholanolone	3α-Hydroxy-5β-androstan-17-one
Epi-aetiocholanolone	3β-Hydroxy-5β-androstan-17-one
Androstanedione	Androstane-3,17-dione
Androstenedione	Androst-4-ene-3,17-dione
Androstenediol	Androst-4-ene-3β,17β-diol
Nortestosterone	17β-Hydroxyoestr-4-en-3-one
Adrenosterone	Androst-4-ene-3,11,17-trione
Androstenol	Androst-16-en-3β-ol
Ethisterone	17α-Ethinyl-17β-hydroxyandrost-4-en-3-one
Cortisone (Compound E)	17α,21-Dihydroxypregn-4-ene-3,11,20-trione
Cortisol (Compound F)	11β,17α,21-Trihydroxypregn-4-ene-3,20-dione
Corticosterone	11β,21-Dihydroxypregn-4-ene-3,20-dione
Deoxycorticosterone (cortexone)	21-Hydroxypregn-4-ene-3,20-dione
Aldosterone	11β,21-Dihydroxy-3,20-dioxopregn-4-en-18-al
Reichstein's Compound S	17α,21-Dihydroxypregn-4-ene-3,20-dione
Reichstein's Compound E	11β,17α,20β,21-Tetrahydroxypregn-4-en-3-one
Reichstein's Compound epi-E	11β,17α,20α,21-Tetrahydroxypregn-4-en-3-one
Tetrahydrocortisone	3α,17α,21-Trihydroxy-5β-pregnane-11,20-dione

Trivial name	Systematic name
Tetrahydrocortisol	$3\alpha,11\beta,17\alpha,21$-Tetrahydroxy-$5\beta$-pregnan-20-one
Allotetrahydrocortisone	$3\alpha,17\alpha,21$-Trihydroxy-5α-pregnane-11,20-dione
Allotetrahydrocortisol	$3\alpha,11\beta,17\alpha,21$-Tetrahydroxy-$5\alpha$-pregnan-20-one
Cortol	5β-Pregnane-$3\alpha,11\beta,17\alpha,20\alpha,21$-pentol
β-Cortol	5β-Pregnane-$3\alpha,11\beta,17\alpha,20\beta,21$-pentol
Cortolone	$3\alpha,17\alpha,20\alpha,21$-Tetrahydroxy-$5\beta$-pregnan-11-one
β-Cortolone	$3\alpha,17\alpha,20\beta,21$-Tetrahydroxy-$5\beta$-pregnan-11-one
Prednisone	$17\alpha,21$-Dihydroxypregna-1,4-dien-3,11,20-trione
Prednisolone	$11\beta,17\alpha,21$-Trihydroxypregn-1,4-diene-3,20-dione
Dexamethasone	9α-fluoro-16α-methylprednisolone
Betamethasone	9α-fluoro-16β-methylprednisolone
Triamcinolone	9α-fluoro-16α-hydroxyprednisolone
Oestrone	3-Hydroxyoestra-1,3,5(10)-trien-17-one
Oestradiol-17β	$3,17\beta$-Dihydroxyoestra-1,3,5(10)-triene
Oestriol	$3,16\alpha,17\beta$-Trihydroxyoestra-1,3,5(10)-triene
Equilin	3-Hydroxyoestra-1,3,5(10),7-tetraen-17-one
Equilenin	3-Hydroxyoestra-1,3,5(10),6,8(9)-pentaen-17-one
Ethinyloestradiol	17α-Ethinyl-$3,17\beta$-dihydroxyoestra-1,3,5(10)-triene
Stilboestrol	4,4'-Dihydroxy-α,β-diethylstilbene

INDEX